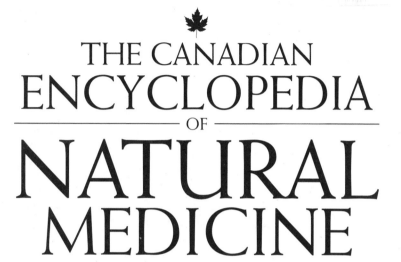

THE CANADIAN
ENCYCLOPEDIA
OF
NATURAL
MEDICINE

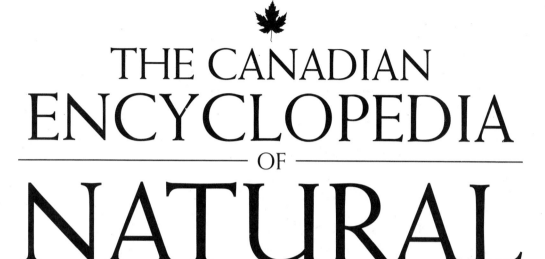

THE CANADIAN ENCYCLOPEDIA
OF
NATURAL MEDICINE

SHERRY TORKOS, B.Sc. Phm.

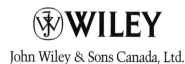

WILEY

John Wiley & Sons Canada, Ltd.

Library and Archives Canada Cataloguing in Publication Data

Torkos, Sherry
    The Canadian encyclopedia of natural medicine / Sherry Torkos.

Includes index.
ISBN 978-0-470-83908-9

    1. Naturopathy—Encyclopedias. 2. Self-care, Health. I. Title.

RZ433.T67 2007   615.5'3503   C2007-900992-1

Production Credits
Cover design: Ian Koo
Interior text design and typesetting: Adrian So
Author photo: Precious LaPlante
Printer: Tri-Graphic

John Wiley & Sons Canada, Ltd.
6045 Freemont Blvd.
Mississauga, Ontario
L5R 4J3

Printed in Canada

This book is printed with biodegradable vegetable-based inks. Text pages are printed on 60 lb. 100% PCW using TG ECO100 by Tri-Graphic Printing, Ltd., an FSC certified printer.

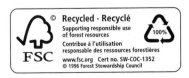

1 2 3 4 5 TRI 11 10 09 08 07

CONTENTS

vi | Contents

Section IV: Appendices

FOREWORD

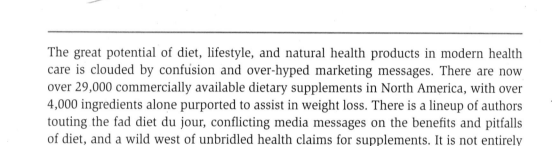

The great potential of diet, lifestyle, and natural health products in modern health care is clouded by confusion and over-hyped marketing messages. There are now over 29,000 commercially available dietary supplements in North America, with over 4,000 ingredients alone purported to assist in weight loss. There is a lineup of authors touting the fad diet du jour, conflicting media messages on the benefits and pitfalls of diet, and a wild west of unbridled health claims for supplements. It is not entirely surprising that consumers, patients, and health care providers alike are all craving sound, unbiased, and scientifically grounded information.

Enter trusted pharmacist Sherry Torkos, a renowned expert and talented writer who has consistently set the gold standard in health promotion literature. Like thousands of others, I have always been impressed by Sherry's books, with their superb coverage of women's health, emotional disorders, anti-aging interventions, and sound, scientifically based measures for the maintenance of a healthy, lean body. It was no shock to me that Sherry would take on the Mount Everest of nutritional projects—the daunting task of covering the need-to-know information regarding nutrition, lifestyle, and supplements in relation to the most common medical disorders and diseases.

In addition to the global aspects of diet and nutrients, lifestyle habits, and stress management for overall health, Sherry provides condition-specific advice on complementary interventions, dietary modifications, and key nutritional and herbal supplements—all without overwhelming the reader. The end result is the ultimate resource for consumers, patients, and health care providers. Pharmacists, doctors and patients will also appreciate the unique and detailed descriptions of the prescription drugs that can deplete vitamins and minerals. This drug–nutrient interaction is an underappreciated factor and a particularly important one when considering that prescription drug usage in Canada now exceeds $20 billion.

It will be obvious and appreciated by readers that this is an exhaustive work, a cross-over book that will be useful and reader-friendly to both consumers and doctors alike. Leaving no stone unturned, Sherry has elegantly put together a book that stands alone. She has filtered out the hype and synthesized thousands of scientific papers from various medical disciplines—there simply is no other book like it. This resource is timely and destined to become one that will be referred to over and over again. Most importantly, it is a resource that allows for informed choice without bias or commercial spin, providing practical advice that is sure to make a difference in the lives of many. The book strikes me as an extension of Sherry herself, a trusted advisor in the otherwise confusing world of nutrition and natural health products.

Respectfully,
Alan C. Logan, ND, FRSH

ACKNOWLEDGEMENTS

There are many people that I would like to thank for their help and support with this book.

To my husband Rick and my family, who have stood by me through this book and many others, I thank you for your patience and understanding of my commitment to this project and all the long hours required.

To my medical advisory board: Dr. Elvis Ali, Jean-Yves Dionne, Rhonda Dorren, Sam Graci, Dr. George Grant, Karlene Karst, Brad King, Dr. Michael Lyon, Tracy Marsden, Dr. Joey Shulman, Lorna Vanderhaeghe, and Farid Wassef, I appreciate your time and expertise in reviewing sections of my manuscript. To Dr. Bryce Wylde, many thanks for providing the chapter on homeopathy and for sharing your knowledge and passion. To Dr. Alan Logan, thank you for your support and enthusiasm with this book. I feel very fortunate to work amongst such brilliant and inspiring people.

To Katherine Zia, my developmental editor and publicist, whom I have had the pleasure of working with for over ten years, a tremendous thanks and much appreciation for all the help you gave me in researching, planning, and staying on track with this book.

To the team at Wiley: Jennifer Smith, Leah Fairbank, Liz McCurdy, Lindsay Humphreys, and the design department, thanks for all your help throughout this project.

To my copyeditor, Valerie Ahwee, I appreciate all your hard work in reviewing my manuscript and your fine editorial assistance.

Finally I would like to thank you, the reader, for your interest in health and wellness and for your desire to read this book.

ADVISORY BOARD

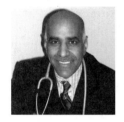

Dr. Elvis Ali B.Sc, F.I.A.C.A., D.Hom., N.D.
Dr. Ali is a licensed naturopathic doctor. He graduated with his first degree, B.Sc. (Biology), in 1979 and received a Doctorate in Naturopathic Medicine in the first full-time undergraduate class (1987) from the Canadian College of Naturopathic Medicine. He has been in private practice for 20 years, specializing in Chinese medicine, sports medicine and nutrition. In 2006 Dr. Ali completed his course on Body/Mind Medicine at Harvard Medical School, and he is a member of the postgraduate association at Harvard.

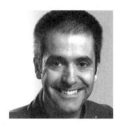

Jean-Yves Dionne B.Sc. Pharm.
Jean-Yves Dionne, pharmacist, is a scientific advisor and natural health products consultant for several companies. He is often called upon to speak to health professionals about complementary medicines. In 2003, he received the Aventis Pharma award for outstanding contribution to teaching for the course Phytotherapy and Natural Health Products at the Faculté de Pharmacie de l'Université de Montréal. Jean-Yves is co-author of *Herbs: Everyday Reference for Health Professionals*, published by the Canadian Pharmacists Association. He contributes to and acts as reviewer for www.passeportsante.net, The Virtual Compendium on Natural Health Products and for various magazines both scientific and lay press. Mr. Dionne sits on the board of the Table Filière des Plantes Médicinales du Québec (medicinal herbs round table), of the Canadian Natural Health Product Research Society and the Canadian Natural Product Association.

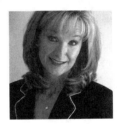

Rhonda Dorren B.Sc. Pharm.

Rhonda Dorren received her Bachelor of Science degree in Pharmacy at the University of Alberta in Edmonton. A licensed pharmacist in Alberta and an author, she has developed a consultation practice in Natural Medicine Pharmacy, utilizing a unique blend of allopathic and biological medicines. See www.rhondadorren.com.

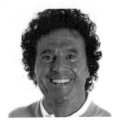

Sam Graci

Sam Graci is a Canadian lifestyle researcher and the author of four #1 best-selling books in Canada. His latest book, *The Bone-Building Solution*, is co-authored with Carolyn DeMarco, M.D. and Leticia Rao, Ph.D. His books are written on 100% recycled paper, with biodegradable vegetable ink. A portion of the proceeds from the sale of his four books are donated to Scouts Canada for their tree-planting program and also donated to non-profit environmental groups.

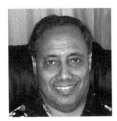

Dr. George Grant M.Sc., Ed.D., C.Chem, R.M.

Dr. Grant is a multi-talented scientist, lecturer, prolific author and Canada's top stress management and wellness coach. He is the founder of the International Academy of Wellness and has pioneered the research on Beta Endorphins, HPLC analysis of B vitamins, and anti-cancer medicines.

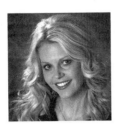

Karlene Karst RD

Karlene Karst is a leading health specialist in nutrition and natural medicine. She is a highly sought-after, passionate speaker who is dedicated to improving the health of society by sharing her knowledge. She is a frequent guest on radio and television shows across North America. Karlene is author of *The Metabolic Syndrome Program* and co-author of the national best-seller *Healthy Fats for Life*.

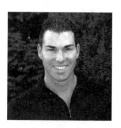

Brad King M.Sc., MFS

Brad King is one of Canada's most sought after authorities on nutrition, obesity and longevity. He is the author of eight books, including the international best-seller *Fat Wars*, and is a 2003 inductee into the Canadian Sports Nutrition Hall of Fame. His free monthly newsletter (*Awaken Your Body*) can be found at www.AwakenYourBody.com.

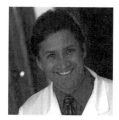

Michael R. Lyon, BSc, MD

Dr. Michael Lyon is the Medical and Research Director for the Canadian Centre for Functional Medicine located in Vancouver, B.C. He heads a team of clinicians and researchers dedicated to biotechnology, nutritional and natural health product research. He is involved in collaborative clinical research with various Canadian universities and the Imperial College of Medicine in London, England, in the field of obesity, diabetes and appetite regulation, and with the University of British Columbia in the area of childhood learning and behavioural disorders. In addition to being published in medical literature, Dr. Lyon is the author of *Healing the Hyperactive Brain Through the New Science of Functional Medicine* and *Is Your Child's Brain Starving?*, and he is the co-author of *How to Prevent and Treat Diabetes with Natural Medicine*, *Beat Diabetes Naturally* and *Hunger Free Forever: The New Science of Appetite Control.*

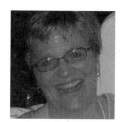

Tracy Marsden

Tracy earned science and pharmacy degrees from the University of Alberta and worked in a community pharmacy setting for over fifteen years. Her enthusiasm for wellness prompted her to obtain additional training in herbals and homeopathy. She worked several years as a Natural Medicine Consultant for a pharmacy chain, where she also helped develop marketing strategies for their natural products department. Tracy has consulted to a number of natural products manufacturers and is a regular columnist for *Pharmacy Post*. She has also written on natural product marketing for *Integrated Health Retailer* magazine. President of the Alberta College of Pharmacists for 2004–2005, Tracy is well respected in the health care field. She is a founding partner of Rocky Mountain Analytical, a private Canadian wellness-focused medical laboratory.

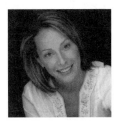

Dr. Joey Shulman

Dr. Joey Shulman is the author of *Winning the Food Fight: Every Parent's Guide to Raising a Healthy, Happy Child* (Wiley 2003) and the national best-seller *The Natural Makeover Diet: 4 Steps to Inner Health and Outer Beauty* (Wiley 2006). As one of Canada's foremost authorities on nutrition and wellness, she is a highly sought-after speaker, inspiring and educating large audiences across North America. Dr. Joey has spoken to numerous large corporations, and was an invited speaker at Dr. Andrew Weil's second annual Nutrition and Health conference in Tucson, Arizona. She is the vice-president of nutrition for Truestar Health, North America's leading online health site, and is a proud spokesperson for Genuine Health supplements. As a new mom, she is also a proud endorser and head nutritionist for Sweetpea Baby Food, a line of top-quality frozen organic baby food. For more information, please visit www.drjoey.com.

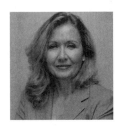

Lorna Vanderhaeghe M.S.

Lorna Vanderhaeghe is Canada's leading women's natural health expert. Lorna has a Masters in Health Studies in nutrition and a degree in biochemistry. She is the author of eight books and thousands of articles. Her latest book is *Sexy Hormones*. Lorna believes in empowering people with health knowledge so they may achieve optimal wellness. She has an award-winning website (www.healthyimmunity.com) and a monthly e-letter and an Internet talk show called "Ask Lorna".

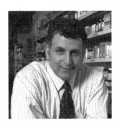

Farid Wassef RPh CCN

Farid Wassef is a clinical pharmacist and nutritionist from Stouffville, Ontario. He frequently lectures to the public and to healthcare professionals, and appears both on television and radio to discuss integrative approaches to health and wellness. In 2003 he co-authored *Breaking the Age Barrier: Strategies for Optimal Health, Energy, and Longevity*. In 2006 he was honoured as the Canadian Pharmacist of the Year for patient care. www.prescription4nutrition.com

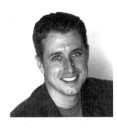

Dr. Bryce Wylde B.Sc., RNC, D.H.M.H.S., H.D.

Dr. Wylde is Toronto's expert homeopathic doctor and functional medicine nutritionist. He is the resident homeopathic doctor on CityTV's Breakfast Television and a regular on a number of other television and radio shows. His practice has a particular motivation towards helping those with autoimmunity, digestive complaints, and the integrative treatment and prevention of cancer.

INTRODUCTION

A PHARMACIST'S PERSPECTIVE:
The Power of Natural Medicine in Modern Health

The history of medicine is a fascinating story of the transition from ancient healing techniques to brilliant scientific and technological advances. We have gone from using medicine men and plant-based remedies to creating pharmaceutical drugs and sophisticated surgical procedures. Undoubtedly, medicine today now provides us with the ability to fight off deadly diseases and live longer lives; however, we must not forget that many solutions can still be found in nature. In fact, many of the prescription medications used today are derived from plants. As well, we must be aware that lifestyle factors—diet, activity level, sleep, and environment—play a critical role in health and disease prevention.

In the last 20 years, we've witnessed a growing desire to look to natural remedies first before taking prescription medications that may have drug interactions, side effects, and high costs. There is increasing interest in prevention for both minor and chronic health concerns and awareness of taking responsibility for one's health. People are no longer satisfied with the idea of taking a pill to fix their problems. They are starting to question the indiscriminate use of prescription drugs and the motivations behind the industry, and they are becoming better educated about their options.

I have also witnessed a growing awareness among doctors, pharmacists, and other health care professionals in holistic therapies, but we still have a long way to go before mainstream medicine and natural medicine are fully integrated. And that's where I come in. As a traditionally trained pharmacist with a complementary background in natural health, nutrition, and fitness, my goal is to bridge the gap between the two worlds and in doing so, help people along their journey to optimal health.

HOW IT ALL BEGAN

My interest in natural medicine came from a personal experience. As a young teen I suffered from undiagnosed celiac disease, a genetic condition in which the body cannot digest gluten, which is a protein found in many grains. For several years, I experienced abdominal pain, bloating, weight loss, fatigue, visual impairment, hair loss, and skin rashes. Despite seeing several doctors, I did not get a proper diagnosis and was instead given large doses of unnecessary prescription medications.

I was sick almost every day for nearly four years. As my health continued to deteriorate, I developed both physical and emotional symptoms. I suffered with depression, poor concentration, and impaired memory. What I didn't know at the time was that gluten was destroying the absorptive surface of my intestines, causing malnutrition, wasting, and damage to vital organs.

Luckily for me, my parents never gave up. Finally, after much searching, we found a doctor who immediately recognized my symptoms as celiac disease and put me on a strict gluten-free diet. My stomach symptoms gradually improved on the restricted diet. However, my health was far from restored. I was still quite fatigued, forgetful, and suffered with eczema, poor night vision, and lack of hair growth. This is when I turned to holistic therapies. I read, researched, and investigated how to improve my health. I began taking therapeutic dosages of vitamins, minerals, and essential fatty acids to correct the deficiencies that I had experienced for so many years. Slowly, but steadily, I began to return to a state of optimal health.

Coping with a health problem at such a young age was a life-altering experience, and filled me with a passion for health and a willingness to look "outside the box" for answers. After high school, I studied science, pharmacy, and nutrition in Philadelphia and went on to build a holistic pharmacy practice in the Niagara area of Ontario. In my practice, I have worked with many people facing serious health challenges, such as heart disease, diabetes, cancer, and depression, and I have seen how remarkably well the body can heal and repair when it is given the proper elements.

My intention with this book is to have people refer to it for both prevention and treatment of health conditions, and then consult with their health care practitioner for proper guidance and monitoring. *I must stress that the information in this book is not intended to diagnose or replace the advice of your doctor or health care provider. Under no circumstances should you stop taking existing medications or combine supplements with existing medications without consulting your doctor first.* I believe that conventional medicine does offer benefits when used appropriately, but I also believe that nutritional therapies, herbs, exercise, meditation, and other holistic measures can provide potential solutions and significant steps toward prevention and as such, should be given equal consideration. Knowledge and understanding about natural therapies is imperative before you can integrate it into your life.

In some cases striking the balance between the two modalities is easier said than done. Difficulties arise because many mainstream health practitioners remain cautious or even skeptical about the benefits of natural remedies. By providing comprehensive, science-based information on natural medicine, I hope to provide you with a sound resource that can be taken to your health care provider when discussing a health concern. As such, the information provided in this book reflects the most recent data from scientific studies, in many cases published in respected medical journals. I refer to research throughout the book, and only recommend supplements and therapies that have been studied and found to be beneficial. I also note drug interactions, contraindications, and side effects where relevant.

HOW TO USE THIS BOOK

My book is divided into five sections:

In Section One, there are six chapters that outline my Prescription for Healthy Living.

- Chapter One outlines the macronutrients—the protein, carbohydrates, and fats that are the basic components of our diet.
- Chapter Two provides details on the micronutrients—the essential vitamins and minerals.
- Chapter Three highlights the functional foods that provide health benefits beyond nutrition.
- Chapter Four will give you my top 10 principles for a healthy diet.
- Chapter Five describes the benefits of physical activity and offers guidelines and tips on incorporating exercise into your lifestyle.
- Chapter Six discusses the importance of sleep and stress management, two often overlooked elements that are essential for health.

In Section Two, you will find The Natural Pharmacy.

- Chapter Seven offers a reference guide to 66 of the most common and widely recommended dietary supplements.
- Chapter Eight provides my principles for safe supplementation—guidelines and recommendations on choosing and using natural remedies, complete with medicine cabinet musts and healthy travel kit ideas.
- Chapter Nine is contributed by Dr. Bryce Wylde, a colleague and well-known homeopathic doctor who discusses the principles of homeopathy and the top 25 conditions that can be helped with homeopathic medicine.

Section Three covers the 87 most common health conditions from A to Z.

- Each condition is described including causes, symptoms, and risk factors. Conventional medical approaches are discussed and then I offer a natural prescription, which includes dietary strategies, lifestyle recommendations, and supplements.

If you are coping with a health condition listed in this book, it is not my intention that you follow every recommendation I make. Instead, implement as many of the lifestyle and dietary strategies as possible and discuss my supplement recommendations with your health care provider. Under my "Top Recommended Supplements" section I list those that are supported by scientific research to offer benefits for the particular condition. Next, I list "Complementary Supplements"—those that offer some benefits or play a supportive role; these would be secondary considerations.

Since many supplements have similar effects on the body, and there are potential interactions between drugs and supplements, it is recommended that you consult with your health care provider before taking a new product. Unlike many drugs, supplements may take weeks to months before the full effect is achieved, so patience is required.

In addition to your primary care provider, you may want to look for additional health care providers that offer different perspectives, such as a naturopathic or homeopathic doctor, registered dietitian, massage therapist, acupuncturist, or chiropractor. When looking for alternative health care providers, make sure they are properly trained and always check references. You may also want to find a pharmacist in your area who, like myself, has a broad range of knowledge in natural medicine. Pharmacists are always available, without an appointment, to answer questions and discuss your concerns, especially about medications.

Section Four contains the appendices—the supplementry charts, tables, and resources that are referred to throughout this book.

Over 20 years ago, I discovered the power of natural medicine for myself. That discovery set a course for my future that has taken me around the world from pharmacies and medical clinics, to lecture halls and conferences, through the writing of several health books, and finally to the publication of this reference guide. This latest book reflects many years of work and hundreds of hours of research, as well as my sincere desire to help Canadians achieve better health.

My message to you is this: Don't wait for health problems to arise. Take a proactive approach now. Learn about the power of nutrition, exercise, supplements, stress management, and other lifestyle factors in the prevention of disease and take the necessary steps today. If you are currently struggling with a health problem, realize that there are options, and that a plan that incorporates a variety of healing modalities will most likely provide you with the best possible outcome.

I hope I've provided you with a useful resource to achieve optimum health for you and your family. I wish you all the best as you create your own prescription for successful and healthy living!

Sherry Torkos

SECTION I

PRESCRIPTION FOR SUCCESSFUL LIVING

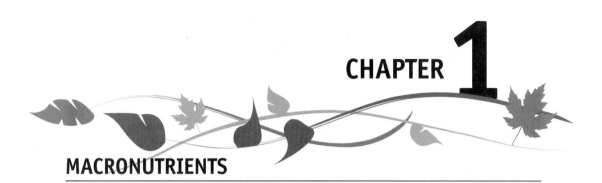

CHAPTER 1

MACRONUTRIENTS

Macronutrients are essential nutrients—carbohydrates, proteins, and fats—that the body needs for energy and proper growth, metabolism, and function. They are called "macro" because we need these nutrients in large quantities compared to the micronutrients (vitamins and minerals), which are needed in smaller quantities. In this section I will explain the various macronutrients, recommended intakes, and the best food sources.

Macronutrients provide us with calories as follows:

Carbohydrate: 4 calories per gram

Protein: 4 calories per gram

Fat: 9 calories per gram

For example:

If a food product contains 10 g of carbohydrate, 2 g of protein, and 1 g of fat per serving, it would provide 10 × 4 = 40 calories from carbohydrate, 2 × 4 = 8 calories from protein, and 1 × 9 = 9 calories from fat for a total calorie count of 57 calories per serving.

PROTEIN

Protein is a necessary component for building, maintenance, and repair of many body systems and processes, including:

- Production of collagen and keratin, which are the structural components of bones, teeth, hair, and the outer layer of skin; they help maintain the structure of blood vessels
- Manufacture of hormones, such as insulin and thyroid hormone
- Production of enzymes that control chemical reactions in the body
- Proper immune function—production of antibodies, white blood cells, and other immune factors
- Transportation of oxygen, vitamins, and minerals to target cells throughout the body

• Source of energy—the liver can use protein to make glucose when there is not enough carbohydrate available, such as when you skip a meal or follow a low-carb diet.

Food Sources

Protein is found in animal products, nuts, legumes, and, to a lesser extent, in fruits and vegetables. When we eat protein the body breaks it down into amino acids, some of which are called *essential* because they must be provided by the food we eat. Others that can be produced by the body are called *non-essential*.

Protein from animal sources contains all of the essential amino acids. Therefore, your best sources of lean protein are chicken, turkey, fish, and eggs. Choose free-range and organic wherever possible to reduce ingesting harmful hormones and chemicals.

Plant proteins do not contain all the essential amino acids and are considered *incomplete* proteins. It is possible, though, to combine various plant proteins to get all the essential amino acids. For example, eating oats, lentils, and sunflower seeds either together or separately throughout the day provides all the essential amino acids. You could also combine whole-wheat pasta with white kidney beans or tofu with brown rice to get all the necessary amino acids. It just requires careful meal planning.

There are certain advantages of eating plant over animal proteins—they provide fibre and phytochemicals (antioxidants), do not contain saturated fat, and may play a role in disease prevention. Soy protein, for example, has been shown to significantly lower cholesterol and triglyceride levels, and protect against bone loss. A number of studies have found lower risk of chronic disease in those who eat a plant-based diet.

....

The Institute of Medicine recommends ranges for macronutrient intake that are associated with a reduced risk of chronic disease while providing adequate intake of essential nutrients. They suggest that adults get 45–65 percent of calories from carbohydrates, 20–35 percent from fat, and 10–35 percent from protein. Ranges for children are similar, except that infants and younger children need a slightly higher proportion of fat (25–40 percent).

....

CARBOHYDRATES

Carbohydrates are the body's main source of fuel—glucose, which is needed by every cell in our body. They also provide valuable nutrients (vitamins, minerals, and essential fatty acids) and fibre, which is important for intestinal health.

Food Sources

There are two classes of carbohydrates—simple and complex. Simple carbohydrates include naturally occurring sugars in milk and fruit, and refined sugars (granulated sugar). There is a major difference among these simple carbohydrates: fruits offer a range of nutrients and fibre, while refined sugars provide empty calories and lack nutritional value. Excess sugar consumption is linked to dental caries, obesity, insulin resistance, high triglycerides, low HDL (good) cholesterol, and compromised immune function. The World Health Organization recommends reducing sugar intake to below 10 percent of total calories. Aside from candy and baked goods, sugar is also found in pop, condiments (ketchup, barbecue sauces), juices, ice cream, and other sweets.

Complex carbohydrates include starches and indigestible dietary fibre. Starches are found in bread, pasta, rice, beans, and some vegetables. Today many of our starches are refined and processed, which strips the food of its fibre and nutrients. For example, white bread, pasta, and rice are much less nutritious, so choose the brown or whole-grain products.

Dietary fibre is found in fruits, vegetables, beans, and the indigestible parts of whole grains such as wheat and oat bran. In addition to supporting intestinal health and proper elimination, fibre also improves blood sugar balance, lowers cholesterol, reduces the risk of colon and breast cancer, and plays a role in weight management.

The recommended intake of fibre for adults 50 years and younger is 38 g for men and 25 g for women; for men and women over 50 it is 30 and 21 g per day, respectively, due to decreased food consumption. Sadly, most people get only one-third to one-half of the recommended amount. To boost fibre intake, incorporate more raw vegetables, fruits, whole grains, and legumes in your diet and consider a fibre supplement.

Glycemic Index

The glycemic index (GI) is a scale that measures how quickly carbohydrates are broken down into sugar. Those that are broken down quickly—such as simple carbohydrates and refined starches—have a high GI. Foods that are broken down slowly—such as most vegetables, fruits, and unprocessed grains—have a low GI.

Numerous studies have linked high-GI diets to obesity, insulin resistance, type 2 diabetes, and increased risk of heart disease. Eating high-GI foods can lead to blood sugar imbalances that may result in fatigue, increased appetite, and food cravings. For these reasons, it is best to minimize high-GI foods and maximize your intake of low-GI foods. See Appendix B for more information on the GI and the rating for common foods.

FATS

"Fat" has become a negative word as it is associated with obesity, yet we do need a certain amount of fat in our diets and on our bodies. The point to keep in mind is that there are *good* fats and *bad* fats.

The good fats are the unsaturated fats, namely, the monounsaturated fats (olive, canola, and peanut oil) and polyunsaturated fats. The polyunsaturated fats provide us with essential fatty acids (EFAs), which are broken down into two groups:

- *Omega-6 fatty acids:* Linoleic acid (LA), which is converted into gamma-linolenic acid (GLA) and arachidonic acid (AA)
- *Omega-3 fatty acids:* Alpha-linolenic acid (ALA), which is converted into eicosapentaenoic acid (EPA) and docosahexaenoic acid (DHA)

The body cannot make EFAs, so they must be obtained through diet or supplementation. They are essential for many body processes and functions, including:

- Growth and development of brain, nervous system, adrenal glands, sex organs, inner ear, and eyes
- Energy (fat is the most concentrated source of energy)
- Absorbing fat-soluble vitamins (vitamins A, D, E, K, and carotenoids)
- Maintaining cell membrane integrity
- Regulation of cell processes such as gene activation and expression, enzyme function, and fat oxidation
- Production of hormones and chemical messengers

Food Sources

Here is a breakdown of the EFAs and their sources:

- *LA:* Found in vegetable oils such as safflower, evening primrose, sunflower, corn, hemp, canola, and olive oil.
- *GLA:* Found in borage, blackcurrant, and evening primrose oils.
- *AA:* Found in meat and eggs. We get adequate AA through diet. Too much of this fat is not good, as it causes inflammation.
- *ALA:* Found in flaxseed and hemp oil and, to a lesser extent, in nuts, green leafy vegetables, wheat germ, and blackcurrant seeds.
- *EPA and DHA:* Found in fatty fish, such as salmon, mackerel, herring, cod, sardines, and tuna.

There is great controversy over what constitutes the optimal dietary intake ratio of omega-6 to omega-3 fatty acids. It is estimated that we currently get around 15:1, whereas leading EFA authorities recommend a ratio closer to 4:1 or even 2:1.

The Institute of Medicine has set an adequate intake level for linoleic acid for adults 19–50 years of age at 17 g/day for men and 12 g/day for women; alpha-linolenic acid at 1.6 g/day for men and 1.1 g/day for women. These levels are lower for younger and older individuals.

Rather than trying to calculate the perfect ratio or intake, aim to have more omega-3s (fish, flaxseed, hemp, and fish oils) and GLA (borage, blackcurrant, or primrose oil) from diet and/or supplements, as these are the beneficial fats that are commonly deficient.

Diets rich in the omega-3 fatty acids offer cardio protection by lowering blood cholesterol and triglyceride levels, reducing blood clotting, and reducing the risk of heart attack and sudden death. These fats also reduce inflammation and are helpful for arthritis and other inflammatory disorders. GLA also reduces inflammation, and prevents clotting, dilates blood vessels, improves skin health, and benefits those with diabetes and arthritis.

SATURATED FATS

Saturated fats are found in animal products such as meat, poultry, milk, cheese, butter, and lard, as well as in tropical oils (such as palm, palm kernel, and coconut oil) and foods made from these oils. These fats are high in cholesterol and linked to heart disease, high cholesterol, obesity, and cancers of the breast, colon, and prostate.

Most people get 38 percent or more of the day's calories from fat while health authorities suggest no more than 20–35 percent of which less than 10 percent comes from saturated fat. To cut your intake of saturated fat, trim fat and skin from meat, choose lean poultry over red meat, and low-fat cheese and dairy (cottage cheese, feta, and hard cheeses have less fat). Butter is fine in moderation (see sidebar).

••

BUTTER VERSUS MARGARINE

For years margarine was considered to be a healthier alternative to butter, however most margarines contain hydrogenated oils (trans fats), which are artificial processed fats linked to heart disease and cancer. The exception is non-hydrogenated margarines, such as Becel, which contain beneficial plant sterols that can help lower cholesterol. While butter contains saturated fats, they are short-chain saturates, which are easily digested and provide a source of useable energy. Butter also contains nutrients: lecithin, vitamins A and E, and selenium. So the bottom line is: Choose butter or a non-hydrogenated margarine.

••

TRANS FATS

Trans fatty acids are naturally found in small amounts in animal products; however, the majority of trans fats in our diet come from the artificial form. Trans fats are created when oils undergo a chemical process called hydrogenation, which solidifies them. This is the process that makes vegetable oil into margarine. Trans fat is also found in cookies, crackers, french fries, baked goods, and other snack foods.

When trans fats were first introduced into our food supply, they were thought to be a healthier alternative to saturated fats. Many years later this was found to be false. Trans fats elevate cholesterol levels, increasing the risk for heart disease and heart attack, and are also linked to cancer, particularly breast cancer. The Institute of Medicine has stated that there is no safe limit for trans fats in the diet and that we should reduce consumption of these dangerous fats. Food companies have been making efforts in this area. You will now see many packaged foods labelled "trans fat free."

CHOLESTEROL

Cholesterol is a waxy substance found in the fats (lipids) in our blood. It is manufactured in the liver and also obtained from consuming saturated and trans fats. Cholesterol is not all bad—the body requires it to produce sex hormones, maintain cell membranes, and for a healthy nervous system.

Aside from diet, cholesterol levels can be elevated by family history, lack of activity, and liver disorders, and cholesterol consumption increases the risk of heart disease.

As with fats, there is good and bad when it comes to cholesterol. The good cholesterol is HDL (high-density lipoproteins) and the bad is LDL (low-density lipoproteins). LDL cholesterol can build up in the artery walls of the brain and heart, narrowing the passageways for blood flow, a process known as atherosclerosis, the precursor to heart disease and stroke.

HDL cholesterol is called good cholesterol because it picks up the LDL deposited in the arteries and transports it to the liver to be broken down and eliminated.

To lower LDL and raise HDL levels, exercise regularly, minimize saturated fats, avoid trans fats, and don't smoke (smoking lowers HDL).

TRIGLYCERIDES

Triglycerides (TG) are the chemical form in which most fats exist in food (both animal and plant fats). They are also present in the blood along with cholesterol.

A diet that is high in fat, sugar, refined carbohydrates, and alcohol can elevate TGs. Overeating also raises TG because excess calories are converted to fat in the liver and then into TG to be transported in the blood. High levels of triglycerides are associated with heart disease and diabetes. It is possible for triglycerides to be high even when blood cholesterol is normal, so get your levels checked regularly. In most cases, TG levels can be effectively managed with diet and exercise.

SUMMARY

In this section we learned that our bodies need a balance of quality protein, carbohydrates, and fats. These macronutrients provide us with the energy and nutrients needed for proper growth, development, and many body processes. In a later chapter I will outline principles for a healthy diet—my top recommendations for a nutritional plan for optimal health and disease prevention.

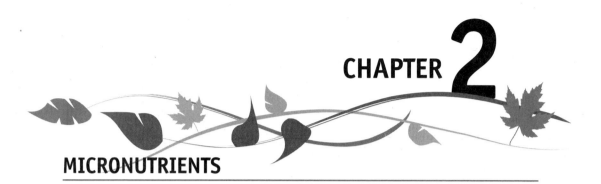

CHAPTER 2

MICRONUTRIENTS

Micronutrients are vitamins and minerals—nutrients required by the body in small amounts—yet have powerful effects. They assist in energy-producing reactions, growth and development, protect against free radical damage, and perform many vital functions. Micronutrients are essential for health, and a deficiency can lead to health problems and disease.

In 2002 the US Food and Nutrition Board, the Institute of Medicine, and Health Canada released a report providing reference values for nutrient intakes for healthy North Americans, including:

- *Recommended Dietary Allowance (RDA):* The average daily dietary nutrient intake level sufficient to meet the nutrient requirement of nearly all (97–98 percent) healthy individuals in a particular life stage and gender group.
- *Adequate Intake (AI):* The recommended average daily intake level based on observed or experimentally determined estimates of nutrient intake of apparently healthy people that are assumed to be adequate. The AI is given when an RDA cannot be determined.
- *Tolerable Upper Intake Level (UL):* The highest average daily nutrient intake level that is likely to pose no risk of adverse health effects for almost all individuals in the general population. As intake increases above the UL, the potential risk of adverse effects may increase.

In this chapter I have outlined the essential vitamins, minerals, and trace elements; their functions in the body; their role in disease prevention and treatment; deficiency symptoms; drugs that deplete; and supplement guidelines.

The table at the end of this chapter summarizes food sources, recommended intake levels, and possible side effects and toxicity for the various nutrients. For some nutrients an RDA has not been established; however, an AI is provided. It is important to note that the RDA is mainly based on information on short-term effects. The optimum nutrient intake for health and disease prevention may be higher than the RDA, and varies with age, state of health, diet, and other factors.

WHO NEEDS SUPPLEMENTS?

There are many factors that cause nutrient depletion, such as poor diet, stress, exercise, use of prescription drugs, environmental toxicity, and excessive alcohol intake. For many micronutrients, deficiency, inadequate intake or nutrient depletion is common relative to the RDA. This is why supplements are so important in making up for shortcomings in the diet and preventing deficiencies.

VITAMINS

There are 13 essential vitamins that our bodies need for proper growth, function, and maintenance of healthy tissues. The vitamins are either water-soluble or fat-soluble. The B-vitamins and vitamin C dissolve in water and are easily eliminated from the body. Adverse reactions, even with high-dose supplements, are rare with these vitamins. Fat-soluble vitamins (A, D, and E) are not readily excreted from the body and have the potential to accumulate in the tissues and cause adverse effects at high doses.

Vitamin A

- Found in animal foods and converted from beta-carotene in plant foods.
- Required for vision, gene expression, reproduction, embryonic development, red blood cell production, and immune function.
- Prescription vitamin A derivatives are used to treat skin conditions (acne) and retinitis pigmentosa (genetic eye disease).
- Deficiency is rare in Canada, but common in developing countries due to malnutrition. It causes night blindness, dry eyes and skin, and impaired growth.
- Drugs that deplete vitamin A: cholestyramine, colestipol, mineral oil, and neomycin.
- Supplements should be avoided by those at risk of lung cancer (smokers) or liver toxicity (alcoholics, liver disease).
- Doses greater than 10,000 IU daily should be avoided by pregnant women due to the risk of birth defects. Most prenatal vitamins provide 5,000 IU.
- Doses greater than 5,000 IU may increase risk of osteoporosis.
- Supplements of vitamin A beyond what is provided in a multivitamin are not recommended due to risk of toxicity. To avoid this risk, choose a multivitamin that contains beta-carotene, which is converted to vitamin A in the liver, but is not associated with health risks.

Vitamin B1 (Thiamine)

- Required for energy production, nerve and muscle function, enzyme reactions, and fatty acid production.
- Deficiency causes beriberi, a disease that affects cardiovascular, nervous, muscular, and gastrointestinal systems.
- Deficiency is common in developing countries; in North America it occurs in alcoholics, those with kidney disease, malabsorption syndromes (celiac disease), and in those with poor diets.

- Drugs that deplete vitamin B1: furosemide, antibiotics, oral contraceptives, and phenytoin.
- Most people get adequate thiamine from diet and/or a multivitamin.

Vitamin B2 (Riboflavin)
- Required for energy metabolism, enzyme reactions, vision, and skin/hair/nail health; functions as an antioxidant; activates vitamin B6, niacin, and folate.
- May play a role in preventing migraine headaches and cataracts.
- Deficiency occurs in alcoholics, the elderly, and those with poor diets.
- Symptoms of deficiency include sore throat; redness/swelling of the mouth, throat, tongue, lips, and skin; decreased red blood cell count; and blood vessel growth over the eyes. Deficiency may impair iron absorption and increase risk of pre-eclampsia in pregnant women.
- Drugs that deplete vitamin B2: antibiotics, chlorpromazine, amitriptyline, adriamycin, and phenobarbitol.
- Most people get adequate riboflavin from diet and/or a multivitamin.

Vitamin B3 (Niacin)
- Required for energy metabolism, enzyme reactions, skin and nerve health, and digestion.
- High doses of nicotinic acid (3 g daily) can lower cholesterol (reduce LDL and triglycerides and increase HDL) and reduce the risk of heart attack and stroke; high dosages should be supervised by a physician.
- Deficiency causes pellagra, the symptoms of which are skin rash, diarrhea, dementia, and death.
- Deficiency may be caused by poor diet, malabsorption diseases, dialysis, and HIV.
- Drugs that deplete vitamin B3: antibiotics, isoniazid, and 5-Fluorouracil (chemotherapy).
- High-dose niacin, taken along with statin drugs (i.e., lovastatin), may increase the risk of rhabdomyolysis (muscle degeneration and kidney disease).
- Most people get adequate niacin from diet and/or a multivitamin; supplements may be recommended for those with high cholesterol.

Vitamin B5 (Pantothenic Acid)
- Required for carbohydrate metabolism, adrenal function, enzyme reactions, and production of fats, cholesterol, bile acids, hormones, neurotransmitters, and red blood cells.
- Deficiency is rare, except in malnutrition, and causes burning/tingling in hands and feet, fatigue, and headache.
- Drugs that deplete vitamin B5: oral contraceptives, amitriptyline, imipramine, and desipramine.
- Most people get adequate niacin from diet and/or a multivitamin.

Vitamin B6 (Pyridoxine)

- Necessary for protein and fat metabolism, hormone function (estrogen and testosterone), and the production of red blood cells, niacin, and neurotransmitters (serotonin, dopamine, and norepinephrine).
- Used therapeutically for PMS, depression, morning sickness, carpal tunnel syndrome, and heart health (lowers homocysteine, an amino acid that, at high levels, can cause arteriosclerosis and build up arterial plaque).
- Deficiency is uncommon, except in alcoholics and the elderly, and causes seizures, irritability, depression, confusion, mouth sores, and impaired immune function.
- Drugs that deplete vitamin B6: antibiotics, oral contraceptives, isoniazid, penicillamine, and Parkinson's drugs.
- Supplements are recommended for the elderly, alcoholics, and those with poor diets.

Vitamin B12 (Cobalamin)

- Required for nerve function, synthesis of DNA and RNA, metabolism of energy, enzyme reactions, and production of red blood cells.
- Used therapeutically for heart health (lowers homocysteine), male infertility, prevention of neural tube defects, asthma, and cancer prevention.
- Deficiency is common among the elderly and those with poor diets, pernicious anemia, depression, Alzheimer's, or malabsorption conditions (celiac disease).
- Deficiency symptoms: anemia, appetite loss, constipation, numbness and tingling in the extremities, and confusion. Pregnant women with deficiency have increased risk of giving birth to a child with neural tube defects.
- Drugs that deplete B12: acid-lowering drugs (omeprazole, lansoprazole, ranitidine), oral contraceptives, antibiotics, cholestyramine, and metformin.
- Supplements are recommended for those over age 50, vegetarians, women planning to become pregnant, those with poor diets, and those at risk of heart disease.

Biotin

- Part of the B-vitamin family; involved in the synthesis of fat, glycogen, and amino acids and enzyme reactions; required for DNA replication; important for healthy hair and nails.
- Used therapeutically to strengthen fingernails.
- Deficiency is rare except in those with hereditary disorders of biotin metabolism, liver disease, and during pregnancy (due to increased needs). It can also occur in those who consume raw egg white for prolonged periods (weeks to years) because a protein found in egg white (avidin) binds biotin and prevents its absorption or in those given intravenous feeding without biotin supplementation.
- Deficiency symptoms include hair loss; scaly red rash around the eyes, nose, mouth, and genital area; depression; lethargy; hallucination; numbness and tingling of the extremities; and impaired glucose utilization and immune system function.
- Drugs that deplete biotin: primidone, carbamazepine, phenobarbital, phentyoin, valproic acid, and antibiotics.
- Most people get adequate biotin from diet and/or supplements.

Folate (Folic Acid)

- Part of the B-vitamin family; known as folate when it occurs in foods, or as folic acid when present in supplements or added to foods.
- Required for cell division, growth, amino acid metabolism, enzyme reactions, and production of RNA, DNA, and red blood cells.
- Used for heart health (lowers homocysteine) and prevention of cancer (colon and cervical) and birth defects (neural tube).
- Deficiency occurs in alcoholics and those with poor diets, and causes anemia, fatigue, weakness, headache, hair loss, diarrhea, and poor immune function. Pregnancy or cancer results in increased rates of cell division and metabolism, increasing the need for folate.
- Drugs that deplete folate: non-steroidal anti-inflammatory drugs (NSAIDs) such as ibuprofen and aspirin, phenytoin, methotrexate phenobarbital, cholestyramine, colestipol, trimethoprim, and sulfasalazine.
- Supplements are recommended for most adults for heart and cancer protection, and especially for pregnant women; multivitamins typically provide the recommended amount of 400 mcg per day.

Vitamin C (Ascorbic Acid)

- Required for synthesis of collagen (structural component of blood vessels, tendons, and bone), norepinephrine (neurotransmitter), and carnitine (amino acid involved in energy production); promotes wound healing; supports immune function and gum health; and has antioxidant properties.
- Used to prevent cataracts, macular degeneration, heart disease, stroke, cancer, and colds; improve wound healing and response to stress; reduce bronchial spasms in asthmatics; and prevent lead toxicity.
- Severe deficiency causes scurvy (bleeding, bruising, hair and tooth loss, joint pain, and swelling), which is rare today.
- Marginal deficiencies are common among the elderly, alcoholics, and those with cancer, chronic illness, or stress. Symptoms include fatigue, easy bruising, poor wound healing and appetite, anemia, and sore joints.
- Drugs that deplete vitamin C: oral contraceptives, aspirin, corticosteroids, and furosemide.
- Large doses of vitamin C (greater than 1,000 mg/day) may reduce the effect of warfarin (blood-thinning drug).
- The Linus Pauling Institute recommends 400 mg of vitamin C daily, which is higher than the RDA, yet much lower than the UL. Most multivitamin supplements provide 60 mg of vitamin C.
- Natural and synthetic forms are chemically identical and have the same effects on the body.
- Mineral salts of ascorbic acid (i.e., calcium ascorbate) are buffered and therefore less acidic and less likely to cause upset stomach.

Vitamin D

- Regulates calcium and phosphorus levels and promotes absorption of these minerals for growth of bones and teeth; involved in insulin secretion; supports immune function; regulates blood pressure.
- Vitamin D can be produced in the skin upon exposure to sunlight or must be obtained from the diet.
- Used to prevent and treat osteoporosis, psoriasis, autoimmune disease, and to reduce the risk of cancer.
- Deficiency occurs with inadequate dietary intake, limited sun exposure, kidney or liver disease, and alcoholism. Elderly, dark-skinned, obese people, or those with inflammatory bowel disease and fat-malabsorption syndromes (celiac disease and cystic fibrosis) are also at greater risk.
- Deficiency causes rickets (weak, deformed bones) in children, osteomalacia (soft bones) and osteoporosis in adults, dental problems, muscle weakness, and tooth decay.
- Drugs that deplete vitamin D: carbamazepine, phenytoin, phenobarbital, cimetidine, ranitidine, cholestyramine, colestipol, orlistat, and mineral oil.
- Since vitamin D is found in few foods and at low amounts, a supplement is recommended for most people. Most multivitamins provide 400 IU (10 mcg). Those with limited sun exposure, osteoporosis, multiple sclerosis, psoriasis, and those over age 65 should consider additional vitamin D.

Vitamin E

- Is an antioxidant (protects cell membranes against oxidative damage; prevents LDL oxidation) that supports immune function, prevents blood clotting, and dilates blood vessels.
- Used to prevent and treat heart disease, cancer, macular degeneration, and cataracts, enhance immune response, reduce oxidative stress, and improve cognitive function.
- Deficiency is rare, except in those who are malnourished or who have fat-malabsorption conditions (celiac disease, cystic fibrosis); however, suboptimal intake is common and associated with increased risk of heart disease.
- Symptoms of deficiency include impaired balance and coordination, damage to sensory nerves (peripheral neuropathy), muscle weakness (myopathy), and damage to the retina of the eye (pigmented retinopathy).
- Drugs that deplete vitamin E: cholestyramine, colestipol, isoniazid, mineral oil, orlistat, sucralfate, phenobarbitol, phenytoin, and carbamazepine.
- Vitamin E may enhance the blood-thinning effects of warfarin.
- It is difficult to achieve the RDA from diet alone; supplements are particularly necessary to achieve amounts needed for disease prevention.
- Look for natural vitamin E (alpha-tocopherol); the synthetic form (dl-alpha-tocopherol) is less bioavailable (i.e., less absorbable) and only half as potent.

Vitamin K

- Essential for blood clotting; required for bone formation and cell growth.
- Useful in the prevention of osteoporosis.
- Deficiency is rare in adults and causes impaired blood clotting; it is more common in newborns and can cause severe bleeding. Injections of vitamin K1 are typically given to newborns.
- Symptoms of deficiency include easy bruising and bleeding (nosebleeds, bleeding gums, blood in the urine or stool, or heavy menstrual bleeding).
- Drugs that deplete: antibiotics, aspirin, phenytoin, phenobarb, cholestyramine, colestipol, orlistat, and mineral oil.
- High intake of vitamin K from foods or supplements can reduce the efficacy of blood-thinning drugs (warfarin).
- Most people get adequate vitamin K from the diet and/or a multivitamin.

MINERALS, TRACE MINERALS, AND ELECTROLYTES

Minerals are elements that originate in the earth. The body cannot make minerals so they must be obtained through the diet and/or supplements. Both plant and animal foods provide minerals. Plants obtain minerals from the soil they are grown in. Animals get minerals from the plants they eat, and then we get these minerals indirectly by eating the animal products. There are also some minerals present in drinking water, but this varies with geographic location, as does the mineral content of plants.

Minerals are categorized according to our daily requirements. Calcium, magnesium, and phosphorus are considered major minerals since we require a substantial amount of these for health and wellness. The trace minerals, which are required in smaller amounts, are chromium, copper, fluoride, iodine, iron, manganese, molybdenum, selenium, and zinc. The minerals potassium and sodium are known as electrolytes, substances that dissociate into ions (charged particles) in solution, making them capable of conducting electricity.

MINERALS
Calcium

- The most abundant mineral in the body; essential for building and maintaining bones and teeth; required for muscle contractions and nerve function; regulates blood pressure, blood vessel contractions, and clotting; involved in enzyme reactions.
- Used for the prevention of osteoporosis, colorectal cancer, pre-eclampsia, and lead toxicity and the treatment of high blood pressure.
- Deficiency can occur with poor diet, abnormal parathyroid function (gland that regulates blood calcium levels), kidney failure, and vitamin D or magnesium deficiency.
- Symptoms of deficiency include bone loss and weakening, muscle cramps, heart palpitations, tooth decay, back and leg pain, insomnia, nervous disorders, and rickets (bone deformities in children).
- Drugs that deplete calcium: cimetidine, ranitidine, omeprazole, aluminum antacids, corticosteroids, cholestyramine, mineral oil, phenytoin, and furosemide.

- A high intake of sodium (salt), protein, phosphorus (soft drinks and food additives), or caffeine (more than 2 cups of coffee or 300 mg caffeine per day) can promote calcium losses.
- Calcium supplements may reduce the efficacy of calcium channel blockers (drugs used to lower blood pressure); use with thiazide diuretics increases the risk of hypercalcemia (high blood calcium levels); calcium supplements may reduce absorption of antibiotics (tetracycline, quinolones), bisphosphonates (osteoprosis drugs), and levothyroxine (thyroid hormone).
- It is difficult to meet the RDA through diet alone unless dairy intake is high. Most multivitamin/mineral supplements provide a small amount of calcium because it is quite bulky. Therefore, a separate calcium supplement may be necessary, especially for those at risk of osteoporosis and those with high blood pressure.
- There are several forms of calcium: Carbonate provides the highest amount of calcium (40 percent) and is inexpensive; citrate provides 21 percent calcium, but may be better absorbed in the elderly and those taking acid-lowering drugs.
- To maximize absorption, take no more than 500 mg of elemental calcium at one time, take with meals, and ensure adequate vitamin D intake (as this is required for calcium absorption).
- Separate calcium-rich foods and supplements by two hours from iron supplements (calcium reduces iron absorption); avoid drinking tea with meals, as the tannins in tea reduce calcium absorption.
- Some vegetables contain chemicals that inhibit the absorption of calcium, such as oxalic acid, which is found in raw spinach, rhubarb, sweet potato, and dried beans. Cooking these foods releases calcium that is bound to oxalic acid, thus improving the amount you can absorb. Phytic acid, which is found in wheat bran or dried beans, also reduces calcium absorption.

Magnesium
- Required for nerve and muscle function, formation of bones and teeth, synthesis of the antioxidant glutathione, cell membranes, and body temperature regulation; involved in energy production, numerous enzyme reactions, and synthesis of DNA and RNA.
- Used to prevent heart disease and in the treatment of high blood pressure, pre-eclampsia, heart disease, diabetes, osteoporosis, migraine headaches, and asthma.
- Deficiency is uncommon, but may occur in those with poor diets, malabsorption syndromes (celiac disease), Crohn's disease, intestinal surgery or inflammation, kidney disease, diabetes, alcoholism, and in the elderly due to reduced absorption.
- Marginal deficiency (consuming less than the RDA) is common and is estimated to affect 75 percent of people.
- Symptoms of deficiency: muscle cramps and spasms, weakness, insomnia, poor appetite, kidney stones, osteoporosis, nervousness, irritability, anxiety, depression, and high blood pressure.
- Drugs that deplete magnesium: furosemide, hydrochlorothiazine, cholestyramine, and oral contraceptives.

- Other interactions: Magnesium reduces absorption of digoxin, nitrofurantoin, anti-malarial drugs, quinolone antibiotics, tetracycline, chlorpromazine, alendronate, and etidronate, so separate intake of magnesium from these foods by two hours.
- High doses of zinc (greater than140 mg/day) reduce magnesium absorption.
- It is difficult to meet the RDA through diet alone; therefore, a multivitamin/mineral supplement is recommended. Certain individuals may require an additional magnesium supplement.

Phosphorus

- Required for structure of bones, teeth, soft tissue, and cell membranes (phospholipids); energy production and storage; enzyme reactions; hormones; formation of DNA and RNA; and maintaining acid-base balance.
- Deficiency is rare except among alcoholics and those with kidney disease, malabsorption syndromes (celiac or Crohn's disease), or poor diets.
- Symptoms of deficiency: poor appetite, anemia, muscle weakness, bone pain, rickets in children, osteomalacia in adults, increased risk of infection, and numbness and tingling of extremities.
- Drugs that deplete phosphorus: aluminum and magnesium (antacids and supplements), cholestyramine, and digoxin.
- Most people get adequate phosphorus through diet; supplements are rarely necessary.

TRACE MINERALS
Chromium

- Involved in glucose metabolism (enhances effect of insulin) and enzyme reactions.
- Used for diabetes and for those with impaired glucose tolerance and to lower cholesterol and triglycerides.
- Severe deficiency is rare, but marginal deficiency is common; it is estimated that 90 percent of adults consume less than the RDA.
- The main cause of deficiency is poor dietary intake (high-sugar diets increase urinary excretion of chromium).
- Deficiency results in impaired glucose utilization and may be a contributing factor to the development of type 2 diabetes; symptoms include elevated blood sugar, numbness, and tingling in the extremities and nerve problems.
- Drugs that deplete chromium: corticosteroids (prednisone).
- Other interactions: Chromium may enhance the blood sugar-lowering effects of insulin and oral drugs (glyburide and metformin), thus requiring a dosage adjustment.
- Since marginal deficiencies are common, a multivitamin/mineral complex containing chromium is recommended. Chromium is available in several forms. Most studies involving chromium were done with the picolinate form, which is readily absorbed and utilized by the body. Certain individuals (diabetics and those at risk for diabetes) may require an additional supplement.

Copper

- A component of enzymes, which are required for energy production, connective tissue formation, iron metabolism, brain and nervous system, synthesis of neurotransmitters, melanin, myelin, hemoglobin, and the antioxidant superoxide dismutase; involved in regulating gene expression.
- Severe deficiency is rare, but marginal deficiencies are common. The typical diet provides about 50 percent of the RDA. Others at risk: Premature and low birth-weight infants with diarrhea; infants fed only cow's milk formula, which is low in copper; those with malnutrition, malabsorption syndromes (celiac disease), cystic fibrosis, and those receiving intravenous feeding.
- Deficiency leads to iron deficiency and anemia, low white blood cell count (increased risk of infection), osteoporosis, loss of skin pigment, and impaired growth in children.
- Drugs that deplete copper: penicillamine, ethambutol, and zidovudine.
- Other interactions: Prolonged high doses of zinc (50 mg daily or more) may result in copper deficiency.
- A varied diet provides adequate copper for most individuals. In addition, taking a multivitamin/mineral complex will provide the RDA.

Fluoride

- Essential for formation of healthy bones and teeth.
- Used to prevent cavities, harden tooth enamel, and strengthen bones (prevent osteoporosis).
- Deficiency causes tooth decay and dental caries (cavities).
- Drugs that deplete fluoride: Calcium supplements and calcium- and aluminum-containing antacids reduce fluoride absorption (separate intake of fluoride from these by two hours).
- Supplements are available by prescription and are recommended only for children living in areas with low water fluoride concentrations; rarely required for adults.
- People who consume well water should have the fluoride content of their water tested.

Iodine

- Required to make thyroid hormones, which regulate metabolism, energy production, and body temperature, and are essential for growth and reproduction.
- Used for prevention of radiation-induced thyroid cancer in those with iodine deficiency and to treat fibrocystic breast disease.
- Deficiency may occur in those who do not consume salt, fish, or sea vegetables and is becoming more common in the general population due to restrictions on salt intake for blood pressure.
- Deficiency reduces thyroid hormone production, causing hypothyroidism, fatigue, weight gain, goiter, miscarriage, birth defects, and stunted growth. It is also the most common cause of brain damage worldwide.
- Drugs that deplete iodine: potassium iodide, possibly resulting in hypothyroidism.

- Other interactions: Amiodarone (heart drug) contains high levels of iodine and may affect thyroid function; potassium iodide may decrease the anticoagulant effect of warfarin.
- A deficiency of selenium, vitamin A, or iron can worsen iodine deficiency.
- Foods containing goitrogens—such as cabbage, broccoli, cauliflower, Brussels sprouts, and soybeans—inhibit the synthesis of thyroid hormone. These foods are a concern only for those who are iodine deficient and consume high amounts of them. Cooking deactivates the goitrogens.
- Supplements are rarely necessary, but should be considered in pregnant and lactating women if dietary iodine is insufficient to meet the RDA.
- A daily prenatal supplement providing 150 mcg of iodine will help to ensure that pregnant and breast-feeding women consume sufficient iodine during these critical periods.

Iron

- Required to produce hemoglobin and myoglobin (proteins involved in the transport and storage of oxygen) and amino acids (carnitine); required for cellular energy production; produces enzymes that have antioxidant effects; supports DNA synthesis and immune function.
- Used for prevention of anemia in pregnancy and in others at risk, and in the treatment of restless legs syndrome.
- Deficiency is common, especially in women with heavy menstrual bleeding and during pregnancy (increased needs for baby), vegetarians, and those with malabsorption syndromes (celiac disease), bleeding ulcers, copper deficiency, and in surgery.
- Deficiency leads to depleted iron stores, impaired red blood cell formation, and anemia. Symptoms include fatigue, paleness, headache, hair loss, brittle nails, rapid heart rate, increased risk of infections, and rapid breathing on exertion.
- Drugs that deplete iron: antacids, cimetidine, ranitidine, omeprazole, lansoprazole, aspirin, anti-inflammatory drugs, and cholestyramine.
- Iron supplements can bind to and reduce absorption and efficacy of levodopa, levothyroxine, methyldopa, quinolones, tetracyclines, bisphosphonates, and zinc and calcium supplements. To avoid this, separate intake of iron supplements from these products by two hours.
- Vitamin C-rich foods and supplements enhance the absorption of nonheme iron (form of iron found primarily in plants).
- A multivitamin/mineral complex providing the RDA is recommended for most premenopausal and pregnant women and those at risk of deficiency.
- Men and post-menopausal women should choose iron-free multivitamin/mineral supplements to avoid iron excess.

Manganese

- Required for the production and activation of enzymes that are involved in energy metabolism; bone, cartilage, and collagen formation; and the production of antioxidants.

- Deficiency is uncommon, but may occur in those with epilepsy, hypoglycemia, diabetes, schizophrenia, and osteoporosis.
- Deficiency symptoms: impaired growth and reproductive function, skeletal abnormalities, impaired glucose tolerance, and altered carbohydrate and fat metabolism.
- Drugs that deplete: magnesium-containing antacids and laxatives and tetracycline.
- Absorption is reduced by calcium, phosphate, and iron.
- Supplements beyond the amount provided by diet and/or a multivitamin and mineral complex are not necessary.

Molybdenum
- Required for the production of enzymes that are cofactors in amino acid metabolism, formation of uric acid, and the metabolism of drugs and toxins.
- Deficiency is extremely rare and may occur in those with a rare genetic condition; deficiency causes seizures, developmental delays in neonates, tachycardia, brain damage, and coma.
- Drugs that deplete: high intakes of copper or sulphate.
- Supplements beyond the amount provided by diet and/or a multivitamin and mineral complex are not necessary.

Selenium
- Component of enzymes that function as antioxidants; involved in detoxification; converts thyroid hormone to its active form; supports immune function; enhances the antioxidant activity of vitamin E.
- Used to strengthen immune function and prevent infection, to protect against colon and prostate cancer, and to prevent oxidative stress and support immune system function in those with HIV/AIDS.
- Deficiency is uncommon, but may occur in those with poor diets, those who live in areas where the soil is depleted in selenium, Crohn's disease, and malabsorption syndromes (celiac disease).
- Symptoms of deficiency: muscular weakness and wasting, cardiomyopathy (inflammation of the heart), pancreatic damage, and impaired immune function.
- Drugs that deplete: valproic acid and corticosteroids (prednisone).
- Supplements beyond the amount provided by diet and/or a multivitamin and mineral complex may be necessary for some individuals.

Zinc
- Involved in numerous enzyme reactions; required for growth and development, immune and neurological function, reproduction and regulation of gene expression; stabilizes the structure of proteins and cell membranes.
- Used to support immune function, reduce severity and duration of the common cold, and delay the progression of macular degeneration.
- Severe deficiency is rare, except in those with a genetic disorder, severe malnutrition or malabsorption, severe burns, or chronic diarrhea.

- Marginal deficiencies are common in malnourished people, vegetarians, pregnant women, the elderly, and those with celiac disease, Crohn's disease, colitis, and sickle cell anemia.
- Symptoms of deficiency include impaired growth and development, skin rashes, severe diarrhea, immune system deficiencies, impaired wound healing, poor appetite, impaired taste sensation, night blindness, clouding of the corneas, and behavioural disturbances.
- Drugs that deplete: diuretics, anticonvulsants, iron supplements, penicillamine, ACE-inhibitor drugs, acid-reducing drugs, and oral contraceptives.
- Zinc supplements can reduce copper levels, so look for a multivitamin that contains copper as well as zinc.
- Zinc supplements can reduce absorption of antibiotics (tetracycline and quinolones), so separate intake of zinc supplements from these products by two hours.
- Since the average zinc intake is below the RDA and many conditions and drugs deplete zinc levels, a supplement should be considered. Most multivitamin and mineral complexes provide at least the RDA for zinc.

ELECTROLYTES
Potassium

- Required to maintain fluid balance; required for nerve conduction and muscle function; cofactor for enzymes involved in energy production and carbohydrate metabolism.
- Used for prevention of stroke, osteoporosis, kidney stones, and in the treatment of high blood pressure.
- Deficiency (hypokalemia) is common and caused by prolonged diarrhea or vomiting, alcoholism, kidney failure, laxative abuse, anorexia, or magnesium deficiency.
- Deficiency symptoms include fatigue, muscle weakness and cramps, bloating, constipation, and abdominal pain. Severe hypokalemia may result in muscular paralysis or abnormal heart rhythms.
- Drugs that deplete: furosemide, hydrochlorothiazide, corticosteroids, pseudoephedrine, caffeine, and high-dose penicillin.
- Drugs that enhance potassium (may cause hyperkalemia): Spironolactone, triamterene, amiloride, ACE-inhibitors, anti-inflammatory drugs (ibuprofen), heaparin, digoxin, and beta-blockers.
- The average dietary potassium intake is about 2,300 mg/day for women and 3,100 mg/day for men. Evidence suggests that diets supplying at least 4,700 mg per day are associated with a decreased risk of stroke, hypertension, osteoporosis, and kidney stones, and this is the AI level set by the Institute of Medicine.
- Multivitamin/mineral complexes typically provide 99 mg of potassium per serving. Depending on dietary intake and personal risk factors, additional potassium supplements may be necessary for some people.
- Take supplements with meals or choose a microencapsulated form to reduce the risk of upset stomach.

Sodium

- Regulates fluid balance along with potassium; required for nerve conduction and muscle function; assists absorption of chloride, amino acids, glucose, and water; regulates blood volume and blood pressure.
- Excess sodium intake is linked to gastric cancer, osteoporosis, high blood pressure, and kidney stones. Reducing sodium intake may help to reduce the risk of these conditions.
- Deficiency is rare; low blood levels of sodium (hyponatremia) may be caused by fluid retention or excess sodium loss (excessive sweating, prolonged exercise, severe and prolonged vomiting and diarrhea, and kidney disease).
- Symptoms of hyponatremia include headache, nausea, muscle cramps, fatigue, confusion, and fainting. Severe cases may lead to swelling of the brain, seizures, coma, and brain damage.
- Drugs that deplete sodium: diuretics, anti-inflammatory drugs, carbamazepine, codeine, morphine, and some antidepressants.
- Supplements are rarely necessary, except in the above-mentioned conditions.
- The AI level for sodium and sodium chloride (salt) is based on the amount needed to replace losses through sweat in moderately active people and to achieve a diet that provides sufficient amounts of other essential nutrients. Most adults consume an amount much greater than the AI.

The table below contains nutrient recommendation for individuals 19 years and older, and women 19 years and older who are pregnant or lactating. To access guidelines for infants, children, and teenagers, refer to the Institute of Medicine's Web site at www.iom.edu.

Vitamins	Food Sources	RDA or AI*	UL	Side Effects/ Toxicity
Vitamin A	Liver, dairy products, and oily fish (Beta-carotene is found in orange and green vegetables and fruit)	(mcg/day) Men = 900 Women = 700 Pregnancy = 770 Lactation = 1,300	(mcg/day) Men = 3,000 Women = 3,000 Pregnancy = 3,000 Lactation = 3,000 Note: 1 mcg = 3.33 IU	Liver toxicity and birth defects (associated with vitamin A, not beta-carotene)
Vitamin B1 (thiamine)	Brewer's yeast, organ meats, whole grains, legumes, and nuts	(mg/day) Men = 1.2 Women = 1.1 Pregnancy = 1.4 Lactation = 1.4	Not determined	No adverse effects known with food or supplements
Vitamin B2 (riboflavin)	Dairy, whole grains, meat, eggs, dark green vegetables, fortified cereals	(mg/day) Men = 1.3 Women = 1.1 Pregnancy = 1.4 Lactation = 1.6	Not determined	No adverse effects known with food or supplements

Vitamin B3 (nicotinic acid, nicotinamide)	Fish, meat, poultry, dairy, nuts, seeds, whole grains, fortified cereals	(mg/day) Men = 16 Women = 14 Pregnancy = 18 Lactation = 17	35 mg/day	No adverse effects from niacin in foods; supplements may cause flushing and upset stomach; higher doses (500 mg/day) may cause liver problems, particularly with time-release products
Vitamin B5 (pantothenic acid)	Liver, kidney, egg yolk, brewer's yeast, broccoli, chicken, beef, whole grains, legumes	(mg/day)* Men = 5 Women = 5 Pregnancy = 6 Lactation = 7	Not determined	No adverse effects known from foods or supplements
Vitamin B6 (pyridoxine)	Fortified cereals, bananas, spinach, chicken, salmon, organ meat	(mg/day) Men and women 19–50 years = 1.3 Men 51+ = 1.7 Women 51+ = 1.5 Pregnancy = 1.9 Lactation = 2.0	(mg/day) Men = 100 Women = 100 Pregnancy = 100 Lactation = 100	No adverse effects from food; high-dose supplements may cause neuropathy (pain and numbness in extremities)
Vitamin B12 (cobalamin)	Meat, poultry, fish, milk, and fortified cereals	(mcg/day) Men = 2.4 Women = 2.4 Pregnancy = 2.6 Lactation = 2.8	Not determined	No adverse effects known from foods or supplements
Biotin	Egg yolk, liver, wheat bran, yeast, oatmeal, soybeans, cauliflower, mushrooms, and nuts	(mcg/day)* Men = 30 Women = 30 Pregnancy = 30 Lactation = 35	Not determined	No adverse effects known from foods or supplements
Folate (folic acid)	Dark leafy vegetables, fortified cereals, citrus fruits, and legumes	(mcg/day) Men = 400 Women = 400 Pregnancy = 600 Lactation = 500	(mcg/day) Men = 1,000 Women = 1,000 Pregnancy = 1,000 Lactation = 1,000	No adverse effects known from foods or supplements
Vitamin C (ascorbic acid)	Citrus fruit, tomatoes, red peppers, broccoli, strawberries, and potatoes	(mg/day) Men = 90 Women = 76 Pregnancy = 85 Lactation = 120	(mg/day) Men = 2,000 Women = 2,000 Pregnancy = 2,000 Lactation = 2,000	Upset stomach, diarrhea, kidney stones (in those at risk), excess iron absorption
Vitamin D	Fatty fish (mackerel, salmon, sardines), fish liver oils, eggs from hens fed vitamin D, and milk	(mcg/day)* Men and women 19–50 years = 5 50–70 = 10 71+ = 15 Pregnancy = 5 Lactation = 5	(mcg/day) Men = 50 Women = 50 Pregnancy = 50 Lactation = 50 Note: 1 mcg = 40 IU	Hypercalcemia (calcium deposits in kidneys, arteries, heart, ears, and lungs, and bone loss); symptoms include headache, weakness, nausea, vomiting, constipation

(continued)

Vitamin E	Vegetable oils (olive, sunflower, safflower oils), nuts, whole grains, and green leafy vegetables	(mg/day) Men = 15 Women = 15 Pregnancy = 15 Lactation = 19	(mg/day) Men = 1,000 Women = 1,000 Pregnancy = 1,000 Lactation = 1,000 Note: 1 mg alphatocopherol = 1.5 IU	No adverse effects from vitamin E-containing foods; supplements may increase the risk of bleeding in some individuals, particularly those taking blood-thinning drugs
Vitamin K	Green leafy vegetables, cabbage, Brussels sprouts, vegetable oils (canola, soybean, cottonseed, and olive)	(mcg/day)* Men = 120 Women = 90 Pregnancy = 90 Lactation = 90	Not determined	No adverse effects known from foods or supplements; those taking anticoagulant drugs should monitor their intake of vitamin K

Minerals	Food Sources	RDA or AI*	UL	Side Effects/ Toxicity
Calcium	Dairy, tofu, cabbage, kale, broccoli, bok choy, and legumes	(mg/day)* Men and women 19–50 = 1,000 51+ = 1,200 Pregnancy = 1,000 Lactation = 1,000	(mg/day) Men = 2,500 Women = 2,500 Pregnancy = 2,500 Lactation = 2,500	May cause kidney stones, hypercalcemia (high blood calcium), and kidney problems in those at risk; high doses may cause constipation and gas
Magnesium	Leafy green vegetables, unrefined grains, nuts, seeds, meat, milk, soybeans, tofu, legumes, and figs	(mg/day) Men 19–30 = 400 Men older than 30 = 420 Women 19–30 = 310 Women 31+ = 320 Pregnancy 19–30 = 350 Pregnancy 31+ = 360 Lactation 19–30 = 310 Lactation 31+ = 320	(mg/day) Men = 350 Women = 350 Pregnancy = 350 Lactation = 350	No adverse effects from magnesium in food; high-dose supplements may cause diarrhea
Phosphorus	Dairy products, meat, fish, eggs, nuts, lentils, cereals, and bread	(mg/day) Men = 700 Women = 700 Pregnancy = 700 Lactation = 700	(mg/day) Men 19–70 = 4,000 Men 70+ = 3,000 Women 19–70 = 4,000 Women 70+ = 3,000 Pregnancy = 3,500 Lactation = 4,000	High doses may cause calcification of soft tissues (kidneys), reduced calcium absorption and bone mass; those with kidney disease are at greatest risk of toxicity

Trace Minerals	Food Sources	RDA or AI*	UL	Side Effects/ Toxicity
Chromium	Whole grains, cereals, green beans, broccoli, meat, poultry, and fish	(mcg/day)* Men 19–50 = 35 Men 51+ = 30 Women 19–50 = 25 Women 51+ = 20 Pregnancy = 30 Lactation = 45	Not determined	Reports of kidney failure and impaired liver function with high doses (greater than 1,200 mcg/day) over long periods of time
Copper	Organ meats, shellfish, nuts, seeds, whole grain, prunes, and dark green vegetables	(mcg/day) Men = 900 Women = 900 Pregnancy = 1,000 Lactation = 1,300	(mcg/day) Men = 10,000 Women = 10,000 Pregnancy = 10,000 Lactation = 10,000	Toxicity is rare and causes abdominal pain, vomiting, liver and kidney damage, and coma; doses up to 10,000 mcg/day are not associated with toxicity, except in those with Wilson's disease, Indian childhood cirrhosis, or idiopathic copper toxicosis
Fluoride	Fluoridated drinking water, marine fish with bones, and tea	(mg/day)* Men = 4 Women = 3 Pregnancy = 3 Lactation = 3	(mg/day) Men = 10 Women = 10 Pregnancy = 10 Lactation = 10	Dental and skeletal fluorosis may occur at doses greater than two times the AI; acute toxicity seen at doses of 5 mg/kg body weight causes nausea, abdominal pain, and diarrhea
Iodine	Salt, seafood, sea vegetables (kelp), and vegetables grown in iodine-rich soil	(mg/day) Men = 150 Women = 150 Pregnancy = 220 Lactation = 290	(mg/day) Men = 1,100 Women = 1,100 Pregnancy = 1,100 Lactation = 1,100	High intakes may cause hypothyroidism and goiter; toxicity is rare and occurs only with very high doses; symptoms include burning of the mouth, throat, and stomach; fever, nausea, and vomiting; those with iodine deficiency, goiter, cystic fibrosis, or thyroid disease may be more susceptible to adverse effects

(continued)

Iron	Fruits, vegetables, fortified bread and cereals, meat, poultry, and fish	(mg/day) Men = 8 Women 19–50 = 18 Women older than 50 = 8 Pregnancy = 27 Lactation = 9	(mg/day) Men = 45 Women = 45 Pregnancy = 45 Lactation = 45	Iron supplements (regular doses) may cause nausea, vomiting, and constipation; overdose can be fatal; individuals with genetic disorders of iron overload (hemochromatosis), alcoholic cirrhosis, and liver disease may experience adverse effects with intakes below the UL
Manganese	Whole grains, nuts, legumes, leafy green vegetables, avocados, egg yolks, and teas	(mg/day)* Men = 2.3 Women = 1.8 Pregnancy = 2.0 Lactation = 2.6	(mg/day) Men = 11 Women = 11 Pregnancy = 11 Lactation = 11	Inhaled manganese dust and high levels in drinking water can be toxic to the brain; those with liver disease may be at increased risk of adverse effects from manganese
Molybdenum	Legumes, nuts, whole grains, liver, and hard drinking water	(mcg/day) Men = 45 Women = 45 Pregnancy = 50 Lactation = 50	(mcg/day) Men = 2,000 Women = 2,000 Pregnancy = 2,000 Lactation = 2,000	Toxicity is rare and may cause gout-like symptoms and neurological problems; those with copper deficiency are at increased risk of molybdenum toxicity
Selenium	Organ meats, seafood, plants, and grains grown in selenium-rich soil	(mcg/day) Men = 55 Women = 55 Pregnancy = 60 Lactation = 70	(mcg/day) Men = 400 Women = 400 Pregnancy = 400 Lactation = 400	Toxicity may occur at doses greater than 400 mcg/day and causes hair and nail brittleness and loss, upset stomach, skin rash, fatigue, and irritability
Zinc	Red meat, shellfish, eggs, whole grains, and fortified cereals	(mg/day) Men = 11 Women = 8 Pregnancy = 11 Lactation = 12	(mg/day) Men = 40 Women = 40 Pregnancy = 40 Lactation = 40	Zinc toxicity causes abdominal pain, diarrhea, nausea and vomiting. High dosages of supplements may reduce copper levels.

Electrolytes	Food Sources	RDA or AI*	UL	Side Effects/ Toxicity
Potassium	Bananas, baked potatoes, oranges and orange juice, raisins, artichokes, avocados, spinach, nuts, seeds, lima beans, meat, cod, chicken, and salmon	(mg/day)* Men = 4,700 Women = 4,700 Pregnancy = 4,700 Lactation = 5,100	Not determined	Adverse effects include nausea, vomiting, abdominal pain, and diarrhea; symptoms of toxicity include tingling in extremities, muscle weakness, temporary paralysis, and abnormal heart rhythm
Sodium	Salt, processed foods (deli meats), soy sauce, pickles, snack foods (chips, pretzels, salted nuts), and canned tomato juice	(g/day)* [Salt] Men and women: 19–50 = 1.5 [3.8] 51–70 = 1.3 [3.3] 71+ = 1.2 [3.0] Pregnancy = 1.5 [3.8] Lactation = 1.5 [3.8]	For all adults: 2.3 g/day of sodium 5.8 g/day of salt *Note:* 2 g of sodium = 5 g of salt (sodium chloride)	Ingestion of a high amount may cause edema, elevated blood pressure, nausea, vomiting, diarrhea, and abdominal cramps

*Adequate Intake (AI) recommendation

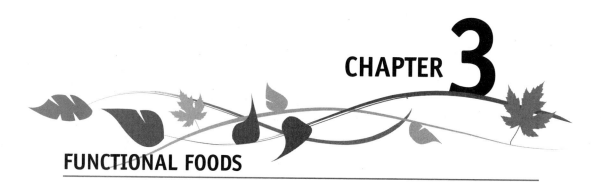

CHAPTER 3

FUNCTIONAL FOODS

Hippocrates wisely stated back in 400 BC, "Let food be your medicine and medicine be your food." Modern research has validated this doctrine. Today we know that what we eat is a major determinant of health, and that food provides both nutritive and healing properties.

Functional foods, as defined by the International Food Information Council, are "foods or dietary components that may provide a health benefit beyond basic nutrition." In other words, these foods provide more than just vitamins and minerals; they contain compounds that have beneficial actions in the body and can reduce the risk of chronic disease. These are foods that you want to include more of in your daily diet. Below are some examples of functional foods and their associated health benefits.

- Apples provide both soluble and insoluble fibre (one medium apple with skin provides about 3 g of fibre). Apple skins are a major food source of a type of flavonoid called quercetin, which is a potent antioxidant that helps protect against heart disease and cancer. These flavonoids, along with vitamin C, give apples immune-bolstering properties. Phenolic compounds found in apple skins provide protection against many chronic diseases and have recently been found to provide UVB sun protection. So there is a lot of truth to the saying, "An apple a day keeps the doctor away." Fuji apples have the highest concentration of phenolic and flavonoid compounds, but Red Delicious apples are also quite high.

- Berries, cherries, and red grapes contain plant pigments called anthocyanidins, which give these fruits their radiant red and purple colour. Anthocyanidins have antioxidant properties, preventing free radical damage and reducing the risk of chronic disease. These compounds are also important for proper brain and blood vessel function.

- Broccoli contains sulphoraphane and indole-3 carbinol, antioxidants that neutralize free radicals, enhance detoxification, and may reduce the risk of cancer. These compounds are found in other cruciferous vegetables, such as kale, cauliflower, and cabbage. Try to have a serving of these foods every day.

- Carrots are an excellent source of many antioxidant compounds, particularly beta-carotene, which is part of the carotenoids. Carotenoids help protect against cardiovascular disease, cancer, macular degeneration, and cataracts, and they also promote good night vision. New research is looking at the effects of another phytonutrient in carrots, called falcarinol, and its ability to reduce the risk of colon cancer. To get the maximum amount of nutrients from carrots, eat them raw or lightly steamed.

- Chocolate and cocoa provide various flavonoids that provide antioxidant benefits for the heart and other organs. Dark chocolate contains more antioxidants and less fat than milk chocolate. Look for products that contain 70 percent or more cocoa.

- Citrus fruits contain flavanones (a type of flavonoid), antioxidants that reduce free radicals, prevent cellular damage, and boost defences against viral infections. Oranges, grapefruit, lemons, and limes offer a wide range of nutrients (vitamin C, folate, and fibre).

- Collard greens and kale contain plant pigments called lutein and zeaxanthin, which are important for eye health and can reduce the risk of macular degeneration (age-related blindness). Supplements of lutein have been shown to improve vision in those with macular degeneration and prevent disease progression. One to two servings of kale or collard greens per week provide the recommended amount of lutein and zeaxanthin. Other food sources include spinach, broccoli, and leeks, but they contain a lesser amount.

- Cranberries contain proanthocyanidins, which have been shown to reduce the risk of urinary tract infections. Preliminary research also shows that these compounds may help lower cholesterol, improve gum health, prevent ulcers, and prevent brain damage after a stroke. The bladder benefits are seen with one to two glasses of juice daily. Look for pure cranberry juice or low-sugar juice cocktail.

- Fish and fish oils contain omega-3 fatty acids (EPA and DHA), which have been found to reduce risk of coronary heart disease. Specifically, they reduce triglycerides, increase HDL (good cholesterol), reduce inflammation, prevent clotting, and reduce blood pressure. They are also known to be beneficial for vision and brain health. Choose wild (not farmed) fish.

GET YOUR OMEGA-3S

The recommended intake of fish oils for heart health is 1–3 g daily from supplements or one to two servings of fish per week. Sadly, our fish supply is contaminated with PCBs, dioxins, and pesticides, which increase the risk of cancer. Farmed fish, especially salmon, contains the highest amount of toxins. Health authorities recommend consuming no more than six meals per year of farmed salmon. Wild Pacific salmon has fewer toxins and can be eaten once or twice a month. You can also get your omega-3s through a fish oil supplement. Look for a quality product that is tested for purity and provides at least DHA and EPA.

••

- Flaxseed provides lignans, plant compounds with antioxidant activity that may protect against heart disease and some cancers. (It lowers LDL cholesterol, total cholesterol, and triglycerides.) Flaxseed is a good source of dietary fibre (14 g of fibre per 50 g serving) and is thus used to relieve constipation and to treat ulcerative colitis and irritable bowel syndrome. Flaxseed also contains beneficial omega-3 fatty acids. To obtain all the benefits, eat the milled flaxseed or get whole seeds and crush them in a food processor or coffee grinder. Take 15 mL (1 tbsp) once or twice daily. Store milled seeds in the refrigerator or freezer in an opaque, airtight container; they will be stable for 90 days.

- Garlic contains sulphur compounds, which offer a number of health benefits. Studies have shown that garlic mildly reduces cholesterol, reduces LDL oxidation (atherosclerosis), prevents blood clotting, and fights cancer. It also possesses anti-inflammatory, antibacterial, and antiviral effects. Studies have found benefits with as little as 900 mg of garlic per day, which is approximately equivalent to one clove.

- Ginger has a long history of use for relieving stomach problems. Clinical studies have validated its benefits for preventing the symptoms of motion sickness (especially seasickness) and in the treatment of nausea and vomiting associated with pregnancy. The active compounds in ginger, called gingerols, have potent anti-inflammatory effects, making it helpful in the treatment of arthritis and other inflammatory conditions. New research suggests that ginger may also help fight cancer. Choose fresh ginger over the dry (powder) form to maximize intake of the active compounds.

- Green tea is rich in catechins (a type of flavonoid) called epigallocatechin gallate (EGCG). This compound has been found to reduce the risk of certain cancers, reduce the size of existing tumours, and inhibit tumour growth. It also supports heart function by lowering blood pressure and reducing the risk of fatal heart attacks. EGCG also supports nerve function and may benefit Parkinson's and Alzheimer's disease. Recently EGCG has been found to reduce body fat and improve metabolism. Most studies evaluating the health benefits of green tea involved drinking 750–2,500 mL daily. Black tea, white tea, Oolong tea, and other teas derived from the plant *Camellia sinesis* may offer similar health benefits but are not as widely researched.

- Oat bran contains a soluble fibre called beta-glucan, which has been shown to lower cholesterol and reduce the risk of heart disease. Studies have found that 3 g of beta-glucan daily can reduce total cholesterol by an average of 5 percent. This amount can be found in approximately 60 g of oatmeal or 40 g of oat bran. Other good forms of soluble fibre are psyllium, apples, and beans.

- Onions contain a variety of nutrients, such as vitamin C and chromium. Powerful sulphur compounds in onions are responsible for their pungent odour and for many of their health benefits. They can help reduce blood sugar, cholesterol, and blood pressure. Onions provide a concentrated source of the flavonoid quercitin, which helps reduce inflammation and may halt the growth of cancer. Cooking meats with onions may help reduce the amount of carcinogens produced when meat is cooked at high heat. There are many varieties of onions. In general, the more pungent an onion, the more active compounds and health benefits it has.

- Soybeans contain isoflavones (daidzein and genistein), which help reduce cholesterol levels, fight cancer, increase bone density, and reduce menopausal symptoms. Research suggests that consuming 25 g of soy protein daily can provide a significant cholesterol-lowering effect. Aside from soybeans and tofu, you can get the benefits of soy protein by eating soy nuts, soy milk, soy yogurt, and bars and shakes containing soy protein.

- Tomatoes contain an antioxidant called lycopene, which has been found to reduce the risk of prostate and colon cancer, support prostate health, reduce blood clotting and inflammation, and reduce heart attack risk. Most studies found health benefits with an intake of 8–10 mg daily. Lycopene is also present in tomato sauce, tomato paste, and ketchup, which contain a higher amount of lycopene than fresh tomatoes. To obtain 10 mg of lycopene, you would have to eat about 10–15 raw tomatoes, 60 mL (2 oz.) of ketchup, or 20 mL (4 tsp) of tomato paste. Lycopene is also found in papaya, strawberries, watermelon, guava, and pink grapefruit.

- Yogurt contains active bacteria cultures known as probiotics or friendly bacteria, which improve gastrointestinal health (digestion and elimination) and immune function. These active cultures also help digest the naturally occurring sugar (lactose) in dairy products that causes bloating and diarrhea in some people. Avoid the "diet" or "light" yogurts, since they are sweetened with aspartame, a chemical whose safety in food is questionable. The amount of probiotics in yogurt varies with brand and storage. For this reason those looking for the consistent benefits of probiotics often opt for supplements.

Many compounds found in functional foods are available in supplement form. Supplements often provide a standardized amount of the active compounds, they are easy to take, and are a great way to complement the diet.

The health benefits make functional foods worthy of inclusion in your daily diet. Try to have a few each day. Look for organic products to reduce your exposure to harmful pesticides.

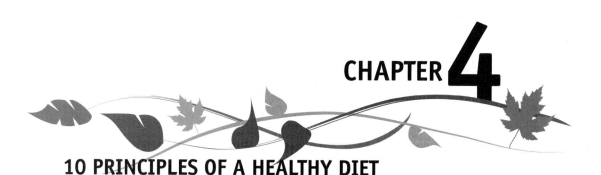

CHAPTER 4

10 PRINCIPLES OF A HEALTHY DIET

In the preceding chapters I discussed the necessary elements of nutrition and good health: the macronutrients, micronutrients, and functional foods.

In this chapter I will share with you my 10 principles for a healthy diet, elements that I recommend based on current science for optimal health, energy, and disease prevention.

1. MAKE QUALITY FOOD CHOICES

Fresh, natural, unprocessed foods should form the basis of your diet. Look for organic produce to reduce ingestion of toxic pesticides. If organic is not available, look for locally grown fruits and vegetables. Items from foreign countries may contain higher levels of pesticides and bacteria. To preserve the nutrients in your food, minimize storage time and cooking or reheating.

Choose whole-grain (brown rice, multigrain breads) over the refined and processed products. Refined grains (white bread) have most of the vitamins, minerals, and fibre removed.

Quality protein sources include free-range and organic meat and poultry, legumes, nuts, seeds, and tofu. If you are following a vegetarian diet, be sure to incorporate a variety of plant-based proteins to ensure that all essential amino acids are consumed.

Consume health-promoting fats from fish, nuts, seeds, and quality oils (hemp, flaxseed, canola, olive, sunflower, and safflower).

Avoid or minimize eating fast/processed foods, as they are typically high in calories, poor in nutritional value, and laden with potentially dangerous chemicals and preservatives. Read your labels carefully.

FORGET THE FADS

Avoid fad diets, which can be hard to follow, have few nutrients, and can even be dangerous. Whether your goal is weight loss or better health, stay away from the latest fad and make healthier food choices.

2. ENJOY VARIETY

To get a broad range of nutrients in your diet, enjoy a variety of foods, rather than sticking to your favourites. This is particularly important with vegetables and fruits, as their nutrient profiles vary greatly. To obtain the many antioxidants, vitamins, minerals, and phytonutrients, eat a variety of plant foods every day. Experiment with new foods and recipes, and try to reintroduce previously disliked foods.

3. MODERATION: KNOW YOUR CALORIE REQUIREMENTS AND PORTION SIZES

Your caloric requirements are dependent upon your age, gender, height, weight, and activity level. The Institute of Medicine provides the following recommendations for adults 30 years and older:

Height/Weight	Gender	Calories (Sedentary)	Calories (Active)
5' 1" 98–132 lbs.	Women Men	1,688–1,834 1,919–2,167	2,104–2,290 2,104–2,290
5' 4" 110–150 lbs.	Women Men	1,816–1,982 2,068–2,349	2,267–2,477 2,490–2,842
5' 7" 125–170 lbs.	Women Men	1,948–2,134 2,222–2,538	2,434–2,670 2,683–3,078
6' 1" 139–187 lbs.	Women Men	2,083–2,290 2,382–2,736	2,605–2,869 2,883–3,325

Those engaged in vigorous physical activity or who are pregnant or lactating have increased calorie requirements.

To figure out how many calories you should consume from carbohydrates, fat, and protein, consider the ranges set out by the IOM. They recommend that adults get 45–65 percent of their calories from carbohydrates, 20–35 percent from fat, and 10–35 percent from protein.

AVOIDING PORTION DISTORTION

Overeating can lead to obesity, high triglycerides, insulin resistance, free radical damage, and shortened life expectancy. To prevent overeating, control your portion sizes and eat slowly. A serving equals one piece of fruit, 1 cup of raw or ½ cup of cooked vegetables, one slice of bread, ½ cup of cooked rice or pasta, or 2–3 oz. of meat. Eating slowly allows your stomach to send a message to your brain that you are full. Chew your food thoroughly and drink water to allow for proper digestion. It should take you 20–30 minutes to eat a meal.

4. EAT SMALL AND FREQUENT MEALS

Try to eat every three hours—three small meals and two snacks daily. This will improve metabolism (calorie burning) and blood sugar balance, which improves energy and mood.

Breakfast is essential to fuel your body. If you aren't very hungry in the morning, then have a light meal such as yogurt and berries or a protein shake. Try not to eat too late in the evening (after 8 p.m.), as this could impact sleep. Don't skip meals, even if you are trying to lose weight, since this causes fatigue, poor concentration, sluggish metabolism, and triggers food cravings.

5. DRINK PLENTY OF WATER

Water is essential to health—it helps regulate body temperature, removes wastes, and transports nutrients throughout the body. A lack of water causes dehydration, which can be deadly. To keep your body well hydrated, drink 2–3 L of water daily. Water purified by reverse osmosis is best because tap water may contain high amounts of chlorine, which can be harmful to the stomach and bladder. Keep in mind that intense physical activity and heat exposure increases water loss and the need for more fluids.

6. BOOST FIBRE INTAKE

Most Canadians are getting only a fraction of the recommended amount of fibre, which is 25–38 g daily for most adults. Fibre is critical because it can reduce your risk of chronic diseases, such as diabetes, heart disease, and certain cancers, plus it keeps your bowels regular, improves blood sugar control, and plays a role in weight management. Dietary fibre is found in fruits, vegetables, beans, seeds, and whole grains such as wheat and oat bran. If your diet is lacking in fibre, look for a supplement.

7. REDUCE THE SALT, AND INCREASE THE POTASSIUM

Salt (sodium) is necessary for health, as it helps maintain fluid balance and aids muscle and nerve function; however, most Canadians consume far too much salt and this can contribute to high blood pressure, especially in older individuals, African Americans, and those with diabetes and kidney disease.

The IOM recommends adults consume 3.8 g of salt daily to replace the amount lost through sweat. The tolerable upper intake level (maximum recommended amount) is 5.8 g per day and most adults regularly consume more than this amount; we need to cut back.

There is naturally occurring salt in dairy, seafood, vegetables, breads, and grains; however, the majority of our salt intake comes from processed and prepared foods, such as deli meats, condiments (ketchup), dressings and sauces (soy), and snack foods (chips, pretzels), so cut back on these foods and season food with herbs or flavoured oils and vinegars rather than using the salt shaker.

Potassium is another important nutrient for regulating fluid balance. It is also important for nerve and muscle function and supports cell structure and integrity. The IOM recommends that adults consume at least 4.7 g of potassium per day to lower blood pressure, blunt the effects of salt, and reduce the risk of kidney stones and bone loss. Most Canadians consume much less than this recommended amount. To boost potassium intake, eat more bananas, oranges and orange juice, avocado, peaches, and tomatoes.

8. MINIMIZE SUGAR

The typical adult consumes about 72.5 kg of sugar each year, which is clearly too much. Excessive sugar intake has been linked to diabetes, obesity, elevated triglycerides, tooth decay, poor immune function, emotional swings, and other health problems. Refined (white) sugar contains propyl alcohol, which cannot be broken down in the body. Accumulation of this chemical in the intestines can disrupt digestion and be toxic to the body.

The World Health Organization recommends restricting consumption of added sugar—including sugar from honey, syrups, and sweetened drinks/juices—to less than 10 percent of calories.

To satisfy a craving for sweets, have fruit (fresh or dried). Fruit contains natural sugar (fructose), but it also provides vitamins, minerals, and fibre. Mashed bananas or apple sauce are great substitutions for sugar in baked goods. Artificial sweeteners such as aspartame and saccharin should be avoided because they have been linked to headaches, mental illness, brain damage, and cancer. Stevia, a natural sweetener obtained from a plant, is a good substitute. It can provide up to 300 times the sweetening power of sugar without the calories.

9. CUT DOWN ON CAFFEINE

A high intake of caffeine can promote calcium loss from bones, increase blood pressure, affect fertility in women, and cause sleep disturbances (insomnia), irritability, anxiety, and tremors. It is also highly addictive—abrupt withdrawal, even if you drink only one cup of coffee daily, can cause headaches, irritability, and fatigue within hours of missing your usual drink.

Drip coffee has the highest caffeine content at 100–200 mg. Black tea and green tea contain approximately 35–45 mg, but the effects of caffeine are blunted by an amino acid (theanine), which has a calming effect. Cola contains about 35 mg per can and chocolate contains 6–20 mg per 30 g piece. Try switching your coffee or cola to tea. If you need a coffee, then limit it to no more than 500 mL (2 cups) daily.

10. LIMIT ALCOHOL

Heavy and chronic drinking (more than three drinks per day) is linked to liver and cardiovascular disease, pancreatitis, immune system depression, increased risk of cancer (esophagus, mouth, liver, breast, and colon), brain shrinkage, sexual dysfunction (impotence), infertility, and malnutrition. Alcohol and what it is mixed with floods the body with excess calories, which can contribute to weight gain.

There are some benefits with moderate alcohol consumption. Research has found that one or two drinks daily reduces the risk of heart disease, likely due to its ability to increase HDL (good) cholesterol, reduce blood clotting, and the increased antioxidant activity, as seen with red wine and dark beer. So the bottom line is to limit your intake to one or two drinks per day.

PUTTING IT ALL TOGETHER

As you read through this chapter, you probably identified some areas where you need to make changes. This is the first step—realization. Next, work on slowly making healthier food choices, such as cutting out fast food, eating more vegetables, drinking more water, or limiting your sugar or caffeine intake. By gradually making changes, you will be more likely to stick with your nutritional plan.

Take time to plan your meals, so that you are not reaching for fast food or un-healthy snacks.

Don't get discouraged by an occasional overindulgence. If you have a bad diet day, don't let it perpetuate. Get back on track the next day. Consistency counts.

By following a healthy diet you will notice that you have more energy, a better mood, and an overall improved sense of well-being.

CHAPTER 5

EXERCISE FOR BETTER HEALTH

There is no getting around it—regular exercise and physical activity are essential for good health and must be part of your daily life. You will notice recommendations throughout this book for exercise, as virtually every parameter of health can be improved with exercise. Numerous studies have shown that regular exercise cuts your risk of chronic, debilitating diseases such as heart disease (by reducing cholesterol and blood pressure), osteoporosis, cancer, diabetes, and prevents premature death! It is also essential to develop and maintain both a healthy body weight and muscular strength. Plus it offers emotional benefits, as exercise reduces stress and anxiety, and improves sleep and overall emotional well-being.

With today's busy, fast-paced lifestyle, exercise usually falls to the bottom of the priority list while it should be at the top. There are plenty of reasons why people don't exercise. Lack of time is the most common excuse, so below I show you how to boost the activity in your lifestyle. Many people find they don't have the energy to exercise, yet they don't realize that exercise actually gives them more energy. Some people have a misconception that exercise is expensive. That is only if you join a fancy health club. There are plenty of activities you can do with little or no cost. Some are concerned about health problems (arthritis and back problems), yet exercise can actually benefit and improve these problems. Regardless of your health status, age, or current fitness level, there are activities that you can do to improve your health. So now that we have put aside the common obstacles, let's take a look at the various types of exercise and how to build them into our lifestyle.

CARDIOVASCULAR (AEROBIC) EXERCISE

Cardiovascular activities involve large muscle groups and increase heart rate for more than a few minutes. Examples include brisk walking, swimming, biking, aerobics, dancing, and rollerblading. These exercises help burn calories, and also improve cardiovascular and respiratory (lung) function by conditioning the lungs to use more oxygen while increasing your heart's efficiency (decreasing heart rate).

Aim for 30 minutes to an hour five times per week. If you are currently not exercising, then start slowly—five minutes on your first day and then increase gradually. With time, endurance improves.

Pick activities that you enjoy and do them in the morning or right after work, preferably on an empty stomach. Morning is best because you will have more energy and will continue to burn calories for several hours afterward.

To determine the intensity level for optimal cardiovascular (and fat-burning) benefits, check your heart rate. The activity should increase your heart rate to 60–80 percent of your maximum rate for 30 minutes or longer. To find your maximum rate, subtract your age from 220. Then calculate 60–80 percent of that figure. Beginners should aim for 60 percent, while more advanced exercisers can aim for 80 percent.

For example, if you are 40 years old:
220 – 40 = 180
60–80 percent of 180 = 108–144

You should keep your heart rate between 108 and 144 beats per minute for 30 minutes.

Other ways to gauge your intensity level are:

Breath sound check: Your breathing should be heavier and audible.
Talk test: You should be capable of talking, but not with great ease.

To increase intensity, add resistance or power to the movements. For example, when a brisk 30-minute walk becomes easy, add hand weights or walk on hills. Moving your arms above your heart will also increase your heart rate.

RESISTANCE TRAINING

Activities that challenge your muscles against resistance increase strength, endurance, and muscle mass, and strengthen bones. This can be achieved with weightlifting, exercise machines, bands/tubes, using your own body weight, or lifting heavy objects. These activities are particularly important for older adults because they help prevent and slow the muscle and bone loss that occurs with aging.

Try to spend 20–30 minutes three to four times a week doing resistance activities. Choose two body parts per workout. For example, do chest and triceps on Monday, back and biceps on Wednesday, and legs and shoulders on Friday. Pick two exercises per body part and do two or three sets of 8–12 repetitions of that exercise. Vary your activities and routine to continually challenge your muscles.

POST-WORKOUT RECOVERY

Research shows that by consuming a high-quality protein shake (especially whey protein isolate) immediately after performing resistance exercise, you can greatly increase your body's ability to recuperate. This is largely due to a very powerful amino acid in protein—essential to early muscle repair—called leucine.

STRETCHING

Stretching after a workout is a great way to improve flexibility and joint health and prevent next-day soreness. Spend about five to 10 minutes stretching all your muscles. Stretch slowly and gently, breathe deeply, and hold each position for at least 10 seconds.

HOW MUCH EXERCISE DO YOU NEED?

Guidelines from the National Academy of Sciences and the Institute of Medicine (used by Canada and the United States) recommend that, regardless of weight, adults and children should spend a total of at least one hour each day in moderately intense physical activity. This recommendation takes into consideration the increased caloric intake of our population, our lack of activity, and our rising prevalence of obesity.

BUILDING ACTIVITY INTO YOUR DAY

If you don't have an hour that you can dedicate to exercise, work on incorporating more activity into your daily routine. Every little bit helps. Studies have actually shown that the benefits of exercise are cumulative (i.e., performing a few minutes of exercise at a time is as effective as performing all the exercise at once). Here are some suggestions:

• Do housework or gardening with vim and vigour.
• Take the stairs instead of the elevator.
• Use your break at work to go for a brisk walk.
• Ride your bike to the store.
• Park your car farther away and walk to your destination.
• Wash your car instead of using the drive-through.

Of course, if you can set aside an hour for exercise each day, that is great. Otherwise, try to set aside an hour three to four times a week and on the other days, use some of the above ideas to work more movement into your day.

EXERCISE FOR WEIGHT LOSS

Regular exercise is essential for losing body fat and maintaining muscle mass. In fact, it has been found that those who work out five times a week lose three times as much fat as those who exercise only two or three times weekly. Exercise supports fat loss by:

• Burning calories and stored fat
• Raising the metabolic rate for four to 24 hours afterward
• Slowing the movement of food through your digestive tract, so you feel full longer
• Balancing blood sugar—exercise pulls stored calories (energy) in the forms of glucose and fat out of tissues, which helps balance blood glucose levels, making you less likely to feel hungry

MORE MUSCLE BURNS MORE CALORIES

It is a common misconception that aerobic exercise is the most effective way to lose body fat. Aerobic activities do burn calories, but resistance training plays a stronger role because it builds lean muscle mass, which boosts your metabolism, burns calories, and encourages the body to utilize fat more efficiently as fuel. The bottom line is the more muscle you have, the more calories you burn. In fact, 1 pound (0.5 kg) of muscle burns roughly 50 calories per day, compared to 1 pound (0.5 kg) of fat, which burns only 2–3 calories per day.

CREATING YOUR FITNESS PROGRAM

If you have been sedentary all your life, the prospect of getting active may be intimidating, so take it slowly. If you do too much too soon, you may injure yourself or become too discouraged to continue. Here are some important points to keep in mind:

- Before you start an exercise program, consult with your doctor, especially if you have any health conditions or are taking medication.
- For guidance on proper exercise technique and help in designing a workout tailored to your needs, see a certified personal trainer.
- To keep your motivation high, get a workout partner, vary your activities, and, most importantly, have fun.
- Don't expect overnight results. Set reasonable goals, be consistent with your exercises, and you will see both the physical and emotional rewards.
- Be sure to drink lots of water during and after your workout, and make time to stretch your muscles.

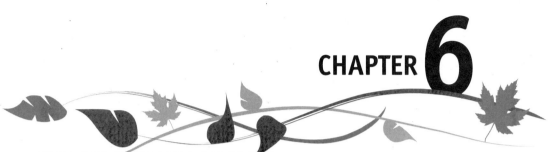

CHAPTER 6

THE IMPORTANCE OF SLEEP AND STRESS MANAGEMENT

Right along with proper nutrition and regular exercise are two other essential elements for healthy living—adequate sleep and stress management. These essential but often overlooked factors are paramount for physical and emotional well-being and disease prevention. In this chapter we take a closer look at the value of sleep, how to get a better night's rest, and how to deal with stress more effectively.

SLEEP

Sleep is one of the body's most basic needs for health and well-being, yet with today's busy lifestyles, sleep deprivation has become all too common. In fact, nearly half of all adults report having difficulty sleeping.

While we think of sleep as a relaxing and passive state, there is actually quite a lot going on in the body during sleep. There are five stages of sleep defined by brain wave activity, muscle tone, and eye movement. Stage one is referred to as drowsy sleep and represents the onset of sleep. During stage two, conscious awareness of the external environment disappears. During stages three and four, the body goes into a deeper sleep, and the brain produces what are called delta waves. Delta sleep is our deepest sleep, the point when our brain waves are least like what they are when we are awake. It is during this time that the body's major organs and regulatory systems are busy working on repair and regeneration and certain hormones, such as growth hormone, are secreted. Stage five, known as REM (rapid eye movement), is the stage during which we dream.

The exact amount of sleep needed varies among individuals, but is thought to be between seven and nine hours. Getting less than six hours is associated with health problems.

An occasional sleepless night is not a concern, but persistent difficulty in falling asleep, waking up too early, awakening frequently during the night, or waking up feeling tired and not refreshed could indicate insomnia. Lack of sleep, particularly deep (delta) sleep, not only makes us feel tired, but it has serious consequences such as memory loss, poor concentration, depression, headache, irritability, increased response to stress, high blood pressure, depressed immune function, and low libido. More recently sleep deprivation has been linked to obesity due to hormonal changes that reduce metabolism and increase appetite. Animal studies have also shown that sleep deprivation can lead to death within two to three weeks—a similar time frame for death due to starvation.

Causes of Insomnia

There are many factors that can affect the quality of sleep such as stress, medical problems (depression, anxiety), medications, alcohol, poor nutrition, noise/light, the need to go to the bathroom during the night, and poor sleep hygiene (going to bed at different times). Insomnia and its causes and treatments are covered in greater detail in Section 3 of this book.

Tips for a Better Night's Rest

For a good night's sleep, consider the following:

- Establish a regular bedtime and wake time.
- Do relaxing activities before bed—read a book, have a warm bath, or meditate.
- Reserve your bedroom for intimacy and sleep only. Don't watch TV, read, or do computer work in your bedroom.
- Make your bedroom dark, quiet, and comfortable.
- Avoid caffeine (coffee, tea, pop, chocolate) and smoking within four hours of bedtime, as this can affect your ability to fall asleep.
- Avoid alcohol; it may help you fall asleep, but drinking alcohol causes nighttime wakening and reduces sleep quality.
- Exercise regularly early in the day. Do not exercise in the evening, as this can be stimulating.
- If you work shifts or travel to different time zones, try a supplement of melatonin (a hormone naturally secreted in response to darkness), as it helps promote good sleep.

STRESS

Stress has become a common complaint of life in the fast lane. We don't have enough time, take on too much, worry about health and wealth, and feel overwhelmed and stressed out on a regular basis. Sound familiar? According to recent reports, 43 percent of all adults suffer the adverse health effects of stress, and stress-related ailments account for 75–90 percent of all visits to physicians. These numbers have been steadily climbing over the past few decades.

Understanding Stress

Stress, as defined by Hans Selye, an Austrian-born Canadian physician who studied the physiological and biochemical results of stress and anxiety, is "the non-specific response of the body to any demand placed upon it." He claimed that it isn't stress that harms us but distress, a phenomenon that occurs when we have prolonged emotional stress and don't deal with it in a positive manner. In other words, stress is not an external force but rather how we react to external stimuli—how we feel and respond to traffic, deadlines at work, or any event that we perceive as stressful.

Stress and Disease

In response to stress, the body releases stress hormones—adrenaline, noradrenaline, and cortisol—to prepare the body to fight, hence this is known as the fight or flight response. Heart rate, blood pressure, and lung tone increase to enhance the function of the heart and lungs. This innate reaction served us well many centuries ago when we had to fight off wild animals and protect our villages. Stress today, however, is very different. It is chronic, pervasive, and insidious because it stems primarily from psychological rather than physical threats and has far-reaching effects on our health.

Numerous studies have linked stress to heart disease, cancer, diabetes, high cholesterol and blood pressure, anxiety, depression, memory loss, insomnia, muscle tension, obesity, fatigue, low libido, erectile dysfunction, menstrual cycle disturbances, and many more problems.

Stress Management

Stress can certainly take a toll on your body and mind, so it is absolutely crucial to find ways to cope effectively. Start by identifying your stressors and then look for ways to change your reaction to those situations. It may be a matter of analyzing and rethinking your natural reaction, avoiding certain situations, or utilizing one of the following stress-reducing strategies. Seeking help from a counsellor or psychologist can be very helpful to learn coping techniques and strategies.

Meditation

Meditation is the practice of focusing the mind and consciously relaxing the body for a sustained period. This is common among Eastern cultures and is gaining popularity in North America. Focusing on a single object or your breath or a sound occupies your mind and diverts it from the problems that are causing you stress. Many studies have found this an effective and practical way to manage stress. All you need is a quiet, comfortable area. Sit down and close your eyes. Relax all your muscles starting with your feet and working up. Focus your attention on your breathing or a calming sight or sound. Breathe in slowly and deeply and then out. Do this for 10 or 20 minutes. You can do this when feeling stressed, or make a habit of meditating once or twice a day for better health and relaxation.

Breathing Techniques

Taking slow, controlled breaths is a great way to promote calming when feeling stressed or anxious. Sit down comfortably and close your eyes. Place the tip of your tongue against the roof of your mouth just behind your front teeth. Begin by exhaling through your mouth around your tongue, then close your mouth and inhale deeply through your nose for four seconds. Hold your breath for five seconds and then completely exhale through your mouth, making a *whoosh* sound. Repeat this cycle four or five times. This technique can be done any time or anywhere.

Exercise

Getting regular exercise is a great way to reduce stress, promote calming, and improve both physical and emotional well-being. Exercise can help elevate your mood, lessen anxiety and anger, and increase blood flow to the muscles, which tend to be tense from stress. Walking, cycling, swimming, and dancing are just a few examples of stress-busting activities. Keep in mind, though, that you also need to find ways to change your reaction to stress (counselling). Yoga and tai chi are excellent forms of exercise to promote relaxation, as they incorporate breathing and visualization.

Visualization

This technique involves concentrating on images in your mind that make you feel calm and relaxed. Close your eyes, take a few deep breaths, and visualize a picture or event that made you feel calm and centred. Focus on the details—the sounds, images, and smells.

Other Considerations

• Massage, acupuncture, and acupressure promote relaxation of the body and mind.
• Supplements that help relieve stress include theanine, B-vitamins, and magnesium. This is discussed further in Section 3 of this book.
• Learn to say no. Taking on too much leads to feeling overwhelmed and pressed for time. Being able to say no (no excuse needed) when asked to take on a new task will make you feel empowered and relieved.
• Avoid negativity, as negative people, places, and events can create stress.
• Channel stress in positive ways—exercise, paint, or clean your house.
• Talk about it—share your feelings and concerns and get support from friends, family, or a therapist.

Improving the quality of your sleep and dealing more effectively with stress will bring many health rewards—fewer physical and emotional ailments and overall improved well-being. Identify the areas where you are struggling, seek help, and work on adopting positive changes.

SECTION II

THE NATURAL PHARMACY

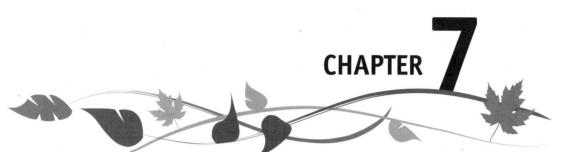

CHAPTER 7

REFERENCE GUIDE TO DIETARY SUPPLEMENTS, HERBAL REMEDIES, AND BRANDED INGREDIENTS

In this section you will find concise information on various nutritional supplements. This list is not all-inclusive—there are thousands of supplements on the market, but I chose to include those with the most research and health benefits. If clinical research has been done on a specific branded product, then I have included that name. As well, I have noted important drug interactions, side effects, and precautions.

You will find other nutritional supplements that have specific uses listed under Section 3. For example, supplements used specifically for weight loss are included in the discussion on obesity.

It is always a good idea to check with your health care provider before taking any new product, particularly if you are taking medications or have a health condition. Dosages are not included here, as they vary with the intended use, age of the person, existing medical problems, and other factors.

AGED GARLIC EXTRACT (KYOLIC)

Garlic is well known for its myriad health benefits and its strong odour. Aged garlic extract is unique in that it is odourless, processed from organically grown garlic, standardized to potent sulphur compounds, and is the most widely researched garlic product available. Studies have shown that aged garlic extract provides benefits for heart protection, liver detoxification, immune enhancement, antioxidant activity, stress management, fatigue, cancer protection, and anti-aging.

ALOE VERA

Aloe vera is a plant that has a long history of use to promote skin healing. It contains amino aids, vitamins C and E, zinc, and essential fatty acids. Research supports the use of topical aloe for genital herpes (to improve healing of lesions), seborrhea, and psoriasis; preliminary research shows benefits with oral aloe to improve blood sugar in type 2 diabetes and for treatment of ulcerative colitis.

ALPHA-LIPOIC ACID

Alpha-lipoic acid, an antioxidant found inside every cell of the body, helps the body convert glucose into energy to meet the body's needs, and is found naturally in liver, yeast, potatoes, spinach, and red meat. Levels may be depleted in those with diabetes, liver cirrhosis, and atherosclerosis. It is used to improve glucose levels in diabetes, treat diabetic neuropathy, and for burning mouth syndrome. Side effects are rare and may include skin rash and upset stomach.

ARGININE

An amino acid found in many foods, such as dairy, meat, poultry, and fish, arginine is involved in cell division, wound healing, removal of ammonia from the body, immunity to illness, the secretion of hormones, and the production of nitrous oxide, a substance the dilates blood vessels. Research supports its use for congestive heart failure, intermittent claudication, angina, impotence, and sexual dysfunction in women; preliminary evidence shows benefits for diabetes and improving recovery from surgery.

BETA-GLUCAN

A type of soluble fibre found naturally in plants such as oats, wheat, and barley, beta-glucan is also available in supplements. Studies have shown that beta-glucan can modestly improve cholesterol levels; it may also reduce blood pressure and improve blood sugar levels in diabetics. There are no known side effects or drug interactions.

BLACK COHOSH (REMIFEMIN)

Black cohosh is an herb used for the treatment of menopausal symptoms; studies show that it can reduce hot flashes and improve mood. Research involving black cohosh, plus St. John's wort, has shown benefits for both hot flashes and depression in menopause. Do not use during pregnancy or breast-feeding; use cautiously with liver disease. High doses may cause upset stomach, nausea, and headache.

BOSWELLIA

An herb with long history of use in Ayurvedic medicine, boswellia is used for arthritis, respiratory diseases, and diarrhea. Its anti-inflammatory properties have been studied and found beneficial for the treatment of rheumatoid and osteoarthritis, asthma, and inflammatory bowel disease. It is generally well tolerated; there are no known drug interactions.

BREWER'S YEAST

A product derived from dried, pulverized cells of the fungus *Saccharomyces cerevisiae*, brewer's yeast is a rich source of B-vitamins, protein, and minerals such as chromium. Supplements are used to treat acute diarrhea and to lower cholesterol and improve blood sugar balance in diabetics. Side effects are rare, but some people are allergic to brewer's yeast.

BROMELAIN

Bromelain is a combination of protein-digesting enzymes (called proteolytic enzymes) found in pineapple juice and in the stem of pineapple plants. It is used to reduce inflammation, treat sinusitis, improve healing from injuries, and support immune function. Side effects are rare, but allergic reactions are possible. It may thin the blood; use cautiously with blood-thinning drugs, such as warfarin, as dosage adjustments may be necessary.

BUTCHER'S BROOM

Butcher's broom is an herb with a long history of use as a diuretic and for urinary problems. Research has demonstrated benefits for reducing the pain, swelling, and fatigue associated with chronic venous insufficiency; it may also be helpful for hemorrhoids, varicose veins, and lymphedema. It is generally well tolerated; there are no known drug interactions.

CARNITINE

Carnitine is an amino acid that the body uses to turn fat into energy. Levels may be depleted in those with kidney, liver, or brain disease, and in those taking anti-seizure drugs such as phenytoin and valproic acid. Research supports benefits for angina, intermittent claudication, congestive heart failure, heart attack recovery, diabetic neuropathy, chronic obstructive pulmonary disease, and male sexual function and infertility. Carnitine is very safe and well tolerated, but should be used cautiously in those with low thyroid hormone.

CAYENNE

Cayenne is a pepper that is part of the capsicum family. Creams containing cayenne are used to reduce pain (arthritis, strains, sprains, fibromyalgia, back pain, headache, and shingles); it helps to reduce the itching caused by psoriasis and the symptoms of neuropathy; it may reduce the stomach irritation caused by non-steroidal anti-inflammatory drugs (NSAIDs). Wash your hands after applying this cream because it can cause burning and stinging if you rub your eyes. Oral cayenne may increase the absorption of theophylline, a drug used for asthma and lung disease.

CELADRIN

Celadrin is a patented blend of esterified fatty acids derived from beef tallow. Studies show benefits for reducing the pain and inflammation associated with osteoarthritis; it may also benefit other inflammatory conditions such as rheumatoid arthritis, eczema, psoriasis, and gout. There are no known drug interactions or side effects. It is available in cream and oral supplements.

CHAMOMILE

An herb popular for its calming properties, chamomile is found in teas, oral supplements, and creams. It is used orally (tea and supplements) to reduce anxiety and promote relaxation. Topical products are used to promote healing. Compounds in chamomile have blood-thinning properties, so it should be used cautiously by those taking warfarin or other blood thinners, as dosage adjustments may be necessary.

CHONDROITIN SULPHATE

Chondroitin sulphate is a naturally occurring substance in the body that is a major constituent of cartilage, the connective tissue found in joints. Oral supplements are used to reduce the symptoms of osteoarthritis (improve mobility and reduce pain); it may also reduce the progression of the disease. Topically it is used to improve wound healing. It is usually well tolerated, although high doses may cause upset stomach.

COENZYME Q10

Coenzyme Q10, an antioxidant naturally found in our bodies, is involved in energy production in every cell. Strong evidence supports supplement use for congestive heart failure; it is also used for high blood pressure, heart attack recovery, mitral valve prolapse, cardiomyopathy, gum disease, diabetes, Parkinson's disease, and migraine headache. Levels may be depleted by statin drugs, beta-blockers, and anti-depressants. Deficiency causes fatigue, gum disease, heart problems, and increased risk of infections.

COLOSTRUM

Colostrum, a component of breast milk, is produced during the first day or two after birth. It provides newborns with a rich mixture of antibodies and growth factors. Supplements are derived from cow colostrums and are used for immune support, diarrhea, and in sports products.

CRAN-MAX

Cran-Max is a whole-berry cranberry supplement that has been found in studies to prevent urinary tract infections. Cranberry contains antioxidants called proanthocyanidins (condensed tannins). Cranberry juice and supplements may also help lower cholesterol and protect against gum disease and *H. Pylori* infection (the cause of ulcers).

CREATINE

Creatine is a naturally occurring substance that plays an important role in the production of energy in the body. Several studies have shown that creatine can increase athletic performance in sports that involve intense but short bursts of activity. It may also offer benefits for weight training and to prevent muscle loss in seniors. Side effects include diarrhea and muscle cramping. It should be avoided by those with kidney disease.

D-GLUCARATE

A supplemental form of glucaric acid, which is a phytonutrient found in fruits and vegetables (apples, Brussels sprouts, broccoli, and cabbage), D-glucarate helps the liver detoxify and eliminate excess hormones (particularly estrogen); it is used for the treatment of PMS, fibrocystic breast disease, uterine fibroids, and other conditions of estrogen excess; it is also used for prevention of hormone-dependent cancers of the breast and prostate. There are no known side effects; there are no known drug interactions. However, many drugs are metabolized in the liver and D-glucarate may enhance the elimination of certain drugs, requiring dosage adjustments.

DIGESTIVE ENZYMES

Digestive enzymes are protein compounds that aid in the breakdown and digestion of food. They are found naturally in raw foods and produced by the body. There are three classes: proteolytic enzymes digest protein, lipases digest fat, and amylases digest carbohydrates. Supplements are used to aid digestion; some people are deficient in digestive enzymes. Proteolytic enzymes may also help reduce pain and inflammation from injuries, osteoarthritis, and surgery. Side effects and allergic reactions are rare.

DIOSMIN

Diosmin is a flavonoid that improves the tone and strength of the blood vessels, reduces swelling, fights free-radical damage, and stimulates lymphatic flow. Over 30 clinical studies have found it effective for improving vein disorders, including varicose veins, chronic venous insufficiency, nighttime leg cramps, and hemorrhoids. It has a quick onset of action (one to two weeks) and is not associated with any side effects or drug interactions. Look for a product standardized to 95 percent diosmin and 5 percent hesperidin.

ECHINACEA

Echinacea is an herb that supports immune function. Most studies have found that it shortens the duration of colds and flus and may halt a cold if it is taken at the first sign of symptoms, but is not effective as a preventative. Side effects are rare; it is not recommended for those with autoimmune disorders such as lupus. Allergic reactions may occur, especially in those with sensitivity to the daisy family.

EVENING PRIMROSE OIL

Obtained from the seeds of the primrose plant, evening primrose oil provides a rich source of gamma-linolenic acid (GLA), which is an omega-6 fatty acid. It has anti-inflammatory properties and is important for brain function. Research supports benefits for the treatment of arthritis, diabetic neuropathy, eczema and dry skin, fibrocystic breast disease, and Raynaud's disease. Side effects (upset stomach) are rare.

FENUGREEK

Fenugreek, an herb used as a medicine and spice for thousands of years in India and Egypt, aids lactation, wound treatment, bronchitis, digestive problems, arthritis, and kidney problems. Studies show that it can reduce blood sugar and cholesterol levels in diabetics; it may also relieve constipation. It is usually well tolerated; high doses may cause upset stomach. It is not recommended during pregnancy. Diabetics may require adjustment in therapy, as fenugreek can lower blood sugar levels.

FEVERFEW

Feverfew is a plant extract that is used for headache prevention. The main active component, parthenolide, prevents platelet clumping and inhibits the release of serotonin and inflammatory chemicals. Several studies have shown that it can reduce the severity, duration, and frequency of migraine headaches; it is not effective as a treatment once a headache occurs. It is well tolerated; there are no known drug interactions.

FISH OIL

Fish oil is a rich source of the omega-3 fatty acids DHA (docosahexaenoic acid) and EPA (eicosapentaenoic acid), which have anti-inflammatory effects. DHA is important for brain function, vision, and joint health. EPA supports immune function, blood clotting, and circulation. Numerous studies have shown that fish oil can reduce the risk of heart attack and stroke; it lowers triglycerides, raises HDL (good) cholesterol, reduces clotting, lowers homocysteine, and may reduce blood pressure. Some research suggests benefits for rheumatoid arthritis, menstrual pain, depression, bipolar disorder, attention deficit disorder, and Raynaud's disease. Side effects are rare; some supplements cause fishy burps.

5-HYDROXYTRYPTOPHAN (5-HTP)

5-HTP is an amino acid that the body uses to make serotonin, a brain chemical that regulates mood, sleep, appetite, pain sensation, and sexual behaviour. Research shows benefits for depression, migraine headaches, weight loss, insomnia, and fibromyalgia. Side effects are rare or minor (upset stomach). Use cautiously with Parkinson's drugs, antidepressants, and drugs that affect serotonin.

FLAXSEED OIL

Flaxseed oil provides both omega-3 and omega-6 fatty acids. The oil is used to reduce inflammation, improve circulation, and for dry skin; however, there is less research to support its proposed health benefits, compared to fish oils. Whole flaxseeds are taken for their laxative benefits. Milled flaxseed provides the beneficial oils, fibre, and lignans (phytoestrogens) that may help in cancer prevention. Flaxseed is generally well tolerated.

FRUCTOOLIGOSACCHARIDES (FOS)

These are short chains of fructose molecules that occur naturally in foods and are also put into supplements. The body cannot digest these substances, but they serve as a food for probiotics (friendly bacteria) in the digestive tract, so are known as prebiotics. Some research shows that FOS lower triglycerides, and preliminary evidence shows benefits for digestion and intestinal health. FOS may cause bloating, flatulence, and upset stomach at doses of 15 g or higher.

GINGER

Ginger is a plant that is used as a spice and therapeutically as an herbal medicine. Research shows benefits for nausea associated with pregnancy, motion sickness, and upset stomach. There are no significant side effects.

GINKGO BILOBA

Ginkgo biloba, a plant, has a long history of use. Ginkgo has undergone extensive research for a variety of health conditions. It is an antioxidant, improves blood circulation by dilating blood vessels, and reduces the stickiness of blood platelets. Research supports benefits for Alzheimer's disease, improving memory and cognitive function, and treatment of intermittent claudication and anxiety. Preliminary research shows benefits for macular degeneration, PMS, Raynaud's disease, and vertigo. Side effects are rare and minor (upset stomach, headaches, and skin reactions); it may enhance the blood-thinning effect of anticoagulants, so dosage adjustments may be necessary.

GINSENG, AMERICAN AND ASIAN

American and Asian ginseng are very similar in composition and properties. Ginseng has adaptogen properties (helps the body deal with stress, whether physical or emotional) and enhances immune function. Research supports benefits for strengthening immunity from colds, flus, and other infections, improving physical performance and a sense of well-being, and enhancing mental function. Preliminary research shows benefits for erectile dysfunction, improving blood sugar control in diabetics, enhancing fertility, and the treatment of attention-deficit hyperactivity disorder (ADHD). Ginseng may enhance the blood sugar-lowering effects of insulin or diabetic medications and may decrease the effect of blood-thinning drugs. It is generally well tolerated, but there are some reports of nervousness, insomnia, and upset stomach. Use cautiously with uncontrolled high blood pressure. It is not recommended during pregnancy, breast-feeding, or by those with breast cancer.

GINSENG, SIBERIAN

Also known as *Eleuthero*, Siberian ginseng is not a true ginseng, but has some similar properties as an adaptogen. It is commonly used to support immune function, mental acuity, and athletic performance and to help reduce the effects of stress. Side effects may include upset stomach, insomnia, and increased blood pressure. It is not recommended for those with uncontrolled high blood pressure.

GLUCOSAMINE

Glucosamine occurs naturally in the body and is a building block used to manufacture components of cartilage, the material that cushions joints. Numerous studies have found that it can improve osteoarthritis symptoms (joint pain, mobility); it may also prevent the progression of the disease. Preliminary research suggests possible benefits for irritable bowel syndrome. It is well tolerated, but may cause mild upset stomach.

GRAPE SEED EXTRACT

Grape seed extract is a source of potent antioxidants called proanthocyanidins, also known as oligomeric proanthocyanidin complexes (OPCs), a type of flavonoid. Research supports benefits for chronic venous insufficiency, varicose veins, prevention of blood clots while flying, and reducing post-surgical edema. Preliminary research suggests benefits for ADHD, PMS, erectile dysfunction, asthma, allergies, hemorrhoids, and prevention of atherosclerosis. It is very well tolerated, but may cause minor upset stomach. It may enhance the effect of blood-thinning drugs.

GREEN TEA

Green tea is derived from the plant *Camellia sinensis*. Unlike black and oolong tea, it is not fermented, which preserves the active constituents. It provides a high level of antioxidants called polyphenols, particularly the catechin called epigallocatechin gallate (EGCG). It is used for heart health, cancer prevention, cervical dysplasia, weight loss, liver disease, and gum health. Green tea contains caffeine, but less so than black tea and coffee. Side effects are rare; large amounts may cause insomnia and nervousness.

HAWTHORNE

Hawthorne is an herb with a long history of use for heart ailments. Research has demonstrated that it can improve the heart's pumping action and is helpful in the treatment of congestive heart failure. It may also lower blood pressure and reduce palpitations and angina. It is generally well tolerated; side effects are minor and may include dizziness, upset stomach, headache, and skin rash.

INDOLE-3 CARBINOL

Indole-3 carbinol is a nutrient found in cruciferous vegetables such as broccoli, Brussels sprouts, cabbage, cauliflower, and kale. It has anti-cancer properties, aids in detoxification of estrogen, reduces the levels of free radicals, and protects liver function. It has been shown in preliminary research to reduce estrogen-promoted cancers (cervical and breast). There are no known side effects.

IPRIFLAVONE

Ipriflavone, a synthetic flavonoid derived from soy, is widely used for osteoporosis (available as a supplement in Canada, yet sold as a prescription drug in many other countries). Many studies have shown that when combined with calcium, it can slow and even reverse bone breakdown; it also helps reduce the pain of fractures caused by osteoporosis. It is generally well tolerated; one study found that long-term use (three years) reduced levels of lymphocytes (white blood cells). Use under doctor's supervision if you have immune deficiency (HIV), kidney disease, or are taking immune-suppressant drugs.

LECITHIN

Lecithin is a source of phosphatidylcholine, a phospholipid (fat-soluble component of all cell membranes). Supplements of lecithin are broken down in the body into choline, which promotes methylation and is used to make acetylcholine, a nerve chemical essential for proper brain function. Some research supports benefits for liver disease; lowering homocysteine; and the treatment of bipolar, Alzheimer's, and other neurological disorders. It is generally well tolerated.

LICORICE

Licorice is an herb with long history of use for digestion and immune support. It contains glycyrrhizin, which causes fluid retention and can raise blood pressure; supplements of deglycyrrhizinated licorice (DGL) do not cause these effects. DGL has been studied for ulcer prevention and treatment, and is generally well tolerated. Licorice is used for cough and asthma; topical products may help relieve eczema. It may raise blood pressure, lower testosterone in men, and have estrogenic effects; it is not recommended during pregnancy, breast-feeding, or for use by those with cancer.

LUTEIN

Lutein, an antioxidant pigment in the carotenoid family, is found in dark green and yellow vegetables. It is highly concentrated in the macula of the eye (behind retina) and plays a role in protecting the retina from oxidative damage and UV light. Research supports benefits for prevention of cataracts and macular degeneration. It is very well tolerated; there are no known drug interactions.

LYCOPENE

Lycopene is a potent antioxidant (carotenoid) naturally present in red vegetables and fruits (tomatoes, pink grapefruit, and watermelon). Research supports benefits for prevention of prostate cancer and pre-eclampsia, and treatment of asthma; it may also help prevent macular degeneration, cataracts, and heart disease. It is very well tolerated; there are no known drug interactions.

LYSINE

An amino acid naturally present in meat, poultry, dairy products, eggs, and beans. Regular supplement use has been shown to prevent cold sores; it may also prevent genital herpes flare-ups. It is generally well tolerated.

MELATONIN

Melatonin, a hormone that is produced in the brain and released in response to darkness, regulates our biological clock (sleep and wake cycles). Supplements have been shown to help shorten the time needed to fall asleep, improve sleep quality, and help with disrupted sleep cycles (such as with travellers and shift workers). It may also help in the treatment of depression, seasonal affective disorder, anxiety, schizophrenia, cluster headaches, and to improve quality of life in cancer patients. Supplements are taken half an hour to one hour before bed to promote better rest. It is well tolerated and does not cause next-day drowsiness; it is not recommended during pregnancy or breast-feeding.

METHYLSULFONYLMETHANE (MSM)

MSM is a naturally occurring sulphur compound in the body; it is also present in certain foods (vegetables). It may be helpful for osteoarthritis, recovery from sports injuries, and for growth of nails and hair, although research is preliminary. It is very well tolerated; there are no known drug interactions.

MILK THISTLE

Milk thistle, an herb with a long history of use for liver and spleen disorders, contains a flavonoid complex called silymarin, which is responsible for its antioxidant, detoxifying, and liver health benefits. Research supports its use for the treatment of viral and alcoholic hepatitis, and liver cirrhosis. Preliminary research suggests that it might protect the liver against drug-induced toxicity caused by acetaminophen (Tylenol) and phenytoin (Dilantin). It is generally well tolerated; there are no known drug interactions.

MODUCARE

Moducare, a patented blend of plant sterols and sterolins (plant fats), helps to restore, strengthen, and balance the immune system. Several studies have demonstrated its immune-modulating effects. It is not recommended for use by those with organ transplants or those taking immune-suppressant drugs; use only under doctor's supervision if pregnant, lactating, diabetic, or if you have an immune disorder.

NETTLE

Nettle is an herb widely used for the treatment of benign prostatic hyperplasia; many studies show benefits for reducing symptoms. Preliminary research suggests benefits for allergies; topical products are used to relieve the pain of osteoarthritis. It may be more beneficial when combined with pygeum and/or saw palmetto, and is generally well tolerated.

PHOSPHATIDYLSERINE

Phosphatidylserine, a phospholipid (fat component of cell membrane) made by the body, performs vital functions such as moving nutrients into cells and pumping waste products out of them. Research shows that supplements can help improve memory, mental function, and depression in the elderly, and it is useful in the treatment of Alzheimer's. It is well tolerated, but may cause mild upset stomach; it may enhance the effect of blood-thinning drugs and supplements, requiring dosage adjustments.

PHYTOSTEROLS/PHYTOSTANOLS

These are naturally occurring compounds (fats) found in almost all plants. Several studies have found benefits with beta-sitosterol (a phytosterol) for reducing symptoms of prostate enlargement. Phytostanols are added to foods (margarine spreads and salad dressings) and sold as supplements; studies have shown that phytostanols and stanol esters can lower cholesterol levels. They are very well tolerated.

POLICOSANOL

Numerous studies have shown that policosanol, a waxy substance obtained from sugar cane, can substantially lower cholesterol, similarly to prescription drugs. It may enhance the effects of blood-thinning drugs and supplements so dosage adjustments may be necessary; it is not recommended during pregnancy or breast-feeding.

PROBIOTICS

Also known as friendly or beneficial bacteria, probiotics are normally present in the mouth, digestive and urinary tracts, and vaginal area. They are also present in some fermented dairy foods (live culture yogurt), although potency and stability is questionable. They provide many health benefits by protecting against infection by harmful bacteria (yeast and bacteria), aiding in detoxification, producing vitamins, aiding digestion, and supporting immune function. Research supports benefits for travellers' diarrhea, constipation, irritable bowel, ulcerative colitis, eczema, allergies, and tooth decay. They also improve immune function, reduce cholesterol, prevent and treat yeast infections, and enhance ulcer treatment. Choose products that are tested for potency and stability, and made from human strains. Probiotics are well tolerated.

PYGEUM

Pygeum is a tree whose bark contains phytosterols and compounds that reduce inflammation and modulate testosterone activity in the prostate. Studies have found it beneficial for improving symptoms of an enlarged prostate; it may also be beneficial for prostatitis (prostate infection). It is often combined with saw palmetto or nettle root, which are also beneficial for reducing prostate symptoms, and is very well tolerated.

RED CLOVER

Red clover is a plant with a history of use for skin disorders, cough, and as a diurectic. Recent research has focused on its isoflavones, which work as phytoestrogens, with possible benefits for menopause. Studies have yielded mixed results for reducing hot flashes. It may help reduce cholesterol levels and protect against osteoporosis by reducing bone loss. It is not recommended during pregnancy, breast-feeding, or for use by those with breast or uterine cancer. It may enhance the effect of blood-thinning drugs, so dosage adjustments may be necessary.

RELORA

Relora, a proprietary blend of extracts of magnolia and phellodendron, has been studied for its stress-relieving properties. It promotes relaxation without sedation, normalizes stress hormones, and reduces stress-related eating. It is generally well tolerated, but may cause mild upset stomach.

RHODIOLA

Rhodiola, an herb classified as an adaptogen, was used historically to combat stress and fatigue and to speed recovery from illness. Studies have demonstrated benefits for reducing fatigue and enhancing mental function. Preliminary research suggests that it may help with altitude sickness and may aid cancer chemotherapy by protecting the liver against drug-induced damage. There are no known side effects or drug interactions.

S-ADENOSYLMETHIONINE (SAMe)

SAMe is a naturally occurring nutrient in the body that is involved in hormone and neurotransmitter production, detoxification, joint health, and many other vital bodily processes. Research shows that supplements can benefit those with depression, osteoarthritis, liver disease, and fibromyalgia. It may also reduce depression associated with Parkinson's disease, and is generally well tolerated, but may cause mild upset stomach. It is not recommended for those with bipolar disorder; use cautiously with other antidepressant products.

SAW PALMETTO

Saw palmetto is an herb that has been widely studied for its benefits for prostate health. Studies show that it can help reduce an enlarged prostate and improve urinary symptoms, similarly to prescription drugs, but it is better tolerated. It may also be helpful for the treatment of prostatitis, and is generally well tolerated.

SOY ISOFLAVONES

Numerous studies have shown that soy foods and supplements can lower cholesterol levels and improve the ratio of LDL to HDL (usual dosage is 47 g per day). Soy isoflavones may help reduce menopausal symptoms (hot flashes); preliminary research suggests it may reduce the risk of breast, uterine, and colon cancer, and benefit those with osteoporosis and osteoarthritis. It is not recommended for those with impaired thyroid function; high supplemental intake is not recommended during pregnancy.

ST. JOHN'S WORT

St. John's wort is an herb with a long history of use for treating emotional disorders. Research supports its use for mild to moderate depression and seasonal affective disorder with effects comparable to those of prescription drugs. Side effects are rare and include skin rash and mild upset stomach. It may cause increased sensitivity to the sun. Use cautiously with other antidepressant products. It may reduce the efficacy of many drugs, including oral contraceptives, organ transplant medications, digoxin, statins, warfarin, proton-pump inhibitors (ulcer drugs), and anaesthetics; consult with your pharmacist before taking this herb.

SUNTHEANINE

Suntheanine is a patented and clinically studied form of the amino acid L-theanine, which is naturally present in green tea. It promotes an alert state of relaxation without drowsiness. Preliminary research suggests benefits for improving the quality of sleep and enhancing learning performance, reducing the symptoms of premenstrual syndrome, heightening mental acuity, promoting concentration, reducing negative side effects of stress and caffeine, and supporting immune function. It is well tolerated; there are no known drug interactions.

TEA TREE

Oil from this tree is widely used for its antiseptic properties; it kills bacteria, viruses, and fungi upon contact. Topical products have been found effective for improving acne and athlete's foot, but may cause skin irritation in some individuals. It may also help in the treatment of gum disease and dandruff.

VALERIAN

Valerian is an herb that is used for its calming and sedating properties. Studies show that it is useful for insomnia and chronic sleep disorders. It may take a few weeks to get the optimal effect. Some studies have found benefits with valerian when it is combined with hops and/or lemon balm. It is generally well tolerated, and does not cause next-day drowsiness when taken at bedtime. It is not recommended for use in conjunction with prescription sleep aids.

WILLOW

Willow is an herb with long history of use for pain and fever. It contains salicin, which is purified to salicylic acid (similar to the active ingredient in aspirin). Research supports benefits for back pain and osteoarthritis. It may also help with dysmenorrhea, tension and migraine headaches, rheumatoid arthritis, tendonitis, and bursitis. It is generally well tolerated, but may cause upset stomach, although not to the same extent as aspirin, which causes stomach irritation and bleeding. It may enhance the effect of blood-thinning products, so dosage adjustments may be necessary.

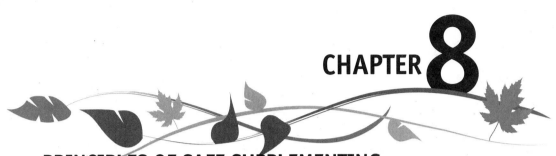

CHAPTER 8

PRINCIPLES OF SAFE SUPPLEMENTING

Mounting clinical research is demonstrating that nutritional supplements can play an important role in health and disease prevention. Every day we are learning of new products, new uses, and new benefits. While these advances in science are exciting and offer great hope, how do we take this information and put it into practical use in our own lives? Choosing an appropriate supplement and creating a supplement program requires careful thought and consideration. In this chapter I outline the role of nutritional supplements, my recommended "foundation" supplements, tips on creating a supplement program, and suggestions for your medicine cabinet and travel essentials.

WHY TAKE SUPPLEMENTS?

You may have heard the phrase, "If you eat a healthy diet, then you don't need to take supplements." If you eat a whole foods diet; with plenty of nutrient-dense fruits and vegetables, whole grains, lean protein, and healthy fats every day, then it may be possible to get what your body needs from diet alone. However, the reality is that most people don't eat healthily on a daily basis. Fast foods and processed foods are prevalent in our diet and these foods are typically devoid of nutrients. Furthermore, there are a number of factors that actually deplete nutrients from our bodies such as stress, environmental toxins and the use of prescription medications.

Nutritional supplements are necessary not only to make up for dietary deficiencies and depletion, but to achieve optimum health and help prevent chronic disease. Throughout this book you will see recommendations for supplements that can help manage or prevent various health conditions. But keep in mind that supplements are intended to complement, not replace, a healthy lifestyle.

CREATING YOUR SUPPLEMENT PROGRAM

There are so many different supplements available and if you took everything that sounds beneficial, you could end up popping pills all day long, which is not necessary to achieve good health. It is important to first look at your diet, lifestyle, and health needs when determining what supplements to take. There are a few supplements that I consider "foundation supplements." These supplements, which include multivitamins and minerals, green foods, and essential fatty acids, should be considered by most people as they offer broad health benefits.

Multivitamins and Minerals

It is my professional opinion that almost everyone can benefit from taking a daily multivitamin. As noted above, even if you eat a healthy diet, you could be lacking in certain nutrients. Aside from diet, there are many factors that increase your need for vitamins and minerals, such as smoking, use of prescription medication, intense exercise, stress, and certain medical conditions such as osteoporosis, heart disease, alcoholism, and malabsorption diseases (celiac and Crohn's diseases). Those on a strict vegetarian diet may also have difficulty in getting enough essential nutrients from diet alone.

Taking a daily multivitamin ensures that your body gets all the essential nutrients it needs to function optimally. Think of a multivitamin as a form of "health insurance."

Since our nutritional needs vary with age and lifestyle factors, it is important to look for products designed for your particular needs. For example:

- Children who are picky eaters could be lacking in various nutrients, such as vitamin C and iron. Those with developmental issues may benefit from essential fatty acid supplements.
- Teenagers who don't eat a healthy diet (too much fast food) may be lacking in vitamins. Growing teens also require extra calcium to build strong bones.
- Women of child-bearing age may need extra calcium and iron, especially if they have heavy menstrual cycles.
- Higher amounts of folic acid—to reduce the risk of birth defects—are recommended for women who plan to get pregnant.
- Women who are pregnant or lactating should take a prenatal supplement, which contains higher amounts of nutrients needed to support a growing baby and the increased demands of breast-feeding. These supplements also contain lower amounts of vitamin A as it can lead to birth defects in high amounts (greater than 5,000 IU daily).
- Athletes require extra antioxidants to compensate for free radicals generated during intense activity.
- Seniors require extra calcium and vitamin D to protect the bones. Vitamin B12 and other B vitamins may be deficient in older individuals depending on diet, medical conditions, and prescription drug use.
- Seniors should not take products containing iron unless advised by their doctor.

Chapter 2 provides extensive information on vitamins and minerals, including dosage ranges based on age and gender, as well as nutrients that may be depleted by prescription drugs or certain health conditions.

Green Foods

Most people find it difficult to consume the recommended seven to 10 servings of fruits and vegetables per day that provide our primary dietary source of vitamins and minerals. To complement your diet, you may want to consider taking a green foods supplement. Green foods such as chlorella, spirulina, barley grass, and wheat grass provide vital nutrients such as antioxidants, minerals, and fibre, which can help boost energy levels, support detoxification, and enhance well-being. There are many green food supplements on the market, which vary in composition. greens + is one of my top recommended brands as it contains the highest quality ingredients and has been clinically studied. You can add your greens + to your morning protein shake, or mix with juice or water. For best results, it is important to take this product daily.

Essential Fatty Acids (EFAs)

EFAs are good fats that are *essential* for health throughout life. They are required for growth and development of the brain, nervous system, adrenal glands, sex organs, and eyes. They maintain the health of cell membranes, produce hormones and brain chemicals, and regulate various cell processes.

The body cannot make EFAs, so they must be obtained through diet or supplementation. As discussed in Chapter 1, the two main classes of EFAs are the omega-3s and omega-6s. Most people get adequate omega-6s as they are found abundantly in vegetable oils. Omega-3s are present in fish and, to a lesser extent, in some plants (flaxseed and leafy green vegetables). Omega-3 deficiency is thought to be quite common, and supplementing with omega-3s offers a number of health benefits, such as reducing the risk of heart attack, and improving brain function and skin health. Omega-3 supplements are also recommended for women who are trying to get pregnant or who are pregnant as these good fats are essential to the growing brain, eyes, and nervous system of the baby.

Fish oil provides the highest amount of omega-3s. Look for a pharmaceutical-grade, cold-pressed fish oil from a reputable manufacturer. Those who cannot tolerate fish oils can take flaxseed or hemp oil. The usual dosage for omega-3s is 1–3 g daily. There are specific formulas for children with improved taste and texture.

BEYOND THE FOUNDATION

Beyond these foundation supplements I would suggest that you look at your particular health needs and any underlying medical problems in determining what other supplements to take. For example, if you have osteoporosis, you may require extra minerals, vitamin D, and other nutrients. If you have heart disease, it would be wise to take coenzyme Q10 along with extra antioxidants. In Section 3 I provide concise guidelines on supplement recommendations for various health conditions. Keep in mind that it is always wise to consult with a professional for advice on which supplements to take, the appropriate dosage, and any precautions.

TIPS ON SELECTING SUPPLEMENTS

There are many factors to consider when choosing a supplement. Before choosing a product, consider my list below of do's and don'ts.

Do's

- Research your options—consult with your pharmacist or health care provider and find out as much as you can about the products you are considering. In particular ask if there are any possible interactions with medications or side effects.
- When buying a multivitamin, look for one that contains a complete array of essential vitamins, minerals, and antioxidants in one formula. This will keep the amount of pills you take to a minimum and will also be easier on your budget. Depending on your diet and needs, you may still need to take additional vitamin C, E, and calcium as it is difficult to fit all of these nutrients into one tablet.
- Buy from a reputable manufacturer. Ask your pharmacist or health food store adviser for a recommendation.
- Remember it may take four to six weeks or longer to notice benefits, and some supplements that are taken for prevention may not offer benefits that you can feel.
- If you are pregnant, nursing a baby, or have a chronic medical condition, be sure to consult a nutrition specialist before purchasing or taking any supplements.
- Read the labels carefully. Look for an expiration date and make sure the product is in good date. If there is no expiration date on the label, don't buy it.
- If you have questions about a certain brand, call the manufacturer and ask your questions.

Don'ts

- Don't take supplements with sugar, starch, corn, wheat, iron, dairy, salt, artificial flavourings and colourings (dyes), and preservatives. These are unnecessary ingredients that can cause allergic reactions in some people.
- Don't choose a supplement based on price. Some vitamins are more expensive due to company marketing and advertising costs and are not necessarily made with better ingredients.
- Don't continue to take a supplement if you have a bad reaction, such as prolonged upset stomach or rash.
- Don't stop taking a prescribed drug or substitute a supplement for a prescribed drug unless under the advice and supervision of your health care provider.
- Don't take a higher dosage of a product than is recommended on the label unless advised to do so by your health care provider.

NATURAL MEDICINE CABINET

Below is a list of certain products that you may want to have on hand to deal with minor ailments.

- Activated charcoal for stomach upset, food poisoning, and drug overdose
- Arnica gel for bruises and injuries

- Lavender oil for relaxation and headache relief
- Magnesium as a natural laxative
- Melatonin as a natural sleep aid
- Tea tree oil as an antiseptic for treatment of minor skin irritations, insect bites, and stings

NATURAL TRAVEL ESSENTIALS

Depending on whether you are travelling north or south, here are some suggestions for remedies to pack for your trip:

- Aloe vera to soothe sunburn
- Activated charcoal for stomach upset, food poisoning, and drug overdose
- Natural insect repellant—look for products that contain eucalyptus oil, catnip oil, garlic, and/or citronella
- Probiotics to take during your trip, especially when travelling overseas, to prevent diarrhea and upset stomach
- Tea tree oil to relieve insect bites and clean wounds
- Zinc oxide for sun protection

So now you may be asking yourself, "Where do I start? How do I begin to include nutritional supplements in my life?" You can begin with my recommended foundation supplements. After that, ask yourself what's missing from your diet and what concerns you the most about your health. Focus on one concern at a time, exploring different nutritional supplements that may offer help. If you invest the time into creating a supplement program that's right for your individual needs, your reward should be improved quality of life.

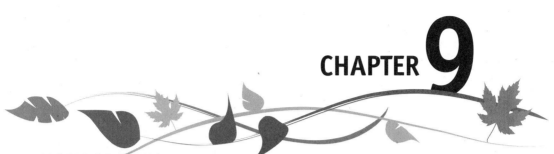

CHAPTER 9

HOMEOPATHY BY BRYCE WYLDE, BSC, RNC, DHMHS, HD

Homeopathy is a branch of natural medicine that has a long history of success. In the last 20 years, there has been a strong resurgence of homeopathy, which has become the fastest-growing field of integrative medicine in Canada, and is the second most popular form of any medicine worldwide.

Even though the nature of homeopathy, its scope, and its applications in health care are less understood in Canada, it remains clear that more than ever, Canadians are turning to homeopathy as an addition to their preventative routines as well as a solution to their most common health complaints. Homeopathy is part of a trillion-dollar, North American natural health care industry. Homeopathic medicine is second in popularity only to mainstream or conventional medicine. Because homeopathy is an inexpensive alternative with little profit margin and no possibility for patenting, its marketability to mainstream practitioners is low, so few are aware of its benefits in a clinical setting.

Homeopathy has long been thought of as "complementary" in the medical field. Contemporary Canadian society's newfound understanding of health care as *prevention of disease* has led to a new perspective of natural approaches like homeopathy as mainstream. In line with this new definition of health care, homeopathy helps the body to do what it should be able to do on its own to keep the body healthy and free of disease. Conventional approaches, such as drugs and surgery, are sometimes necessary, but these approaches should soon become known as the complementary approach!

For over 200 years, Canadians have been using homeopathic medicines successfully to treat acute and chronic illnesses. Interestingly, homeopaths were recognized under government structure before practitioners of conventional medicine. In Upper Canada in 1859, homeopathic doctors were acknowledged and regulated under the Act Respecting Homeopathy. In 1865, An Act to Regulate the Qualifications of Practitioners in Medicine and Surgery in Upper Canada was proclaimed. A clause in this act prohibited any repeal or action that would in any way affect the Homeopathic Act of 1859 and the Eclectic Act of 1861. In 1866, An Act Respecting the Medical Board and Medical Practitioners authorized the formation of a licensing board for conventional doctors, exempting homeopaths and midwives. As a consequence of these two acts, the Council of Education and Registration of Upper Canada was established in 1866, with the authority to grant licences to practise medicine in Upper Canada.

Homeopathic medicines are *micro* doses of plant, mineral, and other naturally occurring substances. They are regulated by Health Canada and are manufactured according to the highest drug safety standards. They carry a drug identification number (DIN), just like any other drug available in local pharmacies. Homeopathic medicines are safe and efficient with no side effects and no drug interactions, allowing people to take conventional medications, if necessary, at the same time as their homeopathic treatment.

HOW HOMEOPATHY WORKS

Simply defined, homeopathic medicines trigger the body's natural defence mechanisms and support systems to manage ailments, as opposed to conventional medicines, which use chemicals to eradicate invading pathogens or change your body's natural chemistry. In this way, homeopathy is able to help the body regain balance by getting it to do better what it is already equipped to do on its own. If necessary, when disease has progressed too far, conventional approaches like drugs and surgery may be prudent to use adjunctively.

Homeopathic medicines work on three basic principles. The first is the law of similars, which states that the same things that cause an illness will ultimately cure it. The second is that infinitesimal doses are all that are needed to trigger the body's natural defence system. The third is that homeopathic medicines are prescribed in a very individualized way, taking into account not only physical symptoms but also the patient's behavioural and mental/emotional condition.

THE SCIENTIFIC PROOF

The international scientific community is quickly becoming interested in studies on homeopathy, many of which are documented in prestigious scientific journals. Scientific studies have demonstrated that highly diluted biological products (homeopathic medicines) can have a verifiable effect on humans. Homeopathy offers a simple, effective, and safe medical therapy free from known side effects. While it is always good to consult with a qualified practitioner, there are many homeopathic remedies that are safe for self-medication.

Research centres around the world are conducting studies of homeopathic medicines and a growing number of these studies are being published in peer-reviewed journals. One of many such studies that has become very well known was published in *The Lancet* in 1997. K. Linde et al. (Munich University) published the results of a meta-analysis of no less than 135 clinical trials that compared homeopathic drugs with a placebo (K. Linde et al., "Are the Clinical Effects of Homeopathy Placebo Effects? A Meta-analysis of Placebo-Controlled Trials," *The Lancet*, 1997, 350; 834–843). The authors concluded that "The results of this meta-analysis are not compatible with the hypothesis that the clinical effects of homeopathy are completely due to placebo."

Another meta-analysis conducted in 2000 on 24 studies relating to controlled, randomized clinical trials concluded that "There is some evidence that homeopathic treatments are more effective than placebo" (M. Cucherat et al., "Evidence of Clinical Efficacy of Homeopathy: A Meta-analysis of Clinical Trials," *European Journal of Clinical Pharmacology*, 2000: 56; 27–33).

Oddly enough, these and other trials and studies have not been given sufficient prominence, either within the scientific community or by media. To get more information on homeopathic research, please call the world leader in homeopathic preparations, Boiron-Dolisos Laboratories (www.boiron.com).

FINDING A GOOD PRACTITIONER

You have attended a workshop, or you may have been given advice by a health store clerk, bought a homeopathic over-the-counter remedy, or investigated the use of a homeopathic medicine on the advice of a friend. You may have already discovered that the remedy Pulsatilla can rid you of your allergy symptoms faster than you could imagine, but you may never have thought of using it for your child's ear infection or your husband's headache. You have had success, but would like to use it to tackle a more important health problem, or perhaps you would like a homeopath to take care of your family. Where do you go from here? How do you find a practitioner? The reality is that your choice of homeopathic practitioner determines the extent of health benefits you are likely to experience when using homeopathic remedies.

Our society has a variety of health care resources, including general practitioners and specialists, pharmacists, nurses and nurse practitioners, and other caregivers in whom we place our trust. But let's not forget the myriad of ancillary practitioners who are just as well educated and ready to treat you for your health concerns using a more natural and gentle approach. These include homeopathic doctors, naturopathic doctors, acupuncturists, traditional Chinese medicine doctors, nutritionists, registered massage therapists, and chiropractors. How do you choose a homeopathic doctor who is qualified to provide safe and effective alternative health care? Are any of these practitioners or their services covered by government health insurance plans? When is it necessary to consult your conventional doctor?

The answers to these questions are actually quite simple. Because there is no provincial regulation regarding homeopathy in any of the Canadian provinces yet (although it is just around the corner in Ontario), before selecting a practitioner, you must make sure that he or she graduated from an institution that provides at least a three-year education (preferably post-graduate), including at least 1,100 hours in a clinic with preceptor and internship. This training is important so that the homeopathic practitioner develops a good understanding of the medical sciences and is equipped to refer you to the appropriate medical practitioner if your problem is beyond his or her particular scope of practice.

Similar to the well-recognized medical system of dentistry (the first ever regulated mainstream form of preventive health care), none of what encompasses homeopathic medicines or its practitioners is covered by provincial health insurance plans in Canada and all expenses incurred by seeing a homeopathic doctor are out of pocket. Although consultations are sometimes expensive, the medicines are not, and the money you save at the end of the day as a result of less time away from work, quicker recovery periods, and not having to purchase expensive drugs will usually be worth the cost of the appointments with a homeopath. Finding a good homeopathic doctor may be a bit of a challenge. There aren't too many of us! Here are a few excellent Web sites that will put you in touch with fully certified homeopathic doctors across Canada:

RESOURCES FOR HOMEOPATHIC PRACTITIONERS IN CANADA

Quebec and Maritimes: http://www.canadahomeopathy.com

Ontario: www.ontariohomeopath.com

Alberta/Saskatchewan/Manitoba: www.wchs.info

British Columbia: www.bcsocietyofhomeopaths.ca

The most important component of treatment by a homeopathic doctor begins with the use of one homeopathic dilution remedy made from a single substance (preferably not a combination remedy). Homeopathic textbooks describe the symptoms associated with one remedy based on human trials of this particular substance, so using a combination of many remedies can make it difficult to evaluate the success of a specific treatment. However, over-the-counter combination remedies, available in Canadian health stores and pharmacies, are excellent for consumers to self-treat minor health conditions, such as allergies, colds and other conditions noted later in this chapter. For advice on more serious health conditions it is important to consult with your health care provider.

As homeopathic practitioners are not yet regulated in any province in Canada, strict criteria for choosing the appropriate practitioner for your family's health care needs are essential. Here are a few tips:

Tip #1: If combination remedies are recommended by your natural health care provider, it indicates that your health issues have not been clearly understood or that the provider's understanding of homeopathic remedies is limited.

Tip #2: Many natural health care providers recommend homeopathic remedies to their patients. Unfortunately, this does not make them a homeopathic doctor, nor does it mean that you are getting optimum health results from the homeopathic remedies you use. Here is an explanation of the various credentials that you may see following a practitioner's name:

CCHC or CCH (Certification in Classical Homeopathy Canada)
Granted by: Canadian Council on Homeopathic Certification. Not a professional organization. Successful candidates are eligible for membership in other organizations. Independent evaluation of an individual's competence to practise homeopathy.

DHANP (Diplomate of the Homeopathic Association of Naturopathic Physicians)

Granted by: Homeopathic Academy of Naturopathic Physicians. Open to naturopathic doctors.

DHt (Diplomate of Homeotherapeutics)

Granted by: American Institute of Homeopathy. Open to licensed medical doctors and osteopathic doctors.

HD (Homeopathic Doctor)

Granted by: Ontario Homeopathic Association. Professional provincial organization with the highest standards in Canada. Successful candidates are eligible for the HD title after completing a minimum of three years of training in medical sciences and homeopathy as well as at least 1,100 hours of clinical internship; must meet the HD requirements and standards of the OHA and be of good moral character.

RSHom (NA) or (UK) (Registered Member of the Society of Homeopaths, North America (RSHom (NA) or (UK))

Granted by: North American (or United Kingdom) Society of Homeopaths. Open to other professional homeopaths.

Tip #3: A professional homeopath will always know that there is virtually a limitless number of treatment plans available, will use a wide range of single homeopathic medicines, and designs a unique treatment plan to ensure you achieve your optimum health benefit from homeopathic treatment. A professional homeopathic doctor will never ignore nutritional and lifestyle factors in your plan of action.

Tip #4: The first interview should always be an in-depth appointment (on average about 1.5 hours in length) covering your chief complaint(s), full health history, your family history (genetic), physical examination (on indication), laboratory workup (or review of existing), your general nature (mental, emotional characteristics), and detailed symptom compilation related to your main body systems and predispositions.

Tip #5: A professional homeopath will know when to make a good referral to a specialist or medical doctor and will not ignorantly insult conventional medicine or its practitioners regardless of his or her current opinion.

HOMEOPATHIC TREATMENTS

Each health concern below has two single homeopathic remedies and one combination remedy that are most successful in treating that particular complaint. Of the two single remedies, select the remedy that most closely matches your symptoms.

For conditions where self-treatment is appropriate, unless otherwise directed by a physician, use potencies 6X through and up to 30CH or simply follow the instructions on the label. Do not purchase a homeopathic medicine without a DIN number.

Take one dose and wait for a response. Depending on the condition it may take several hours to a few days to notice benefits. If there is improvement, continue to take the remedy. If there is no improvement, then consider another remedy or seek medical attention depending on the severity of the health condition.

The frequency of dosage varies with the condition and the individual. Usually a lower dose is required several times an hour; higher doses (given when indication is especially clear) are usually given several times a day; and in some situations, one dose per day can be sufficient. Occasionally, under the care of a homeopathic doctor, only one dose is ever given.

Acne

Silicea: Silicea is given to a person with deep-seated acne along with a general low immune resistance and swollen lymph nodes. Infected spots are slow to come to a head, and also slow to resolve, so may result in scarring. A person who needs this remedy is generally very chilly, but inclined to sweat at night.

Sulphur: Sulphur is for itchy, sore, inflamed eruptions with reddish or dirty-looking skin. Itching may be worse from scratching, and worse from any form of heat, especially bathing or washing. Individuals who need this remedy often have unusual philosophical notions and tend to give hygiene a low priority.

Combination recommendation: Acne Formula R53 by Reckeweg

Allergies (seasonal, hayfever)

Allium cepa: Indications for this remedy include watery eyes and a clear nasal discharge that irritates the upper lip, along with sneezing and a tickling cough. The person usually is thirsty, and feels worse indoors and in warm rooms, and is much better in fresh air.

Sabadilla: Frequent and persistent spasms of sneezing, itching in the nose with irritating runny discharge, a feeling of a lump in the throat, and watery eyes will all suggest a need for this remedy. The person may feel nervous during allergy attacks, and trying to concentrate can bring on drowsiness or a headache.

Combination recommendation: Euphorbium Compositum (nasal spray) by Heel

Anxiety

Argentum nitricum: This remedy can be helpful when anxiety develops before a big event such as an exam, an important interview, a public appearance, or a social engagement. People who need this remedy are often suggestible and impulsive. Often a craving for sweets and salt is strong, which usually makes their symptoms worse.

Gelsemium: Feelings of weakness, trembling, and mental dullness as if paralyzed by fear suggest the need for this remedy. It is often helpful when a person has stagefright about a public performance or interview, or feels anxious before a test, a visit to the dentist, or any stressful event. Chills, perspiration, diarrhea, and headaches will often occur with nervousness. Fear of crowds, a fear of falling, and even a fear that the heart might stop are giveaways that you need this homeopathic remedy.

Combination recommendation: Sedalia by Boiron

Arthritis (Rheumatoid) and Inflammatory Disorders

Bryonia: This remedy can be helpful for stiffness and inflammation with tearing or throbbing pain, made worse by even the smallest motion. The condition may have developed gradually, and is worse in cold, dry weather. Discomfort is aggravated by being touched or bumped, or from any movement. Pressure brings relief because it stabilizes the area. Typically, the person wants to stay completely still and not be interfered with.

Rhus toxicodendron: Rheumatoid arthritis, with pain and stiffness that is worse in the morning and worse on first motion, but better from continued movement, is the indication for Rhus tox. Hot baths or showers and warm applications improve the stiffness and relieve the pain. The condition is worse in cold, wet weather. The person may feel extremely restless, is unable to find a comfortable position, and needs to move constantly.

Combination recommendation: Zeel by Heel

Chronic Fatigue Syndrome

Causticum: Soreness, weakness, and stiffness in the muscles, which feel worse from being cold and overused, suggest a need for Causticum. The forearms often feel stiff, unsteady, and very weak. The muscles of the legs can feel contracted and raw. Problems tend to be worse when the weather is dry and better in rainy weather, but the person doesn't like getting wet. Warm applications often relieve discomfort.

Ranunculus: This remedy is often helpful with inflammation of muscle tissue resulting in stiffness, especially when the neck and back are involved. Stabbing pains and soreness may be felt near the spine and shoulder blades, especially on the left. Problems may be aggravated by cold, damp weather, walking, and alcoholic beverages.

Combination recommendation: Sportenine by Boiron

Cold Sores

Natrum muriaticum: This remedy sometimes stops a cold sore outbreak if it is taken in the early, tingling stage. Eating too much salt (which the individual typically craves) and being in the sun sometimes aggravate the symptoms.

Rhus toxicodendron: Herpes (cold sore virus) outbreaks in any location, especially around the lips, the corners of the mouth, or on and near the genitals and inner thighs, may respond to this remedy. Eruptions, which are red and swollen with burning pain and itching, are relieved by hot water or warm applications. The person feels a constant need to move around.

Combination recommendation: Herpezostin R68 by Reckeweg

Colic

Chamomilla: This remedy is indicated when a baby is hypersensitive to pain. It is especially helpful when there are desperate screams or shrieks and the child wants to be constantly coddled and carried. The abdomen may be distended with gas, and pain can be focused in the navel region. Facial flushing (often on only one cheek) is a common presentation.

Colocynthis: Cramping, cutting pain that makes the baby curl up is a strong indication for this remedy. Pressing hard against the abdomen usually brings relief. Babies who need this remedy look extremely anxious and often feel relief when carried tummy-down on someone's arm.

Combination recommendation: Cocyntal by Boiron

Constipation

Graphites: This remedy is indicated when large stools look like little round balls. An achy feeling in the anus after the bowels have moved is commonly reported.

Lycopodium: A person who needs this remedy has frequent indigestion with gas and bloating, and many problems involving the bowels. Rubbing the abdomen or drinking something warm may help to relieve the constipation.

Combination recommendation: Laxative Combination R68 by Reckeweg

Cough and Cold

Aconite napellus: This remedy is excellent at the onset of a cold, denoted by symptoms that are intense and that come on suddenly. Exposure to cold and wind, stress, or traumatic experience may precipitate the illness. Symptoms include a dry, stuffy nose with a hot, thin discharge; tension in the chest; a scratchy throat; and choking cough. The person often feels thirsty, chilly, anxious, and agitated.

Kali bichromicum: This remedy is usually indicated for later stages of a cold with thick, stringy mucus that is difficult to clear from the nose and throat. The person typically experiences hoarse coughing with persistent phlegm.

Combination recommendation: Coryzalia by Boiron

Depression (It is very important to see your family doctor about this situation.)

Aurum metallicum: This remedy can be helpful for serious people, who are strongly focused on work and achievement, and who become depressed after a strong sense of failure. Discouragement, self-reproach, humiliation, and anger can lead to feelings of emptiness and worthlessness. This symptom picture is usually accompanied by nightmares and oversleeping that fluctuates with insomnia.

Staphysagria: This is used for feelings of hurt, shame, resentment, and suppressed emotions that can lead to depression. If under too much pressure, they can sometimes lose their natural inhibition and fly into rages or throw things. A person who needs this remedy may also have insomnia (feeling sleepy all day, but unable to sleep at night), toothaches, headaches, stomach aches, or bladder infections that are all stress related.

Combination recommendation: There is no effective combination remedy known; use Rescue Remedy by Bach for short periods when feeling overwhelmed.

Diarrhea

Arsenicum album: Diarrhea accompanied by anxiety, restlessness, and exhaustion is the indication. Burning pain is felt in the digestive tract, and the person may be thirsty for frequent small sips of tea or water. Simultaneous vomiting is another strong indication. Arsenicum is often useful when diarrhea has been caused by food poisoning.

Podophyllum: Profuse, watery diarrhea, typically without pain, suggests this remedy will be helpful. The stomach gurgles and grumbles before the diarrhea begins, and there is a frequent feeling of urging.

Combination recommendation: Diarrhea Formula R4 by Reckeweg

Ear Infections

Chamomilla: A sudden intolerable outburst of pain suggests a need for this remedy. Children may seem angry and beside themselves, and often become violent. They need to be carried constantly and walked around or rocked. Ear pain and other symptoms are worse from heat and wind, and the cheeks (often only one) may be hot and red.

Pulsatilla: This remedy is often indicated for ear infections that accompany a cold. Symptoms include a stuffy nose and yellow or greenish mucus. The ear is hot and swollen, and the person feels that something is pressing out of it. Pain is usually a pulsing sensation that gets worse at night.

Combination recommendation: Earache relief drops by Similasan

Eczema

Mezereum: This remedy is indicated when there are intense and itchy eruptions that start as blisters, then ooze and form thick crusts. Scratching leads quickly to thickened skin. The person who requires Mezereum is usually very anxious and has a strong craving for fat.

Sulphur: This remedy is very useful for those who have repeatedly used cortisone on eczema without success. Intensely burning, itching, inflamed eruptions that are worse from warmth and bathing suggest a need for this remedy. Affected areas are red, with scaling or crusted skin.

Combination recommendation: Calendula Gel by Boiron

Flu

Gelsemium: Symptoms of fatigue and aching that come on gradually, increasing over several days, may indicate a need for this remedy. The face feels heavy, with droopy eyes. A headache may begin at the back of the neck and skull, and the person may feel chills and heat running up and down the spine. Anxiety, trembling, dizziness, perspiration, and moderate fever are other indications for *Gelsemium*.

Oscillococcinum: Oscillococcinum is the Boiron brand of a remedy widely used in Canada, the US, and Europe for treating flu symptoms. Lots of good research has shown that it has strong antiviral effects. Use this at the first sign of flu symptoms that include fever, chills, body aches and pains, and headaches.

Combination recommendation: PascoLeucyn by Pascoe

Headache

Belladonna: Major throbbing or pounding head pain that starts at the back of the skull or upper neck and spreads to the forehead and temple (especially on the right) may indicate a need for this remedy. Pain is worse from jarring, light, and noise. For some reason, headaches that require Belladonna are worse around 3 p.m. Pupils may be dilated, with sensitivity to light, and the person may either feel delirious or drowsy.

Spigelia: Excruciating headaches usually present on the left side of the head, with violent throbbing, or stabbing pains above or through the eyeball. Pain extends through the face and is worse from any movement or touch. The person may feel better from lying on the right side with the head supported, and keeping very still.

Combination recommendation: Antimigren by Pascoe

Infertility

Folliculinum: Women who have challenges getting pregnant could find success with this remedy if they have irregular menstrual cycles that are often weeks delayed, with a heavy, clotty flow. Often women in this state feel a loss of will and are full of self-denial. As the exception to the dosing recommendations for the rest of the homeopathics listed in this chapter, dissolve three pills of Folliculinum 30CH under your tongue once daily on days 0 to 10 unless otherwise recommended by a homeopathic doctor.

Luteinum: Infertile women who need this remedy typically have either polycystic ovaries, fibroids, or endometriosis and often have estrogen dominance without even knowing it. Strong indications that this remedy is appropriate are early menstruation and short cycles, which represent a possible luteal phase defect. As the exception to the dosing recommendations for the rest of the homeopathics listed in this chapter, dissolve three pills of Luteinum 30CH under your tongue once daily on days 16 to menses unless otherwise recommended by a homeopathic doctor.

Combination recommendation: None known

Menopause

Lachesis: Intense hot flashes with purple-red flushing, palpitations, and feelings of pressure, congestion, and constriction may indicate a need for this remedy. Tight clothing around the neck and waist may be impossible to tolerate. The unique symptom of this picture is loquacity (extremely talkative), with a strong tendency to feel suspicious.

Sepia: This remedy can be helpful if a woman's periods are sometimes late and scanty. It is best used from the middle to the end of menopause (12–24 months after the last period). During the wind-down, menses can be heavy. The uterus feels weak and saggy, and there may be cravings for vinegar and sour foods. Women who need this remedy usually feel dragged-out and weary, emotionally distraught, and fatigued.

Combination recommendation: PascoeFemin by Pascoe

Sprains/Strains

Arnica montana: This is the most popular remedy in homeopathic literature and is best for recent traumatic injuries. It is brilliant for bruises, sprains, and concussions. Arnica can be helpful for soft tissue damage caused by surgery and dental work. It can also be given preventatively before an anticipated injury (i.e., sports), and used to treat the soreness afterward. It is also helpful in preventing shock.

Bellis perennis: This remedy is useful for deeper tissue injuries from falls, car accidents, and major surgery. Often the patient has a feeling of stiffness or coldness in the injured area. If Arnica has been given for an injury—especially a strain or bruise—but has not had much effect, try Bellis perennis next.

Combination recommendation: Traumeel by Heel

Urinary Tract Infections

Berberis vulgaris: This remedy is for severe cutting or burning pain that extends to the urethral opening, which may also burn at times when there is no attempt at urination. After emptying the bladder, the person feels as if some urine still remains inside. Urging and discomfort are often worse from walking.

Cantharis: A strong urge to urinate accompanied by cutting pains that are felt before the urine passes is a sign that this remedy is appropriate. Some describe the cutting feeling as a scalding sensation when only a few drops of urine pass at a time. The person often feels as if the bladder has not been emptied.

Combination recommendation: Pascosabal by Pascoe

Varicose Veins

Carbo vegetabilis: When varicose veins are accompanied by general poor circulation with icy coldness of the extremities, and a bruised or marbled look, use Carbo veg. The person's legs feel weak and heavy, and often itch and burn.

Hamamelis: This remedy can help when varicose veins are large and sore, and very weak and easily damaged, with a tendency to bleed. The pain is described as a bruise or sometimes a stinging sensation. The muscles of the legs feel tired.

Combination recommendation: Endangitin R63 by Reckeweg

SECTION III

COMMON HEALTH CONCERNS AND CONDITIONS

ACID REFLUX (GERD)

Acid reflux, known medically as gastroesophageal reflux disease (GERD), is a disease in which stomach acid flows back (refluxes) into your esophagus (food pipe). This causes burning and pain, which is commonly known as heartburn. Many people experience an occasional episode of heartburn, which is usually not a cause for concern, but when it occurs continually, it could indicate GERD.

GERD is a common disorder, affecting up to 60 percent of people at some point during the course of a year, and 20–30 percent of people at least weekly.

Normally when you swallow, the lower esophageal sphincter, which is a circular band of muscle around the bottom of the esophagus, relaxes to allow food and liquid to flow down into your stomach. Then it closes again. If this valve becomes weakened or relaxes when it shouldn't, stomach acids can flow up into the esophagus, causing heartburn.

When stomach acids continually reflux upward, it can cause irritation and inflammation of the lining of the esophagus, which is known as esophagitis. This can cause chest pain after eating, difficulty swallowing, and breathing problems.

Although GERD is uncomfortable, there are a number of dietary and lifestyle modifications that can help relieve symptoms.

SIGNS & SYMPTOMS

- Chest pain that may be worse when lying down

- Coughing, wheezing, asthma, and sore throat

- Difficulty in swallowing

- Heartburn, a burning in the chest that may go up into the throat

- Regurgitating food

- Sour taste in mouth

If left untreated, GERD can lead to other conditions such as esophageal narrowing (due to formation of scar tissue) and esophageal ulcer.

RISK FACTORS

- Asthma: Coughing and laboured breathing put pressure on the stomach; asthma medications may relax the esophageal sphincter.

- Connective tissue disorders (scleroderma) and diseases that affect the muscles.

- Diabetes: Gastroparesis (delayed stomach emptying) is a complication of diabetes.

- Hiatal hernia: The stomach protrudes into the lower chest, worsening heartburn and weakening the esophageal sphincter.

- Obesity: Excess weight puts pressure on the stomach, forcing open the esophageal sphincter and allowing stomach acids to back up.

- Overeating and eating high-fat meals puts pressure on the lower esophageal sphincter, allowing stomach acids to back-up.

- Peptic ulcer can affect stomach emptying, causing a buildup of acids.

- Pregnancy: The growing belly puts pressure on the stomach; higher progesterone levels relax the muscles (esophageal sphincter), allowing stomach acids to reflux.

- Smoking increases stomach acid, weakens the esophageal sphincter, and dries up saliva, which helps dilute the stomach acid.

DOCTOR'S ORDERS

Most cases of heartburn and GERD can be treated effectively with over-the-counter (OTC) and prescription medications. The most commonly used classes of drugs include the following:

- Alginic acid forms a protective seal at the top of the stomach to prevent acid reflux. It is found OTC in a product called Gaviscon.
- Antacids contain ingredients such as magnesium, aluminum, and calcium, which work quickly to neutralize stomach acids. However, they do not reduce inflammation or promote healing. Antacids are available OTC and include Tums, Rolaids, Maalox, and Mylanta.
- H2 receptor blockers reduce the production of acid and reflux. They take longer to work, but provide longer relief. Side effects include dry mouth, bowel changes, dizziness, and drowsiness. Examples include famotidine (Pepcid) and ranitidine (Zantac). They are available full strength by prescription, or in lower dosages OTC.
- Proton pump inhibitors block acid production and allow the damaged esophagus to heal. These are long-acting products and the most effective medical treatment for GERD. Examples include Losec (omeprazole), Pantoloc (pantoprazole), and Prevacid (lansoprazole). These products are well tolerated; side effects are rare and include headache and dizziness.

SHERRY'S NATURAL PRESCRIPTION

Dietary Recommendations

Foods to include:

- Drink caffeine-free herbal teas that contain chamomile, ginger, marshmallow, and slippery elm, herbs that are soothing and help relieve heartburn.

- Drinking fluids between meals rather than with meals will also help prevent reflux.

- Eat vegetables, non-citrus fruits, whole grains, beans, fish, and lean meat.

- Eating small, frequent meals (instead of one or two large meals) will prevent excess production of stomach acid and is also less stressful to the esophageal sphincter. Eat slowly and chew your food thoroughly.

- Small amounts of olive and vegetable oils are fine.

- Stay upright after eating and don't eat within three hours of bedtime.

Foods to avoid:

- Alcohol, carbonated beverages, spicy foods, tomatoes, citrus fruits, spearmint, peppermint, and onions are irritating to the esophagus.

- Chocolate and coffee relax the esophageal sphincter and increase the risk of reflux.

- High-fat foods worsen symptoms because they stay in the stomach longer and increase the time the esophagus is exposed to stomach acids. Avoid or minimize cream, butter, ice cream, gravy, oils, fried foods, sausage, and processed fatty meats and cream soups.

Lifestyle Suggestions

- Lose excess weight by eating healthy and exercising regularly.

- Do not bend over, lie down, or exercise right after eating. Wait two hours after eating to exercise and three hours after eating before lying down.

- Do not wear tight belts or pants that are tight at the waist.

- Don't smoke.

- Raise the head of your bed—use pillows or a block under the head of your bed. Keeping your head higher than your stomach will help prevent acids from refluxing.

• •

Several studies have shown a link between elevated body mass index (a scale used to determine overweight and obesity) and symptoms of GERD. The risk of GERD symptoms, such as heartburn and acid reflux, rises with BMI. Studies have also shown that losing excess weight can reduce symptoms.

• •

Top Recommended Supplements

Calcium carbonate: This is the main ingredient in many OTC heartburn products and is also available as a supplement. Calcium helps to neutralize stomach acid and provides short-term relief. Dosage: 500 mg three times daily with meals and before bedtime.

Deglycyrrhizinated licorice (DGL): This herb soothes and coats the mucous membranes of the stomach. It helps restore the mucous lining that protects the stomach from hydrochloric acid (stomach acid). Dosage: Two to four tablets before meals and at bedtime.

Complementary Supplements

Aloe vera juice: Helps reduce acid output and is soothing to the mucous membranes. Research is limited at this point, but it is widely used by naturopathic physicians. Dosage: 1 tbsp two or three times daily.

Digestive enzymes: Improve digestion and may help reduce reflux. Dosage: One capsule with each meal.

Probiotics: Contain friendly bacteria, which improve digestion. Dosage: One capsule twice daily.

FINAL THOUGHTS

To prevent or relieve the symptoms of acid reflux, consider the following:

1. Work on losing excess body weight.
2. Don't smoke.
3. Raise the head of your bed.
4. Avoid high-fat and spicy foods, alcohol, and other triggers, and don't overeat.
5. Consider supplements of calcium and DGL.

ACNE

Acne is a chronic disorder of the skin's sebaceous glands (oil glands), leading to the development of comedones, also known as pimples, or more commonly "zits." Almost every teenager will have an occasional acne outbreak, and approximately 40 percent of teens have severe cystic acne. Even those 30 and older are affected. Acne is not life threatening, but it can leave physical and emotional scars.

During puberty hormones called androgens trigger the sebaceous glands to grow and produce more sebum (oil). Irregular shedding of skin cells lining the hair follicle can lead to clumping and cause the pores to clog. A type of bacteria called *Propionibacterium acnes*, which normally lives in the skin, invades the clogged pore and begins to grow, creating inflammation and irritation. The result is a plugged, inflamed follicle that develops into a pimple.

There are many myths surrounding acne. It is not contagious; you can't catch it from someone else. Acne is also not caused by eating chocolate—unless you are allergic.

SIGNS & SYMPTOMS

- Cystic acne is marked by clusters of deep, painful, fluid-filled cysts; areas of the skin appear red or purple and are inflamed.

- Pitting, pockmarks, and scarring can occur with severe forms of acne, or if the lesions are picked or squeezed and become infected.

- Whiteheads, blackheads, red spots, and white, pus-filled pimples appear primarily on the face, but also on the shoulders, neck, back, chest, and buttocks.

RISK FACTORS

- Allergies: Reactions to foods, medications, or environmental chemicals

- Cosmetics or exposure to airborne grease (working in a fast-food restaurant)

- Exposure to extreme temperatures

- Family history: Having a parent with acne

- Friction and sweating caused by wearing headbands, helmets, or tight collars

- Hormonal changes in teenagers, premenstrual women, and during pregnancy

- Medications: Use of hormones such as testosterone or cortisone

- Race: Caucasians are more affected than African Americans or Asians

- Stress

DOCTOR'S ORDERS

Drugs used for acne work by inhibiting sebum and keratin production, reducing bacterial growth, or encouraging shedding of skin cells to unclog the pores. Most over-the-counter products contain salicylic acid, benzoyl peroxide, or sulphur. Benzoyl peroxide is the most effective. All of these products may cause redness, burning, stinging, and scaling of the skin.

Creams and gels containing tretinoin (vitamin A derivative) or tazarotene (synthetic vitamin A) are used to slough off dead skin, clear pores, and dry acne. Accutane is an oral medication derived from vitamin A; it reduces sebum production and swelling, and minimizes acne-causing bacteria. It is effective, but must be taken for several months and may cause dry mucous membranes, muscle aches, and liver problems. It must be avoided by women who are pregnant or trying to conceive as it can cause severe birth defects.

Antibiotics (tetracycline, erythromycin, or minocycline) are sometimes prescribed for mild to moderate acne. They work for some people, but their use is limited by side effects such as upset stomach, diarrhea, sun sensitivity, and yeast infections.

Birth control pills are prescribed for women with menstrual-related acne. They reduce androgen levels and sebum production. Side effects include blood clots, bloating, cramps, spotting, liver and gallbladder disease, and increased risk of breast cancer.

SHERRY'S NATURAL PRESCRIPTION

Dietary Recommendations

Foods to include:

- Fibre supports detoxification and elimination; flaxseed is particularly helpful as it is high in both fibre and essential fatty acids.

- Yogurt contains beneficial bacteria, which is especially important for those who have taken antibiotics.

Foods to avoid:

- Food allergies can trigger acne breakouts. Refer to that section of this book for more information.

- Sugar reduces immune function and may increase bacterial growth.

Lifestyle Suggestions

- Drink eight to 10 glasses of water daily.

- Wash your face morning and evening with warm water and a gentle cleanser.

- Do not scrub hard or use abrasive cleaners as this can irritate acne.

- Go for regular facials as estheticians can cleanse, exfoliate, and extract pores.

- Sauna or steam help to clear pores and aid in detoxification.

- Resist the temptation to pick or squeeze, which can cause tissue damage, infection, and scars.

- Minimize wearing cosmetics. Use only water-based and hypoallergenic skin care products. Products containing lavender, chamomile, and tea tree are beneficial.

- For severe cases, where there are multiple lesions or cysts, consult a dermatologist.

Top Recommended Supplements

Tea tree oil: A natural antibiotic and antiseptic; try a lotion or cream with 5–15 percent tea tree oil. Studies have found it just as effective as benzoyl peroxide, but it is better tolerated.

Vitamin A: Essential for skin health; regulates sebum and keratin production. Dosage: 5,000–10,000 IU daily. Higher doses should be taken only under medical supervision. Women who are pregnant or trying to conceive should not exceed 5,000 IU daily.

Zinc: Promotes tissue healing, balances hormones, and reduces inflammation. Dosage: 25–50 mg daily. Choose a supplement that also contains copper (3–5 mg) because chronic use of zinc can reduce copper absorption.

Complementary Supplements

B-vitamins: Deficiencies are associated with acne, so supplementing may reduce breakouts. Try a B-complex that provides 50–100 mg of the B-vitamins.

Chasteberry (Vitex): May help premenstrual acne in women. There is limited research, but this herb is well known to help balance hormones. Try 160 mg or 40 drops of tincture daily.

Essential fatty acids: Reduce inflammation and repair damaged skin cells. Try 1–3 g of fish oil daily.

Vitamin C: Aids skin repair and improves collagen production. Take 500–2,000 mg daily.

Vitamin E: Essential for skin health, and may help prevent scarring. Dosage: 400 IU daily.

FINAL THOUGHTS

To improve acne and overall skin health, consider the following:

1. Nourish your body and skin with a healthy diet, including lots of fibre, good fats, and water.
2. Keep your skin clean and avoid picking blemishes.
3. Skin products containing tea tree can improve acne.
4. Supplements of vitamin A and zinc are helpful.
5. Those with severe acne should consult a dermatologist.

ALLERGIC RHINITIS

Approximately 20 percent of Canadians—about seven million adults and children—suffer from seasonal allergies, also known as hay fever. These allergies occur when the immune system overreacts upon exposure to allergens, substances such as trees, grass, or flower pollen. Some people have persistent, year-long allergies that are triggered by environmental factors such as house dust, mould, animal dander, dust mites, and air pollution.

The immune system responds to these otherwise harmless substances as invaders, similar to how it would react to viruses or bacteria. It produces an antibody against the allergen called immunoglobulin E (IgE), which triggers the release of inflammatory chemicals—histamine, leukotrienes, and prostaglandins. Histamine is responsible for the notorious allergy symptoms of itchy, runny eyes and nose, and sneezing; leukotrienes cause excess mucus production; and prostaglandins trigger inflammation.

Researchers do not completely understand why some people get allergies while others don't, but there are a few theories. One is the overuse of antibiotics, which causes destruction of the normal flora (bacteria) in the gut. Another is the ultra-hygienic society that we live in. With little exposure to dirt and bacteria, our immune system is primed to respond when faced with a foreign invader.

THE ORIGIN OF "HAYFEVER"

Despite the common name of "hayfever," allergies are rarely triggered by hay. The name originated in the 1800s when British doctors found that people living in rural areas experienced sneezing and itching with exposure to cut hay or grass. This reaction caused nervousness, which was referred to as "fever," hence the name "hayfever."

SIGNS & SYMPTOMS

- Cough

- Fatigue

- Headache

- Irritability

- Itchy eyes, nose, roof of mouth, or throat

- Sinus pressure and pain

- Sneezing

- Runny nose and congestion

- Watery eyes

Having allergies increases your risk of developing other inflammatory diseases such as asthma and eczema. Prolonged sinus congestion can increase the risk of sinusitis (infection or inflammation of the sinuses).

RISK FACTORS

- Exposure to cigarette smoke during first years of life
- Exposure to indoor allergens (dust or pet dander)
- Family history of allergies
- Firstborn child
- Gender (men are at greater risk)

DOCTOR'S ORDERS

There are several different types of medications that are used to manage allergy symptoms. Antihistamines block histamine release and improve symptoms of itching, runny nose, and sneezing. Benadryl (diphenhydramine) and Chlor-Tripolon are older antihistamines, which cause substantial drowsiness and are taken every six hours. Newer products cause less drowsiness and are taken once daily. Examples include Claritin, Aerius, Allegra, and Reactine. Side effects include dry eyes, mouth, and nose.

Decongestants relieve sinus congestion (feeling of fullness and pressure). Examples include Sudafed (pseudoephedrine) and phenylephrine. Side effects include insomnia, racing heart, increased blood pressure, and irritability. Avoid use with high blood pressure, glaucoma, or prostate enlargement. Note: Decongestant nasal sprays can cause rebound congestion if used longer than three days.

Cromolyn is a drug that prevents the release of histamine. It is most effective as a preventative (before symptoms start) and is available in eyedrops and nasal spray. Singulair is a prescription drug that blocks the action of leukotrienes. It is taken once daily and may cause headache.

Allergy shots are helpful for some people. These injections contain purified allergen extracts, which desensitize you to allergies. They are given yearly, prior to the allergy season.

SHERRY'S NATURAL PRESCRIPTION

Dietary Recommendations

Foods to include:

- Fruits and vegetables provide antioxidants that support healthy immune function.
- Fish, seeds, and nuts contain healthy fats that help reduce inflammation.
- Peppers, onions, and garlic help thin and reduce mucus.
- Wasabi (Japanese horseradish) clears the sinuses.

Foods to avoid:

- Mucus-forming foods such as dairy products, refined flours, and saturated and hydrogenated fats can trigger inflammation and should be avoided.

Note: People who have seasonal allergies often have food allergies as well. Refer to Appendix D for information on how to do an elimination diet.

Lifestyle Suggestions

- Know your triggers and try to avoid them—pollen production is highest between 5 a.m. and 10 a.m., so avoid the outdoors during this time.

- Heavy rain reduces pollen in the air, making post-shower outings safer.

- Wear a mask when cutting the grass or gardening.

- Don't dry your clothes outside, as they can collect pollen.

- Use an air purifier to remove allergens from your home.

- Keep your windows closed to prevent pollen from blowing into your home.

- Use a high-efficiency particulate air (HEPA) filter on your air conditioner and furnace and change it monthly.

- Use a vacuum with a double bag and a high-efficiency particulate air (HEPA) filter.

- Don't keep cut flowers in the house and minimize indoor plants. Wet dirt allows mould to grow.

Top Recommended Supplements

Aller-7: A combination of seven plant extracts that reduces allergy symptoms when taken regularly. Dosage: 660 mg twice daily for six to 12 weeks, then 330 mg twice daily thereafter. There are no serious side effects or interactions.

Butterbur: An herb that reduces inflammation and has antihistamine effects. Dosage: 50 mg twice daily. Studies used a standardized extract providing 8 mg of petasine (an active chemical) three times daily.

Nasaleze: A nasal powder that is inhaled and forms a barrier in the nostrils against allergens. It has no side effects or drug interactions and is safe for children and pregnant women. Several studies have shown that it reduces allergy symptoms and the need for medication. One or two inhalations are used daily as a preventative.

Complementary Supplements

Moducare: A mixture of plant sterols and sterolins (plant fats) that helps balance the immune system. One clinical trial found it reduced allergy symptoms. Dosage: One capsule three times daily.

Probiotics: Help replenish gastrointestinal flora, which is important for immune function. Preliminary research shows benefits for allergies. Dosage: One to three capsules daily.

Quercetin: A flavonoid with antihistamine properties. Dosage: 500 mg three times daily.

Vitamin C: Helps reduce histamine production and works well with quercetin. Dosage: 1,000 mg three times daily.

Vitamin E: Has antioxidant effects and has been shown to reduce allergic response and nasal symptoms (sneezing, itching, stuffiness, and runny nose). Dosage: 400 IU daily.

FINAL THOUGHTS

To keep allergies at bay, consider the following:

1. Eat plenty of antioxidant-rich fruits and vegetables, especially garlic, onions, and peppers, nuts, and seeds.
2. Minimize being outdoors in the early morning.
3. Use an air purifier in your home.
4. For prevention, use Nasaleze and/or Aller-7 regularly.
5. To reduce symptoms once they appear, try Butterbur.

ALZHEIMER'S DISEASE

Alzheimer's disease is a chronic, degenerative disease of the brain that impairs thinking, memory, and cognitive function. It is the most common form of dementia. It is estimated that 280,600 Canadians over 65 and 50 percent of people over age 85 have Alzheimer's disease. These numbers are expected to rise substantially over the next few decades due to our aging population.

Alzheimer's is not a normal part of aging, but it is more common in people as they age. The actual cause is not known, but its effect on brain tissue is clear. The disease causes damage and death to brain cells.

In a healthy brain, there are billions of neurons (nerve cells) that generate electrical and chemical signals, which help us think, remember, and feel. In those with Alzheimer's the neurons begin to die, affecting the normal signalling in the brain. A key feature of this disease is the development of plaques and tangles in the brain. The plaques consist of normally harmless proteins called beta-amyloid. It is thought that a genetic defect in these proteins may be involved in the development of the disease. Tangles refer to a twisting of internal support structures of the brain, which causes damage and death of the neurons.

Research has shown that Alzheimer's disease involves oxidative and inflammatory processes, although it is not known whether these processes are a cause or effect of the disease or both. The ultimate result, however, is disruption of neuronal cell functioning and signalling, leading to neuronal cell death, which impairs memory and other mental abilities. There also are lower levels of some neurotransmitters, chemicals in the brain that carry messages back and forth between nerve cells. This also results in impaired thinking and memory.

Although there's no cure for Alzheimer's disease, a number of medical advances in recent years and the use of natural supplements can delay the progression of the disease and improve symptoms and quality of life.

• •

Alzheimer's was first identified by Dr. Alois Alzheimer in 1906. He described the two hallmark features of the disease—plaques (tiny dense deposits scattered throughout the brain) and tangles (structures of the brain that are twisted)—which interfere with normal brain processes and cause death of brain cells.

• •

SIGNS & SYMPTOMS

- Confusion and disorientation

- Depression

- Difficulty performing familiar tasks (cooking, tying your shoes)

- Difficulty with abstract thinking (for example, dealing with numbers)

- Gradual memory loss

- Increasing forgetfulness

- Loss of judgment (difficulty solving everyday problems)

- Paranoia

- Personality changes (mood swings)

Symptoms and the progression of the disease vary among individuals. As the disease progresses, there is a decline in language skills and the ability to perform tasks. The average length of time from diagnosis of Alzheimer's to death is about eight years, but some people live beyond 10 years.

RISK FACTORS

- Age: It is most common in those over 65, but can rarely affect those younger than age 40.

- Environmental toxicity: Pollution and smoking generate excess free radicals. Some research has connected aluminum and mercury exposure to the disease.

- Family history: Having a parent or sibling with the disease increases your risk as there are genetic mutations that may be inherited.

- Gender: Women are at greater risk.

- Head injury: Some studies show that trauma to the head increases risk of Alzheimer's.

- Hormone replacement therapy: Results from one large-scale study suggested that women taking estrogen after age 65 are at increased risk of Alzheimer's (*JAMA,* 2004: 291; 1701–1712).

- Lifestyle: Inactivity, obesity, poor diet, and smoking increase risk.

- Poorly controlled diabetes increases risk.

DOCTOR'S ORDERS

There are a variety of drugs that can help reduce symptoms of insomnia, anxiety, and agitation.

There are no drugs that can reverse the disease, but there are a few that can help improve cognitive function and slow the cognitive decline associated with Alzheimer's, such as Aricept, Reminyl, and Exelon. These drugs improve the levels of neurotransmitters (chemical messengers such as serotonin and acetylcholine) in the brain and can delay the onset of Alzheimer's in those with mild cognitive impairment. Not everyone responds positively to these drugs; some people have to stop because of side effects such as nausea, vomiting, and diarrhea.

SHERRY'S NATURAL PRESCRIPTION

Dietary Recommendations

Foods to include:

- Fish (wild, organic salmon, halibut, sole, and cod) provide good sources of omega-3 fatty acids, a polyunsaturated fat that has been found to reduce Alzheimer's risk by reducing inflammation and protecting the nerve cell membranes.

- Olive oil is a monounsaturated fat that is also helpful.

- Vitamin E-rich foods such as whole grains, vegetable oils, nuts, seeds, and egg yolks are good. Two studies have found a lower risk of Alzheimer's disease with a higher food intake of vitamin E.

- Zinc may be deficient in those with Alzheimer's. Boost your intake by eating pumpkin seeds, black-eyed peas, wheat germ, tofu, and seafood.

FISH AND YOUR BRAIN

Two prominent clinical studies have demonstrated that eating one fish meal a week was associated with a 60 percent reduction in the risk of developing Alzheimer's disease (*JAMA*, 2002: 288; 2266–2268 and *Archives of Neurology*, 2003: 60; 940–946).

Foods to avoid:

- Aluminum has been associated with an increased risk, although the evidence is not conclusive. However, it may be wise to avoid aluminum food additives, which are found in some baked goods, processed foods, and beverages.

- Saturated and trans fats raise blood cholesterol levels, and are associated with an increased risk of Alzheimer's. Avoid fast foods, deep-fried foods, and baked goods and margarine containing hydrogenated oils; minimize saturated fat (red meat and high-fat dairy).

Lifestyle Suggestions

- Maintain a healthy body weight. Being obese and its consequences of high blood pressure and cholesterol are risk factors for Alzheimer's.

- Exercising regularly helps with weight management, and also increases blood flow to the brain. According to one study, regular exercises (walking 15 minutes three times per week) reduced the risk of Alzheimer's and dementia by 40 percent in individuals over age 65.

- Mental exercises: Some studies have shown that keeping your brain active, especially in later years, reduces the risk of Alzheimer's. The theory is the more you use your brain, the more synapses you create, which provide a greater reserve as you age. Read, do cross word puzzles, and play memory games.

- Minimize aluminum exposure—do not cook foods in aluminum pots, and minimize foods that come into direct contact with aluminum foil and beverages stored in aluminum cans.

- Eliminate risky situations at home that may cause injury or falls, such as clutter and floor mats. Grip rails in the bathroom can be helpful.

- Interact with others as much as possible to enhance communication and get necessary assistance from support groups and health care aides.

Top Recommended Supplements

Acetyl-L-carnitine: An amino acid derivative that crosses into the brain and increases the levels of acetycholine, a brain neurotransmitter that is depleted in those with Alzheimer's. Several studies have shown that it can delay the progression of the disease. Dosage: 1 g three times daily.

Bacopa monnieri: An herb that has been shown to enhance several aspects of mental function. It increases availability of acetylcholine in the brain, which improves memory and cognition. Antioxidant properties help protect brain cells. Dosage: 200–450 mg daily, standardized to contain bacosides.

Ginkgo biloba: An herb that improves memory and cognitive function and slows the progression of Alzheimer's. Four studies have found it helpful in those with early stages of the disease. Dosage: 120–240 mg daily, standardized to 6 percent terpene lactones and 24 percent flavone glycosides. It may take six weeks to notice benefit.

Phosphatidylserine: A nutrient that is related to lecithin, which is naturally occurring in the brain. It helps support the structure and health of cell membranes. Several studies involving more than 1,000 people suggest that phosphatidylserine is an effective treatment for Alzheimer's disease and other forms of dementia. It improves both behaviour and mental function and reduces symptoms of depression. The form used in these studies was from a bovine source. Dosage: 300 mg daily.

Complementary Supplements

B-vitamins: Support neurotransmitter function. Vitamin B1 is involved in nerve transmission and may be deficient in those with Alzheimer's. Two small studies found benefits in mental function with B1 supplements. Dosage: Take 40–100 mg as part of a B-complex as they work together.

Fish oils: Reduce inflammation and protect the nerve cell membranes. Regular consumption of fish reduces Alzheimer's risk and is important for brain function. Those who do not eat fish should consider supplements. Dosage: 1–3 g daily.

Vitamin E: A potent antioxidant that protects the brain from damage due to oxidative stress and inflammation. Higher blood levels of vitamin E are associated with better brain function in older adults and some research has shown that supplements can lower the risk of Alzheimer's. Higher dosages have been found to slow cognitive decline. Dosage: 1,000–2,000 IU daily.

FINAL THOUGHTS

To improve cognitive function and delay the progression of Alzheimer's, consider the following:

1. Eat more fish, whole grains, vegetables, nuts, seeds, and olive oil.
2. Avoid saturated, trans fats, and aluminum-containing food ingredients.
3. Get regular exercise such as walking.
4. Keep your brain active with games, puzzles, and exercises.
5. Consider supplements of acetyl-L-carnitine, bacopa, ginkgo, phosphatidylserine, and fish oils.

ANEMIA

Derived from the Greek, meaning "without blood," anemia is a deficiency of red blood cells and/or hemoglobin. Every cell in our body requires oxygen to function normally. Anemia impairs the ability of blood to transfer oxygen to the tissues throughout the body. Either the body produces too few healthy red blood cells, loses too many, or destroys them faster than they can be replaced. This makes one feel very tired, both mentally and physically.

There are various forms of anemia. The most common form is iron-deficiency anemia. This affects about one in five women, most often during pregnancy. The body needs iron to produce hemoglobin, the oxygen-carrying component of red blood cells. Without adequate iron, hemoglobin levels are low. This form of anemia can result from poor diet (inadequate iron), blood loss (menstruation, surgery, or hemorrhoids), malabsorption diseases such as celiac, or increased iron needs during pregnancy.

In addition to iron, the body needs folate and vitamin B12 to produce healthy red blood cells. B12 deficiency anemia is called pernicious anemia. It is more common among the elderly and those with intestinal disorders, which impair B12 absorption. Bariatric surgery, gastric ulcers, stomach tumours, and excessive alcohol consumption are other known risk factors for the development of pernicious anemia.

Certain chronic diseases such as cancer, Crohn's disease, kidney failure, rheumatoid arthritis, and other inflammatory disorders can impair red blood cell production, which results in anemia.

Aplastic anemia is a rare, life-threatening disease caused by a decrease in the bone marrow's ability to produce blood cells. This may result from chemotherapy, radiation, exposure to environmental toxins, pregnancy, and lupus.

Hemolytic anemia is a condition in which the red blood cells are destroyed faster than they can be produced in the bone marrow. This may result from autoimmune disease and use of certain medications, such as antibiotics.

Sickle cell anemia is an inherited form of anemia caused by a defective form of hemoglobin that causes the red blood cells to become an abnormal (sickle) shape. These cells die prematurely, resulting in a deficiency. This form is most common among Blacks and Arabs. Thalassemia is another form of anemia caused by defective hemoglobin.

SIGNS & SYMPTOMS

- Difficulty in thinking
- Fatigue and weakness
- Frequent infections
- Headaches and dizziness
- Menstrual irregularity
- Numbness in extremities
- Pale skin and lips
- Shortness of breath

If left unchecked, anemia can lead to a rapid or irregular heartbeat (arrhythmia) because the heart works harder to compensate for the lack of oxygen in the blood. This can even lead to congestive heart failure. Untreated pernicious anemia can lead to nerve damage and decreased mental function, as vitamin B12 is important not only for healthy red blood cells but also for optimal nerve and brain function.

Some inherited anemias, such as sickle cell anemia, can be serious and lead to life-threatening complications. Losing a lot of blood quickly results in acute, severe anemia and can be fatal.

RISK FACTORS

- Alcoholism: Alcohol interferes with the absorption of folic acid

- Anorexia or bulimia

- Blood loss: Surgery, heavy menstrual periods, ulcers, and hemorrhoids

- Family history: Sickle cell anemia and thalassemia

- Medical conditions: Kidney or liver disease, cancer, autoimmune disease, and malabsorption disorders, such as Crohn's or celiac disease, and bariatric surgery

- Medications: Non-steroidal anti-inflammatory drugs such as aspirin and ibuprofen can cause stomach bleeding

- Poor diet: Inadequate intake of iron, folate, and vitamin B12

- Pregnancy: Iron stores are depleted by the growing baby

DOCTOR'S ORDERS

The treatment of anemia depends upon the underlying cause. Iron-deficiency anemia is treated with supplemental iron. It may take several months to build back iron stores. Pernicious anemia is treated with injections of vitamin B12, and folate deficiency is treated with folate supplements. Aplastic anemia is very serious and may require blood transfusion or bone marrow transplant. Hemolytic anemia is managed with medications that suppress the immune system so that it stops attacking the red blood cells. Sickle cell anemia is treated with oxygen, intravenous fluids, and sometimes blood transfusions.

SHERRY'S NATURAL PRESCRIPTION

Anemia can be a serious condition and requires medical attention. Do not self-diagnose or begin taking iron supplements unless advised by your doctor.

The recommendations for anemia vary upon the underlying cause. The following information is provided for anemia due to iron, folate, or vitamin B12 deficiency.

Dietary Recommendations

Foods to include:

- Iron-rich foods such as organic beef (calf liver), beans, lentils, fortified cereals, figs, eggs, blackstrap molasses, brewer's yeast, nuts, and seeds

- Folate-rich foods such as dark green citrus, legumes, and fortified cereals

- Dark-green leafy vegetables (except spinach) are good sources of iron and folate

- B12 is found in meat and dairy products, fish, and eggs

- Foods rich in vitamin C, such as citrus, peppers, and berries, improve iron absorption

Foods to avoid:

- Star fruit, rhubarb, spinach, chard, beets, chives, parsley, and chocolate are high in oxalic acid, which inhibits iron absorption

- Coffee reduces iron absorption (more than 3 cups per day)

- Tea contains tannins, which inhibit iron absorption

Lifestyle Suggestions

- Have regular medical checkups and report any changes to your doctor.

- If you have iron-deficiency anemia, cook your food in cast-iron pots and pans as the food will absorb some of the iron from the cookware.

Top Recommended Supplements

Folate: Supplements are required by those deficient and women trying to get pregnant. Dosage: 800–1,200 mcg daily.

Iron supplements: Should be taken only if you have deficiency anemia as excess iron can be dangerous. Usual dosage: 50–100 mg two to three times daily. Look for iron chelates, which are well absorbed and tolerated. Other good choices include iron citrate, gluconate, and fumarate.

....

Fibre can significantly reduce the absorption of iron from foods. Take iron supplements on an empty stomach or with a small snack of low-fibre food, such as crackers, and if taking fibre supplements, separate by three hours.

....

Liver extracts: Made from beef, they provide a rich natural source of iron and vitamin B12, folate, and other nutrients. Dosage varies.

Multivitamin and mineral complex: Highly recommended because there are many nutrients required for healthy blood cells. Aside from iron, B12, and folate, a deficiency of vitamin A, C, E, B2, B6, or copper can lead to anemia.

Vitamin B12: Supplements are required by those who are deficient or at risk of deficiency such as the elderly, vegetarians, and those with malabsorption conditions (celiac and Crohn's). Look for a B-complex supplement that provides 1,000–2,000 mcg daily. Those with malabsorption may benefit from sublingual B12 (small tablet placed under the tongue), which is more readily absorbed. Individuals with pernicious anemia may require B12 injections from their doctor.

Complementary Supplements

Vitamin C: Increases the absorption of iron from food. It also supports absorption of other nutrients. Dosage: 100–500 mg. Take with your iron supplement for best results.

FINAL THOUGHTS

Inherited forms of anemia can't be prevented, but can be managed with medical treatments. Iron and vitamin deficiency anemia can be managed well with the following:

1. Eat more leafy green vegetables, nuts, seeds, whole grains, beans, and legumes.
2. Consider beef and calf liver if you are deficient in iron.
3. Reduce coffee and tea intake.
4. If deficient, supplement with iron, B12, and folate, along with a complete multivitamin and mineral complex.
5. See your doctor and have your blood checked regularly.

ANXIETY

Everyone experiences occasional feelings of anxiety when, for example, starting a new job or speaking in front of a crowd. The excitement brought on by these situations is normal, and can actually help improve performance. However, feeling anxious with no reason, or having excessive worry that affects your quality of life could signify generalized anxiety disorder (GAD). This condition is among the most common psychiatric ailments, affecting 12 percent of Canadians.

Feelings of anxiety trigger the body to release stress hormones that prepare you to react to a threat. This is called the fight-or-flight response. The heart pumps stronger, breathing is increased, blood is shunted to the extremities to increase strength in the arms and legs, and digestion slows down so the body can reserve resources. Hundreds of years ago, this response was experienced occasionally and was vital to our survival. Today, however, stress and anxiety can be persistent and debilitating, with far-reaching consequences on health, leading to high blood pressure and cholesterol, insomnia, mood swings, depression, and other health problems.

Some people experience extreme states of anxiety and worry, called panic attacks, which cause heart pounding, shortness of breath, chest pain, sweating, dizziness, and weakness. This can be scary, as the symptoms mimic the early signs of a heart attack.

There are various lifestyle strategies and supplements that can be helpful in reducing anxiety and improving emotional well-being.

TYPES OF ANXIETY

Generalized anxiety disorder is one type of anxiety disorder. Others include:

Obsessive-compulsive disorder: Obsessions are persistent thoughts, ideas, impulses, or images that are intrusive and inappropriate and cause anxiety or distress. Compulsions are repetitive behaviours (such as hand washing or checking things) or mental acts (such as counting or repeating words) that occur in response to an obsession or in a ritualistic way.

Phobias: A phobia is a significant and persistent fear of objects or situations, such as flying.

Post-traumatic stress disorder: Symptoms of post-traumatic stress disorder include flashbacks, persistent frightening thoughts and memories, anger or irritability in response to a terrifying experience in which physical harm occurred or was threatened (such as rape, child abuse, or war).

SIGNS & SYMPTOMS

Signs and symptoms vary among individuals and in severity, and may include:

- Diarrhea
- Difficulty concentrating
- Edginess

- Excessive worry

- Fatigue

- Headache

- Irritability

- Muscle tension

- Racing heart, palpitations

- Restlessness

- Shortness of breath

- Sleep disturbance

Generalized anxiety disorder is diagnosed when there is excessive anxiety and worry about a number of events or activities over a period of at least six months.

RISK FACTORS

- Alcohol or drug abuse

- Diet (excessive sugar and caffeine)

- Chronic illness (diabetes, low blood sugar, depression, thyroid disorder)

- Family history of anxiety disorder

- Food allergies

- Personality disorders

- Smoking

- Stress (family, work, financial problems)

- Trauma

DOCTOR'S ORDERS

Doctors typically prescribe medications and/or psychotherapy to treat anxiety disorder. Benzodiazepines are the main class of anti-anxiety drugs and include alprazolam (Xanax), clonazepam (Rivotril), diazepam (Valium), and lorazepam (Ativan). These drugs work quickly (30–60 minutes) to ease anxiety and promote relaxation. However, they are addictive and have numerous side effects, including drowsiness, loss of coordination, dizziness, and impaired memory. Buspirone (Buspar) is a different type of anti-anxiety drug that is less addictive, but that still has side effects, including headache, nervousness, and insomnia.

Antidepressants may be used for anxiety that is associated with depression. They work by altering the activity of neurotransmitters (chemical messengers) in the brain. Examples include fluoxetine (Prozac), paroxetine (Paxil), and venlafaxine (Effexor). These drugs may take four to six weeks to work, and are not effective for everyone (some experience worsened anxiety). Other side effects include nervousness, headache, nausea, sexual dysfunction, sleep disturbance, and changes in appetite and weight.

Professional counselling can help a person develop tools and coping skills to deal with stress and anxiety. One form of therapy that is highly effective for anxiety disorder is cognitive behaviour therapy. A therapist works with you to identify distorted thoughts and beliefs that trigger anxiety and you learn to replace negative thoughts and reactions with more positive ones, so that you view and cope with life's events differently.

SHERRY'S NATURAL PRESCRIPTION

Dietary Recommendations

Eating small frequent meals will help promote good blood sugar balance. Drink lots of water and decaffeinated beverages such as herbal teas (lemon balm, passion flower, and chamomile are known for their calming properties), or vegetable juices. Green tea is also helpful, as it contains theanine, an amino acid that has a calming effect.

Foods to include:

• Complex carbohydrates (whole grains such as brown rice, wheat bran, and oats) provide serotonin, a brain chemical that induces a calm feeling.

• Whole grains and leafy green vegetables contain B-vitamins, which are essential to the nervous system and help the body with stress.

• Foods rich in magnesium (brewer's yeast, broccoli, sea vegetables, nuts, salmon, and molasses) promote calming and muscle relaxation.

Foods to avoid:

• Caffeine and alcohol can trigger and worsen anxiety. Go off caffeine slowly to avoid withdrawal symptoms, which can worsen anxiety.

• Sugary foods cause fluctuations in blood sugar, which may cause mood swings and worsen symptoms of anxiety. Cut down on candy, baked goods, condiments (ketchup, salad dressings, and peanut butter), and snack foods.

Note: Food allergies can trigger symptoms of anxiety disorder. An elimination diet can help identify food allergies. Refer to Appendix D.

Lifestyle Suggestions

• Don't dwell on the past and things you can't change. Learn to let things go.

• Look for the positive in a situation rather than focusing on the negative.

• Practise positive affirmations, messages that make you feel empowered and good about yourself. Say them to yourself and post them on your fridge or mirror as a reminder.

• When feeling anxious, calm yourself by going for a walk; closing your eyes and taking slow, deep breaths; meditating; or having a bath with mineral salts.

• Get adequate rest, which is crucial for the nervous system.

• Spend time with family and friends who are supportive. Talk about your fears and problems, as sharing your feelings can be relieving.

- Get regular exercise. Walking, cycling, yoga, tai chi, and Pilates are great ways to reduce stress and anxiety.

- Acupuncture helps promote calming and relaxation.

HOW TO REDUCE ANXIETY

Controlled breathing techniques can help ease anxiety and panic attacks. When feeling anxious, go to a quiet place where you can sit down and close your eyes. Take a slow, deep breath and hold it for four seconds, then exhale slowly for four seconds. Repeat this several times until you feel calmer and more relaxed.

Top Recommended Supplements

B-vitamins: Essential for nervous system function; a deficiency can cause depression and anxiety. Look for a product that provides 50–100 mg of the B-vitamins. Some studies have found benefits with higher doses of a vitamin B3 derivative (niacinamide). Dosage: 500 mg four times daily.

Magnesium: Promotes calming and relaxation; levels may be depleted in those with stress and anxiety. Dosage: 200 mg three times daily. It may cause loose stools, so combine with calcium. A 2:1 calcium to magnesium ratio is recommended to offset that effect.

Suntheanine: A patented extract of theanine, an amino acid present in green tea. It promotes calming and relaxation without drowsiness or addiction. Dosage: 50–200 mg daily.

Complementary Supplements

Passion flower: An herb that promotes relaxation; studies support benefits for reducing anxiety and nervousness. Dosage: 4–8 mg of dried herb daily or 5–10 mL of tincture three to four times daily.

Relora: A combination of magnolia and phellodendron that reduces stress without causing drowsiness. It is non-addictive. Dosage: 250 mg three times daily.

Valerian: An herb with relaxing and calming properties. It causes drowsiness, so it can be helpful for those with insomnia due to anxiety. Dosage: 300–500 mg of an extract an hour before bed.

FINAL THOUGHTS

1. Adopt a positive attitude and practise positive affirmations.
2. Eat a healthful diet with whole grains, vegetables, and magnesium-rich foods.
3. Get adequate rest and exercise regularly to reduce stress and anxiety and improve mood.
4. Take a supplement with B-vitamins and magnesium regularly.
5. To prevent and control anxiety attacks, try Suntheanine, passion flower, or Relora.

ARTHRITIS (RHEUMATOID)

"Arthritis" is a term used to describe conditions that cause joint inflammation. There are over 100 forms of arthritis. Rheumatoid arthritis (RA) is the second most common form of arthritis and affects about 300,000 Canadians, or one in 100.

RA is an autoimmune disease. The immune system produces antibodies that attack healthy joints, causing inflammation in the lining of the joints and pain. Chronic, uncontrolled inflammation leads to damage and destruction of the cartilage and joint tissues (bones, tendons, and ligaments) and the formation of scar tissue. Those with severe RA often suffer with deformity, reduced joint mobility, and pain that limits normal daily activities.

There are several lifestyle modifications and supplements that can help ease the pain and inflammation of RA and improve quality of life.

SIGNS & SYMPTOMS

The symptoms of RA vary from person to person, but typically affect the fingers, wrists, knees, ankles, and toes. It may start gradually or as a sudden, severe attack causing:

- Flu-like symptoms (fatigue, weakness, and loss of appetite)

- Joint pain, stiffness, and warmth

- Swollen, red joints

Some people have continuous symptoms and others go through periods of remission followed by flare-ups. Severe cases of RA can cause red skin lumps (rheumatoid nodules) on the elbows, ears, nose, knees, toes, or scalp and deformity of the joints.

RISK FACTORS

- Age: It can strike at any age; however, most people develop it between ages 25 and 50.

- Gender: Women are three times more likely than men.

- Family history: This may increase risk, but is not absolute; some people with a family history never get the disease, and others with no history will get it.

- Smoking cigarettes over a long period of time

- Environment: Infection (bacterial or viral), stress, food allergies, or toxin exposure may trigger the onset in those who are susceptible.

DOCTOR'S ORDERS

Non-steroidal anti-inflammatory drugs (NSAIDs), such as ibuprofen, naproxen, and indomethacin, are commonly prescribed to reduce pain and inflammation, yet their popularity is waning as many serious side effects have emerged. Ironically, long-term use of these drugs can worsen joint health by accelerating the breakdown of cartilage.

Corticosteroids such as prednisone are used to reduce pain and inflammation, but are not recommended for long-term use as they can cause bruising, thinning of bones, cataracts, weight gain, a round face, and diabetes.

Disease modifiers such as methotrexate, Plaquenil, and Imuran are taken to halt inflammation, slow the progression of RA, and control the immune system response. These drugs can cause serious side effects, such as nutrient deficiencies, blood disorders, and increased risk of infection.

Surgery to remove inflamed tissue and replace joints may be done for severe cases.

....

CAUTION: NSAIDs can cause serious and life-threatening side effects such as stomach ulcers and bleeding, increased gut permeability, water retention, and kidney damage. One class of these drugs (COX-2 inhibitors) has been linked to an increased risk of heart attacks. Use the lowest possible dose for short-term relief. Contact your doctor if you have stomach pain or cramping or dark stools as these are signs of stomach bleeding.

....

SHERRY'S NATURAL PRESCRIPTION

Dietary Recommendations

An elimination diet as outlined in Appendix D can help identify food allergies that could be triggering inflammation.

Foods to include:

• Cold-water fish, olive oil, flaxseed, and hemp, which are rich in essential fatty acids, can help reduce inflammation.

• Asparagus, cabbage, garlic, and onions contain sulphur, which is beneficial for the joints.

• Pineapple contains the enzyme bromelain, which can help reduce inflammation.

• Green tea: Several studies have found that the antioxidants in green tea (catechins) can reduce chronic joint inflammation and slow cartilage breakdown.

Foods to avoid:

• Nightshade vegetables (potatoes, tomatoes, peppers, eggplant) contain a substance called solanine, which can trigger pain and inflammation; preliminary studies have found benefits in avoiding these foods.

• Processed, fast, and deep-fried foods contain trans-fatty acids, which trigger inflammation.

• Red meat, milk, cheese, and deep-fried foods contain saturated fats, which trigger inflammation.

• Sugar, refined carbohydrates, alcohol, and caffeine may worsen symptoms.

Lifestyle Suggestions

• Acupuncture reduces pain and stress.

• Physical therapy, such as ultrasound and laser therapy, is beneficial for pain and inflammation.

- Exercise: Light activities that are not stressful on the joints, such as swimming, cycling, and stretching (yoga), help to improve joint mobility and overall health.

- Hot paraffin baths, therapeutic mud treatments, baths with Epsom/mineral salts, and sauna can reduce pain and inflammation.

- Apply hot or cold compresses to the affected joints. Both are helpful.

- Light massage with botanical oils (camphor, eucalyptus, pine needle or rosemary) can help reduce pain and promote relaxation.

- Assistive devices, such as canes, walkers, and joint supports, offer support and reduce joint strain.

Top Recommended Supplements

Celadrin: A patented blend of fatty acids, Celadrin reduces inflammation and pain, lubricates joints, and promotes healing. Several clinical studies have shown benefits. Celadrin is available in capsules and cream. Dosage: 1,500 mg daily; apply the cream twice daily.

Fish oil: Contains beneficial omega-3 fatty acids (EPA and DHA) which have been shown in studies to reduce the pain and inflammation associated with arthritis. These "good" fats work in part by boosting levels of prostaglandins, which are hormone-like substances that have anti-inflammatory activity. Dosage: the typical dosage is 3 to 9 grams of EPA and DHA daily, although higher amounts have been used in some studies. Look for a product that provides at least 400 mg EPA and 200 mg DHA per capsule.

Multivitamin and minerals: Studies have found certain nutrients are depleted in those with RA, including antioxidants, B-vitamins, copper, selenium, and zinc. These nutrients help reduce free radical damage and inflammation; and support cartilage, bone, and joint health. Refer to Section 2 for information on selecting a product.

Complementary Supplements

Boswellia: A tree resin used in traditional Indian medicine; some studies show that it reduces pain and inflammation, similarly to NSAIDS, but does not cause stomach irritation. Dosage: 400 mg three times daily

Bromelain: An enzyme with anti-inflammatory activity and improves joint mobility. It is well tolerated, and may thin the blood, so use cautiously along with blood-thinning medications. Dosage: 2,000–6,000 MCU daily.

Capsaicin: A hot pepper extract that reduces pain, capsaicin is available in creams; look for a product with 0.025–0.075 percent capsaicin (Zostrix or Menthacin); wash hands after application to avoid getting in the eyes.

Curcumin: A spice from the turmeric plant, curcumin is an antioxidant and has been shown in studies to have anti-inflammatory effects comparable to cortisone; no side effects. Dosage: 400 mg three times daily.

FINAL THOUGHTS

RA is a chronic condition with many underlying factors. The key is to control inflammation and pain, which will help to prevent joint damage and loss of mobility. The main points to keep in mind are:

1. Eat more fish, flaxseed, olive oil, and pineapple and drink green tea.
2. Minimize red meat, dairy, sugar, and refined/processed foods.
3. Do light exercises and stretching daily.
4. Reduce stress and pain with acupuncture, mineral baths, paraffin treatments, and massage.
5. Take a good multivitamin/mineral complex and consider Celadrin and/or fish oils.

ASTHMA

Asthma is a chronic inflammatory disease of the bronchial tubes (airways) of the lungs. Exposure to an asthmatic trigger causes the lining of the airways to become inflamed and irritated, and the cells in the lungs to produce extra mucus, narrowing the airways. The muscles that surround the bronchial walls start to twitch and tighten, further narrowing the airways and causing difficulty breathing. In some cases, breathing may be so laboured that an asthma attack becomes life-threatening. Asthma affects about three million Canadians and every year about 500 people die from asthma.

Researchers believe that asthma results from a combination of environmental and genetic factors. You are more likely to develop asthma if you have a parent with the disease and if you're sensitive to environmental allergens. Common allergens include pollen, animal dander, dust mites, smoke, and chemicals, such as dyes, perfumes, and preservatives in food. Having a respiratory infection, exercise, stress, and exposure to cold air can also trigger an attack.

Asthma is a chronic but manageable condition. While medication may be necessary, there are also lifestyle approaches and nutritional supplements that can help reduce the severity and frequency of attacks.

SIGNS & SYMPTOMS

- Disturbed sleep

- Shortness of breath and difficulty breathing

- Tightness in the chest

- Wheezing and coughing

The signs and symptoms can range from mild to severe. You may have only occasional asthma attacks that are mild and short-lived and between episodes you may feel normal and have no problems in breathing. Some people experience chronic coughing and wheezing and severe attacks.

ASTHMA AND ALLERGIES

Many people with allergies also have asthma and vice versa, but they are different conditions. An allergy is a reaction to a substance that is normally harmless, such as reacting to flower pollen or house dust. Being exposed to an allergen may cause irritation and swelling in various areas of the body, such as the nose, eyes, lungs, and skin. Allergens can make asthma symptoms worse by increasing the inflammation in the airways and making them more sensitive. The best way to find out if you are allergic to something is to be tested by an allergist.

- Exposure to occupational triggers, such as chemicals used in farming and hairdressing, and in paint, steel, plastics, and electronics manufacturing
- Exposure to second-hand smoke
- Family history
- Gastroesophageal reflux disease (GERD)
- Having a respiratory infection as a child
- Living in a large urban area (exposure to environmental pollutants)
- Low birth weight
- Obesity
- Taking antibiotics before one year of age (nearly doubles the risk of asthma by age seven)

DOCTOR'S ORDERS

The medical treatment of asthma often involves use of bronchodilators, which relax the bronchial muscles and open up the airways and anti-inflammatory drugs to reduce swelling in the airways.

Quick-acting brochodilators, also called "rescue" medications, include salbutamol (Ventolin) and ipratropium (Atrovent). These drugs can stop an asthma attack and relieve symptoms of coughing, wheezing, chest tightness, and shortness of breath. These medications should be carried with you at all times so that you have them handy when you feel an attack coming on. There are also long-acting bronchodilators, such as salmeterol (Serevent Diskus), which are used to control moderate and severe asthma and to prevent nighttime symptoms.

Anti-inflammatory medications (steroids), which help relieve the swelling of tissue, are used for those with moderate to severe asthma. They are available in tablets (prednisone) and inhalers such as fluticasone (Flovent), budesonide (Pulmicort), and beclomethasone (Beclovent). They may take a few hours or even days to work, so they are not to be used as rescue medications. Long-term use of these drugs can cause serious side effects, including cataracts, osteoporosis, muscle weakness, decreased resistance to infection, and thinning of the skin. The inhalers are safer than oral steroids, but they may still increase risk of osteoporosis when taken over the long term and can cause thrush and coughing. Using a spacer device (Aerochamber) will help improve delivery of the medication to your lungs and can reduce the risk of thrush and mouth irritation. Other drugs used to reduce inflammation include montelukast (Singulair), nedocromil (Tilade), and cromolyn (Intal).

Those with exercise-induced asthma may need only a bronchodilator when exercising. For asthma triggered by allergies, injections to desensitize you to the allergen can be given. There is also a new drug in Canada called omalizumab (Xolair), which blocks allergy-causing antibodies.

SHERRY'S NATURAL PRESCRIPTION

Dietary Recommendations

Foods to include:

• Dark green, yellow, and orange vegetables and fruits contain antioxidants (carotenoids) that help reduce inflammation and allergies. Citrus fruits and berries contain vitamin C, which also reduce inflammation.

• Eat small frequent meals to keep pressure off your diaphragm.

• Fish and flaxseed contain beneficial fatty acids that can help reduce inflammation.

• Garlic and onions have anti-inflammatory properties.

• Green tea contains antioxidants that reduce inflammation.

Foods to avoid:

• Dairy products can increase mucus formation, which can affect breathing.

• Food additives, dyes, and preservatives can trigger asthma attacks in certain people.

• Frozen drinks and extremely cold foods can cause the muscles in your airways to tighten.

• Salt has been shown to worsen asthma.

Lifestyle Suggestions

• Identify and avoid indoor and outdoor allergens and irritants. Keep your house clean and as dust-free as possible. Control pet dander by having your pets groomed regularly and vacuuming your carpets and furniture.

• Avoid second-hand smoke.

• Manage your stress as stress can trigger an attack. Try yoga, tai chi, stretching, and breathing exercises.

• Monitor your breathing using a peak flow meter and treat an attack as soon as possible to prevent it from becoming severe.

• Maintain a healthy body weight as being obese can impair lung function.

• Regular exercise can strengthen your lungs so that they don't have to work so hard. Aim for at least 30 minutes of moderate intensity activity each day. Gradually build up your intensity level. During cold months, exercise indoors or wear a face mask to warm the air you breathe. Be aware that if your asthma is not under control, exercise can trigger an attack.

• Use an air purifier with a HEPA filter to clean the air you breathe and remove allergens. Change the filters in your furnace and air conditioner regularly.

• Keep the humidity in your home and office low as high humidity can increase the growth of moulds.

Top Recommended Supplements

The supplements listed here can be helpful for managing mild to moderate cases of asthma. However, you should never stop taking your asthma medications unless advised to do so by your doctor.

Magnesium: Helps relax the bronchial tubes and improve lung function. Studies have found that asthmatics have low levels of this mineral. Supplements may help to prevent asthma attacks by reducing bronchial spasms. Dosage: 300–400 mg daily with meals. Doctors also give magnesium by injection to halt an acute attack.

Pycnogenol: An extract from pine bark that has potent antioxidant and anti-inflammatory properties. Some research has shown that it can significantly improve lung function and asthma symptoms. One of these studies involved children and found that it reduced the need for rescue medication. Dosage: Adults should take 100 mg daily; children should take 1 mg per pound of body weight per day.

Vitamin C: Reduces bronchial inflammation, spasms, and the response to allergies. Several studies have shown benefits for reducing the severity and frequency of asthma attacks. Dosage: 1,000 mg daily. To avoid upset stomach, choose a buffered vitamin C such as calcium ascorbate.

Complementary Supplements

Boswellia: An herb that reduces inflammation. Some research has shown that it can reduce the frequency of asthma attacks and measurements of breathing capacity. Dosage: 300 mg three times daily.

Ephedra (Ephedra sinica): Ephedra contains alkaloids, ephedrine, and pseudoephedrine, which are used in decongestants. Dosage: No more than 8 mg per dose or 24 mg in 24 hours should be used. Ephedra can raise blood pressure and heart rate, and may cause insomnia, irritability, and anxiety. Take only under the advice of your health care provider.

Vitamin B6: Deficiency is common in asthmatics. Some research has found that supplements can decrease the frequency and severity of asthma attacks. Dosage: 50 mg twice daily as part of a B-complex or multivitamin.

FINAL THOUGHTS

To improve the management of asthma, consider the following:

1. Eat more fruits, vegetables, garlic, onions, and fish, and drink plenty of water to stay hydrated.
2. Get regular exercise and manage your stress.
3. Monitor your breathing with a peak flow meter and see your doctor regularly for checkups.
4. Use an air purifier and keep your home as clean as possible. Avoid second-hand smoke and other known irritants.
5. Consider supplements of magnesium, pycnogenol, and vitamin C.

ATHLETE'S FOOT

Athlete's foot (*Tinea pedis*) is a common fungal infection that affects 20 percent of the population at any given time. These fungi, called dermatophytes, infect the skin of the foot, which may result in an intensely itchy, red, scaly rash on the soles of the feet and between the toes. The fungi that cause athlete's foot grow in warm, moist environments, so it may be picked up easily by walking barefoot in public areas such as bathrooms, swimming pools, saunas, showers, and locker rooms. Athlete's foot is difficult to get rid of because in socks and shoes, feet provide the same ideal environment for the fungi to thrive. If you are exposed to the fungi that cause athlete's foot, you may be contagious, even if you don't develop athlete's foot. Once you have had athlete's foot, you are more susceptible to reinfection.

RINGWORM NOT A WORM

Contrary to its name, ringworm is not a worm. It is a fungal infection, the same type of fungal infection that causes athlete's foot. Ringworm may be found on any part of the body, and is more common among children and teens. It can be spread through person-to-person contact or by sharing personal items such as clothes and towels. Ringworm earned its name because it causes a distinctive circular patch of itchy, red, raised, or bumpy skin.

SIGNS & SYMPTOMS

- Degree of discomfort can range from mild to severe
- Heels that crack, scale, or peel
- Infected toenails that may thicken, yellow, flake, or crumble
- Intense itching, inflammation, or stinging on the soles of the feet or between the toes (usually the third, fourth, and fifth toes)
- Painful sensations when rubbed or scratched
- Sores or blisters
- Thick, dry skin on the feet

RISK FACTORS

- Affects adults and children, and men more often than women
- Direct contact with fungi in public area
- Person-to-person contact with affected skin
- Warm, moist environments such as wet socks, tight shoes, and sweaty feet will encourage growth
- Weakened immunity such as diabetes or HIV/AIDS

ATHLETE'S UNDERARM?

Because the fungi that cause athlete's foot can grow on human skin, this type of fungal infection may spread to other parts of the body such as the groin (known as jock itch), scalp, and underarm. This is most likely to happen when people touch or scratch the infected area and then touch another part of their body without washing their hands. Be sure to wash your hands regularly while treating an athlete's foot infection. Also, after a bath or shower, use a different towel to dry an infected area than for the remainder of your body. Hot-water wash and dry towels immediately after each use.

DOCTOR'S ORDERS

Although athlete's foot has obvious signs and symptoms, consult with your doctor for a proper diagnosis because symptoms may be masking another condition.

Most cases of athlete's foot may be treated with a prescription or over-the-counter antifungal medication in the form of an ointment, lotion, powder, or spray. For mild conditions, a cream such as terbinafine (Lamisil), clotrimazole (Lotrimin), or miconazole (Micatin) may be used. Even in mild cases, athlete's foot can be difficult to kill. Most antifungal medicines only limit the growth of the fungal infection, which then allows the fungus to gradually die out as the body sheds infected skin. Follow the medication's instructions precisely for optimum effect.

For severe cases, such as when the fungal infection spreads below the surface of the body, a doctor may prescribe an oral medication such as itraconazole (Sporanox), fluconazole (Diflucan), or terbinafine (Lamisil).

SHERRY'S NATURAL PRESCRIPTION

Some people seem to be naturally resilient to athlete's foot while others find it to be a persistent problem. A diet that promotes immune system health and proper hygiene will go a long way toward prevention.

Dietary Recommendations

The body's ability to ward off infections depends on the health of the immune system. While there are no foods that directly treat athlete's foot, eating a healthy diet that supports the immune system and detoxification is crucial to prevention and effective treatment.

Foods to include:

- Fibre-rich foods such as whole grains and ground flaxseed support detoxification.

- Filtered water, green tea, and green drinks support detoxification.

- Garlic helps fight fungal infections.

- Yogurt with active cultures provides beneficial bacteria that help prevent overgrowth of fungus.

Foods to avoid:

- Alcohol weakens the immune system.

- Sugar hampers immune function, so limit candy, sweets, and soft drinks as well as refined starches.

Lifestyle Recommendations

• Wear waterproof shoes or sandals in all public places such as swimming pools and showers.

• Dry your feet and toes thoroughly.

• Wear cotton socks and change socks frequently. Sprinkle baby powder or cornstarch between toes to prevent moisture.

• Wear comfortable, well-ventilated shoes or sandals.

• Avoid socks and shoes made of synthetic materials, which promote sweaty feet.

• Don't wear someone else's shoes.

• Wash all clothes, towels, and bed linens in hot, soapy water.

• For sweaty feet, soak daily for 30 minutes in a footbath with baking soda or salt.

Top Recommended Supplements

Tea tree oil: Has a long history of use for treating skin infections. It contains compounds that have disinfectant, antibacterial, and antifungal properties. It is used topically as a solution or in a cream. Three studies have shown that it is effective for treating athlete's foot. Dosage: Apply a topical solution that contains 25–50 percent tea tree standardized to contain 10 percent cineole and at least 30 percent terpinen-4-ol. Use twice daily for four weeks. Creams containing tea tree can also be used at a 10–50 percent concentration. Do not take tea tree orally. Discontinue use if skin becomes irritated.

· ·

TEA TREE RESEARCH HIGHLIGHT

In a double-blind study, 158 people with athlete's foot were treated with placebo, 25 percent tea tree oil solution, or 50 percent tea tree oil solution, applied twice daily for four weeks. Both tea tree oil solutions were more effective than placebo at eradicating infection. In the 50 percent tea tree oil group, 64 percent were cured; in the 25 percent tea tree oil group, 55 percent were cured; in the placebo group, 31 percent were cured. Most people did not experience any significant side effects. (*Australasian Journal of Dermatology*, 2002; 43: 175–178).

· ·

Complementary Supplements

Garlic: Has antifungal properties. Dosage: 600 mg of aged garlic extract daily.

Vitamin C: Supports proper immune function. Dosage: 500 mg twice daily.

FINAL THOUGHTS

To prevent and manage athlete's foot, consider the following:

1. Eat a healthful diet, including whole grains, yogurt, and garlic.
2. Wear waterproof shoes in public areas and don't share shoes or socks.
3. After bathing, dry your feet thoroughly and apply powder.
4. Wear cotton socks and properly fitted shoes that don't promote sweaty feet.
5. Consider tea tree oil solution for the treatment of athlete's foot.

ATTENTION-DEFICIT/HYPERACTIVITY DISORDER (ADHD)

Attention-deficit/hyperactivity disorder (ADHD) is a chronic neurobehavioural disorder that arises in childhood and may continue into the teen years and adulthood. Children and adults with ADHD may appear inattentive or distracted, hyperactive, and/or impulsive (act without thinking). These symptoms affect the way they interact with the world, negatively impacting their ability to function, concentrate, and excel in school or at work, and affect their efforts to form strong personal relationships. Because the symptoms of ADHD are disruptive and difficult to deal with for other people, children and adults with ADHD are often unfairly judged and suffer from low-self-esteem as a result. Children with ADHD are more likely to have a learning disorder and develop a behavioural disorder. Teens and adults with ADHD are at greater risk for self-destructive behaviours.

ADHD is the most commonly diagnosed mental health problem among children. It is estimated that up to 6 percent of Canadian children show symptoms of ADHD, with males outnumbering females three to one. (Boys tend to be more hyperactive while girls tend to be more inattentive.) Children with ADHD begin to show signs of their condition before the age of four, but it is often not diagnosed until the school years when their inability to conform to school expectations and achieve academic standards becomes apparent.

There has been a great deal of research on ADHD, but the actual cause is not known. There are many misconceptions about the disorder. It does not result from poor parenting skills or low income status. It is thought that ADHD may result from structural changes in the brain, alterations in neurotransmitter levels, and environmental and dietary factors.

Brain scans of some people with ADHD have shown smaller basal ganglia and reduced frontal lobe activity. Basal ganglia, or nerve clusters, are involved in routine behaviours, and the frontal lobes are involved in planning and organizing, attention, impulse control, and inhibition of responses to sensory stimulation.

It is thought that those with ADHD may have low levels of neurotransmitters (chemical messengers) such as dopamine and norepinephrine. Dopamine is involved in controlling emotions and reactions, concentrating, reasoning, and coordinating movement. An abnormally low level of dopamine can cause the three primary symptoms of ADHD: inattention, impulsiveness, and hyperactivity.

· ·

"Learning disabilities are the only major disability area where the existence of the condition is treated with skepticism and where the person who has the condition is blamed for his or her situation."

—ADHD Foundation of Canada Web site

· ·

SIGNS & SYMPTOMS

The hallmark symptoms of ADHD, whether in children or adults, are hyperactivity, impulsiveness, and inattention. Children may be diagnosed with ADHD if they exhibit significant and disabling symptoms at home and at school for at least six months. Not all children with ADHD are hyperactive or impulsive but may have disabling inattentiveness or easy distractibility. Girls are more likely to suffer from the primarily inattentive form of the disorder (often referred to as ADD) and are often never diagnosed. Many adults with ADHD were never properly diagnosed as children and they often suffer serious problems in their life if they don't obtain proper treatment.

Signs of hyperactivity:

- Cannot play independently or quietly
- Cannot sit still or fidgets when sitting
- Restless, jittery, and always moving
- Talks excessively in a loud voice

Signs of impulsiveness:

- Frequently interrupts and blurts out responses
- Impatient, cannot tolerate waiting or line-ups, becomes agitated
- Unable to control impulses, and acts before thinking (such as crossing the street without looking, making rude comments, or exhibiting dangerous or inappropriate behaviour)
- May not be able to control frustration and anger

Signs of inattentiveness:

- Cannot focus or concentrate; easily distracted
- Does not pay attention to what he or she has been told
- Has a hard time finishing large or involved tasks without frequent reminders to stay on task
- Is not well organized; may appear forgetful or careless
- May appear to daydream and not listen

The above symptoms mean a child with ADHD may have difficulty developing healthy social skills and friendships. Other symptoms may include mild to severe sleeping and eating problems.

LOOKING FOR ADHD IN ADULTS

The symptoms of hyperactivity, impulsiveness, and inattentiveness are present in adults, but may be more difficult to identify. Here are some of the criteria that doctors use when diagnosing ADHD in adults:

- A childhood history of ADHD
- Anger and stress management issues

- Difficulty having strong personal relationships, or frequently has negative interactions with people and co-workers

- Difficulty in controlling impulsive behaviour (reckless driving, drug and alcohol abuse, other addictions, frequent job changes, financial problems)

- Difficulty in relaxing; is restless

- Inability to focus on tasks, and cannot make deadlines or complete assigned work

- Forgetful about daily activities (failure to make appointments and commitments)

RISK FACTORS

- Heredity: There are known genes associated with ADHD; having a parent with ADHD triples your risk of developing the disorder; identical twins are both likely to be affected.

- History of antibiotic use

- Illness or infection (Strep, ear infections)

- Imbalance of neurotransmitters

- Infant or childhood exposure to environmental toxins: preservatives, food additives, heavy metals (lead and mercury)

- Infants who experience brain trauma during pregnancy, delivery, or after birth are at greater risk of ADHD.

- Maternal smoking, drug or alcohol use, or exposure to toxins

- Poor nutrition during childhood

- Poor nutrition of mother during pregnancy

ENVIRONMENTAL TOXINS AND ADHD

Preschool children exposed to certain environmental toxins, particularly lead and PCBs, are at increased risk of developmental and behavioural problems, many of which are similar to those found in children diagnosed with ADHD. Exposure to lead, which is found mainly in paint and pipes in older buildings, has been linked to disruptive and even violent behaviour and to a short attention span. Exposure to PCBs in infancy may also increase a child's risk of developing ADHD.

DOCTOR'S ORDERS

There is no definitive way to diagnose ADHD. If a child exhibits symptoms of ADHD, the parents, caregivers, and teachers involved with the child will be asked to fill out a variety of questionnaires regarding the child's behaviour. A complete physical examination is also done to rule out other conditions. In some cases, a psychological assessment is done.

The typical medical approach to the management of ADHD is the use of psycho-stimulant drugs, which boost levels of neurotransmitters (dopamine) in the brain. Although these drugs help relieve symptoms in some children, they don't cure ADHD and they can cause troubling side effects, such as difficulty falling or staying asleep, loss of appetite and weight, and upset stomach. Some children develop jerky muscle movements, such as grimaces or twitches (tics). These drugs may also cause reduced growth rate in children and may negatively impact brain development.

The most commonly prescribed medications for treating ADHD include:

- Dextroamphetamine/amphetamine (Adderall)
- Dextroamphetamine (Dexedrine)
- Methylphenidate (Ritalin or Concerta)

Atomoxetine (Strattera) is a non-stimulant medication for ADHD that is believed to provide the brain with a steady supply of norepinephrine.

Sometimes children with ADHD are prescribed antidepressants if they do not respond to stimulants. These drugs also cause a variety of unpleasant side effects such as sleeping problems, dry mouth, irregular heartbeat, and changes in appetite. The younger the child, the more susceptible he or she is to the side effects.

Counselling and family and school support are other key parts of treatment. It can be demanding and frustrating for parents dealing with a child with ADHD and equally difficult for the child. A holistic strategy that incorporates counselling along with nutritional and lifestyle strategies, patience, and perseverance are essential. Drug therapy should be considered only as a last resort.

SHERRY'S NATURAL PRESCRIPTION

Dietary Recommendations

A nutritious, whole foods diet is essential for the management of ADHD. Some individuals with ADHD have food allergies or sensitivities that can cause inflammation in the gut and worsening of ADHD symptoms. The most common allergens are wheat, yeast, dairy, corn, soy, and food additives (preservatives, dyes and chemicals). To determine potential food allergies, consider an Elimination Diet as outlined in Appendix D.

Foods to include:

- Cultured dairy, such as yogurt and kefir, contains beneficial bacteria that support intestinal health, immune function, and aid in the elimination of toxins.

- Eat fresh organic fruits and vegetables as tolerated, and whole grains (brown rice, whole oats, millet, amaranth, and quinoa).

- Ensure adequate protein intake. Choose free-range poultry, wild fish, beans, and legumes.

- Include healthy fats such as extra-virgin olive oil, hemp oil, or flaxseed oil. Coconut oil is suitable for cooking. Use ghee (clarified butter) instead of regular butter or margarine.

- Medicinal food blends, such as Learning Factors (by Natural Factors), contain a blend of essential nutrients and protein to help support proper brain function and overall health.

Foods to avoid:

- Fast foods, processed foods, and junk foods, such as hot dogs, burgers, french fries, snack cakes, cookies, sugary breakfast cereals, which are high in sugar, refined starch, saturated and trans fats, and preservatives and are also low in nutritional value.

- Read labels and avoid foods that contain ingredients such as additives, flavour enhancers (MSG), artificial sweeteners (aspartame, saccharin), colourings, dyes, and preservatives such as nitrates, sodium benzoate, sulfites, BHA, and BHT. If you have trouble reading or pronouncing an ingredient, chances are you should avoid that food.

Lifestyle Suggestions

Here are some suggestions for helping children with ADHD both at home and at school:

At home:

- Provide support, patience, and love. Children with ADHD exhibit behaviour that can be trying. Despite this, they need as much positive feedback as possible as they work toward correcting these problems.

- Provide structure and realistic expectations. Children with ADHD need to know what's expected of them and they need these expectations to be enforced. Be consistent.

- As your child develops better coping mechanisms and social skills, he or she will be better able to cope with demanding situations. Until then, avoid triggers for bad behaviour such as line-ups, restaurants, etc.

- Avoid overstimulation or keep stimulating activities to under two hours.

- Provide support at home for organizing personal belongings. Keep bins clearly labelled, and a white board with the weekly agenda in plain sight.

- Make physical activity a priority and limit their TV, video game, and computer times to less than two hours per day.

- Keep any discussions clear and brief.

At school:

- Discuss your child's ADHD with school administration and all teachers or aides who interact with your child. If the school or teacher is unresponsive, do not give up.

- Be assertive. You are your child's best advocate. Don't be shy to ask the school for what your child needs such as reading or writing aids or occupational therapy.

- Create a personal learning program suited to your child. School boards call these programs by different names, but they describe what accommodations your child warrants in the classroom, and also typically function to enable the school to apply for financial support for resources and teaching aids.

- Have your child sit close to the front of the class or teacher's desk, beside model students and away from distractions.

- Have the teacher give your child responsibilities in the classroom, which allow him or her to move around with purpose.

- Break large tasks down into manageable assignments. Have a daily agenda and create clear expectations and consequences for classroom behaviour.

Top Recommended Supplements

There are many supplements that can provide nutritional support to children with ADHD. These supplements may be taken in conjunction with prescription medications, but always discuss any supplements with your doctor or pharmacist before giving to a child on medication.

Essential fatty acids: Essential for proper brain development and function; deficiency is common in children with ADHD. The omega-3 fatty acids EPA and DHA (from fish oil) are particularly important for brain function and the proper release of dopamine. Some studies have also shown benefits with evening primrose or borage oil supplements, which provide GLA (an omega-6 fatty acid). Typical dosage: 600 mg EPA and 175 mg DHA. If borage or evening primrose oil is added the typical daily dosage is enough to supply 60 mg GLA.

Multivitamin and mineral formula: Children with ADHD may be deficient in certain nutrients, which can hamper proper brain function and affect behaviour. In particular, the B-vitamins, vitamin C, magnesium, selenium, iron, and zinc are necessary for the brain and nervous system and production of neurotransmitters. Choose a product that is free of chemical additives and dyes.

Probiotics: Beneficial bacteria that support intestinal health, aid digestion of nutrients and elimination of toxins, and support immune function. Children with ADHD may be depleted in beneficial bacteria and have overgrowth of the fungus *Candida albicans*, which can affect behaviour and cognitive function. Dosage: For children over four, give a product that provides at least 10-20 billion live cells daily. Use half that amount for those under age four. Probiotic supplements are available in capsules, chewable tablets, and powders. Many require refrigeration, except Kyo-Dophilus.

Complementary Supplements

American ginseng: Has antioxidant properties, supports immune function, improves resistance to stress, and supports cognitive function (learning, attention, and memory). One study looked at the effects of a product called AD-fX that contains American ginseng extract (HT-1001) providing no less than 15 percent ginsenosides along with an extract of Ginkgo biloba containing 24 percent flavone glycosides and 4 percent total terpenelactones in a group of 36 children with ADHD. This formulation was found to improve behaviour in at least three parameters of ADHD symptoms in 85 percent of human subjects tested (*Journal of Psychiatry & Neuroscience,* 2001: 26(3); 221–228). Dosage (AD-fX): For adults and children seven years and older, one to two capsules twice daily for two months, then one capsule twice daily thereafter.

L-theanine: An amino acid present in green tea that can reduce anxiety, improve concentration and sleep quality and stabilize mood. It is widely used in Japan and Europe for the treatment of ADHD and gaining popularity in North America. Typical dosage: 200 mg two to three times daily for children eight years, and half this dosage for children as young as four years.

RESEARCH HIGHLIGHT

In association with the University of British Columbia, Dr. Michael R. Lyon, MD, author of *Is Your Child's Brain Starving?*, recently completed a double-blind, randomized study on the use of L-theanine (branded ingredient Suntheanine) for 100 boys with ADHD ages eight to 12. The objective of this study was to measure the potential benefits of L-theanine on behaviour, cognitive performance, and sleep quality. This study found that 200 mg of L-theanine chewable tablets twice daily improved sleep quality, reduced hyperactive behaviours and improved short-term memory function.

FINAL THOUGHTS

To improve the management of ADHD, consider the following:

1. Encourage a healthful diet of organic vegetables and whole grains, free-range poultry, wild fish, beans, healthy oils, and cultured dairy.
2. Avoid or minimize fast foods, processed foods, junk foods, preservatives, and other chemicals.
3. Counselling and school support can help both the family and child.
4. Consider supplements of essential fatty acids, multivitamin/minerals, and probiotics.
5. Give a child with ADHD patience, support, and love.

AUTISM (AUTISM SPECTRUM DISORDERS)

Autism is a neurodevelopmental disorder marked by mild to severe delays in communication and social skills. There is a broad range of symptoms and degree of severity with autism, hence the medical name autism spectrum disorders (ASDs). Signs and symptoms usually appear before age three and continue throughout life. Some children learn to cope with their unique needs while others need a lifetime of support.

In addition to problems with communication and general social interactions, children with autism are often disengaged from the world around them and may develop unusually focused interests. Intelligence also greatly varies with children with autism, from below average to genius.

Autism is the most common neurological disorder affecting children and one of the most common developmental disabilities affecting Canadians. Statistics suggest that autism strikes one in every 150 children, and occurs three to four times more often in boys than in girls.

The actual cause of autism is not known, but there appear to be abnormalities in several regions of the brain that affect behaviour and communication. This may result from a combination of genetics and environmental factors, such as toxins and heavy metals, which cause inflammation and oxidative stress in the brain.

Researchers are also looking into the gut-brain link. Many children with autism have digestive problems (diarrhea and constipation) and there are reports showing that symptoms of autism are worsened by certain dietary factors, particularly milk or wheat products. It is thought that food sensitivities may cause alterations in the normal gut flora (bacteria), which impair the absorption of essential nutrients, thus affecting normal development.

Another possible factor involved in ASD is the use of vaccines, particularly those containing thimerosal, a preservative that contains mercury. The measles-mumps-rubella (MMR) vaccine has been implicated in many cases. Overall, the issue of vaccination has been a subject of great debate, with studies both supporting and denying the connection.

There is no cure for autism, but early diagnosis and treatment can help improve quality of life for children with an ASD. There are a variety of specialists that can help children with learning and communication disabilities. Proper nutritional support is essential, and supplements can also be helpful.

SIGNS & SYMPTOMS

The signs and symptoms of autism vary widely and are grouped into three different areas: behaviour, language, and social skills.

Behaviour

- Inability to cope with changes in routines or unexpected situations

- May fidget or exhibit repetitive movements, such as head banging or rocking

- May become inconsolable or explosive

- May develop strict patterns of behaviour and become upset if they can't be followed precisely

- May develop narrow interests that exclude them from others
- May be unusually fixated on or highly sensitive to noise, light, movement, sound, touch, and textures
- May use toys, books, and games in unusual ways
- May have picky eating habits
- May suffer from digestive problems such as upset stomach and diarrhea

Language
- Abnormal tone or rhythm (may speak in a robotic way)
- Cannot participate in a conversations; most expression is one-way
- Delayed or non-existent use of language
- Inappropriate language and expressions; makes odd noises
- Loss of previously acquired words
- Unusual speech patterns, repeated words or phrases

Social Skills
- Cannot maintain eye contact
- Difficulty making and keeping friends
- May be inattentive or appear to not be listening
- May prefer to be alone, engaged in solo play longer than is age appropriate
- May react negatively to being in large group settings, or being touched or bumped
- May not understand or be able to correctly interpret non-verbal communications such as facial expressions
- May blurt out inappropriate comments; appears thoughtless, insensitive
- Rigid; may have strict rules of conduct and react negatively when parents, siblings, or others "break the rules"

SIGNS OF AUTISM IN INFANTS AND TODDLERS

Be on the lookout for the following signs. If your infant or toddler does the following, see your doctor:

- Does not make eye contact and/or interact as expected with parents, family, pets, or surroundings
- Does not make baby noises by the first year
- Does not make hand gestures, point, or wave by the first year
- Does not say single words by 16 months
- Does not make two-word phrases by two years of age

- If your child experiences loss of language or social skills at any time

- If your child reacts in an unusual way or negatively to touch, sounds, movement, or light

RISK FACTORS

- Difficulty or trauma during pregnancy or childbirth (breech position); premature birth

- Digestive system problems

- Environmental exposure: Heavy metals such as lead and other toxins

- Heredity: Those who have a child with ASD have a one in 20 chance of having a second child with the disorder

- Low Apgar score after birth (a test done right after birth that measures a baby's heart rate, breathing, activity and muscle tone, grimace response, and appearance)

- Parental history of schizophrenia, depression, or bipolar disorder

- Vaccination (not a proven risk factor, but several reports have linked the measles-mumps-rubella vaccine to autism)

DOCTOR'S ORDERS

Currently, there is no definitive way to diagnose autism. If signs and symptoms exist, a doctor will do a complete examination and medical history of the child and family. If no other condition is found, the child is usually sent to a developmental specialist or team of specialists that include doctors, psychologists, physiotherapists, speech and language therapists, and occupational therapists. Usually the child is screened over the series of appointments, and parents, caregivers, and teachers are asked to fill out a variety of questionnaires regarding language and social interactions.

Treatments for autism may include special schools or programs tailored for children with autism; behavioural therapy and social skills training; speech, occupational, and physical therapy; and prescription medications that address symptoms such as anxiety, anger management, and repetitive movements.

SHERRY'S NATURAL PRESCRIPTION

Intervention at a young age can help a child with autism to break out of his or her inner world and participate in social interactions. Nutrition and supplements can also offer support.

Dietary Recommendations

Children with autism vary so greatly that broad dietary recommendations are not possible. However, it is critical to try to get these children to eat a healthy diet with as much nutrition and variety as possible. This is easier said than done because they can be highly sensitive to taste and texture and eat only a handful of foods. Be patient and prepared for a lot of experimenting. Exposing children to different foods and encouraging trying new foods is an important social skill for them to learn.

Foods to include:

- Cultured dairy, such as yogurt and kefir, contains beneficial bacteria that support intestinal health, immune function, and aid in the elimination of toxins.

- Ensure adequate protein intake. Choose free-range poultry, wild fish, beans, and legumes.

- Include fresh organic fruits and vegetables as tolerated, and whole grains (brown rice, whole oats, millet, amaranth, and quinoa).

- Include healthy fats such as extra-virgin olive oil, hemp oil, or flaxseed oil. Coconut oil is suitable for cooking. Use ghee (clarified butter) instead of regular butter or margarine.

- Medicinal food blends, such as Learning Factors (by Natural Factors), contain a blend of essential nutrients, protein, and neutraceuticals to help support proper brain function and overall health.

Foods to avoid:

- Processed, refined, and fast foods contain lots of sugar, starch, saturated and trans fats, and are low in nutritional value.

- Read labels and avoid foods that contain ingredients such as additives, flavour enhancers (MSG), artificial sweeteners (aspartame, saccharin), colourings, dyes, and preservatives such as nitrates, sodium benzoate, sulphites, BHA, and BHT. These chemicals can be a problem for those with autism. If you have trouble reading or pronouncing an ingredient, chances are you should avoid that food.

- Food allergies may contribute to symptoms of autism. Common allergens include: gluten (a protein found in wheat, rye and barley) and casein (found in dairy). Many children with autism improve significantly on a strict gluten and casein free diet. To rule out potential sensitivities, try an elimination diet as outlined in Appendix D.

Lifestyle Suggestions

- Social skills training is imperative; visit your local Learning Disability Association for guidance.

- Social skills opportunities; find daycares, schools, camps, and clubs for children with autism spectrum disorders.

- Massage and acupuncture may be helpful.

- Regular exercise is important to developing gross and fine motor skills (though autistic children may not cope well in a typical sports team, so look for individual sports such as martial arts and swimming).

- Water therapy and the use of animals, under supervision, to draw out children are encouraged.

- Music and art may be helpful.

- Exposure to new activities in safe settings (always prepare your child for a new activity and advise the teacher or coach of your child's needs).

- Family support—this cannot be overemphasized; families of children with autism need a huge amount of emotional support.

- Seek out as many government support programs as your province has available.

Top Recommended Supplements

Essential fatty acids: Essential for proper brain development and function; deficiency is common in children with autistic spectrum disorders. The omega-3 fatty acids EPA and DHA (from fish oil) are particularly important for brain development and function. Some studies have also shown benefits with evening primrose or borage oil supplements, which provide GLA (an omega-6 fatty acid). Typical dosages: 600 mg EPA and 175 mg DHA. If borage or evening primrose oil are added, the daily dosage is enough to supply 60 mg of GLA.

Multivitamin and mineral formula: Children with autism may be deficient in certain nutrients, which can hamper proper brain and nervous system function. In particular, the B-vitamins (especially B6), vitamin C, magnesium, selenium, and zinc are necessary for the brain and nervous system and production of neurotransmitters. Choose a product that is free of chemical additives and dyes.

Probiotics: Beneficial bacteria that support intestinal health, aid digestion of nutrients and elimination of toxins, and support immune function. Children with autism may be depleted in beneficial bacteria and have overgrowth of the fungus *Candida albicans*, which can affect behaviour and cognitive function. Dosage: For children over four, give a product that provides at least one billion live cells daily. Use half that amount for those under age four. Probiotic supplements are available in capsules, chewable tablets, and powders. Many require refrigeration.

Complementary Supplements

Carnosine: A substance manufactured in the human body, it is composed of the amino acids alanine and histidine. Carnosine is highly concentrated in the brain, nervous system, eyes, and muscle tissue. On preliminary study found that supplements of 400 mg twice daily significantly improved symptoms of ASD.

Phosphatidylserine: An essential component of all cell membranes that is highly concentrated in the brain and supports proper function of the brain and nervous system. Dosage: 300–500 mg daily.

FINAL THOUGHTS

To improve the management of ASDs, consider the following:

1. Encourage a healthful diet of organic vegetables and whole grains, free-range poultry, wild fish, beans, healthy oils, and cultured dairy.
2. Avoid or minimize fast foods, processed foods, junk foods, preservatives, and other chemicals.
3. Encourage regular exercise and try massage and acupuncture.
4. Counselling, social skills programs, and school support can be very helpful.
5. Consider supplements of essential fatty acids, multivitamin/minerals, and probiotics.

BACK PAIN

Back pain is one of the leading reasons for doctor's visits and missed workdays. Over 80 percent of adults experience low back pain sometime during their life and it can range from mildly uncomfortable to completely debilitating.

We rely on our back for almost every move we make. It takes a great deal of stress and is particularly vulnerable to injury. The area most at risk of injury is the lower back, or lumbar region, because it has the greatest curve and supports most of the body's weight. Because the back is a complex network of bones, joints, muscles, ligaments, disks, and nerves, inflammation or injury to any of these parts can cause acute or chronic pain. The most common cause of back pain is improper or heavy lifting or a sudden awkward movement.

Often back pain will resolve within a few weeks, with or without medical attention. There are numerous drugs that are used to reduce pain and inflammation, but they can cause a range of unpleasant side effects. There are also many natural treatments, including supplements, acupuncture, and chiropractic, that can offer significant benefits for reducing pain and improving healing.

SIGNS & SYMPTOMS

- Pain, aching in the lower or middle back
- Radiating pain to the hips or neck

RISK FACTORS

- Arthritis: Spondylosis is a type of arthritis affecting the spine as a result of the degenerative changes in the spine that often come with aging
- Constipation
- Heavy or improper lifting
- Herniated disc occurs when a disc in the spinal column bulges out and presses on a nerve; if the disc impinges the sciatic nerve, the condition is called sciatica, which causes sharp, shooting pain through the buttocks and back of the leg
- Inactivity (poor muscle strength and flexibility)
- Injury (car accident or a fall)
- Obesity and pregnancy
- Osteoporosis
- Tumour or infection of the spine

DOCTOR'S ORDERS

The treatment of back pain depends on the underlying cause. If it is acute pain due to strain or lifting, a short period of rest may help. However, being inactive for longer than that can do more harm than good. Light activity, such as walking and stretching, can actually speed healing and recovery.

Depending on the cause and severity of your pain, your doctor may recommend physiotherapy. Physiotherapists offer a range of treatments, such as heat, ice, ultrasound, electrical stimulation, and muscle-release techniques, to reduce pain. They also advise on specific exercises to increase your flexibility, strengthen your back and abdominal muscles, and improve your posture. Exercise can help pain from recurring.

Medications, such as pain relievers, anti-inflammatories, and muscle relaxants, may be recommended. Always use the lowest possible dose to minimize side effects and don't rely on medications over the long term unless you have a chronic problem and are under close medical supervision.

Surgery is always considered a last resort for dealing with severe back pain caused by a herniated disk.

SHERRY'S NATURAL PRESCRIPTION

Dietary Recommendations

Foods to include:

• Eat a high-fibre diet, as constipation can worsen back pain.

• Fish and flaxseed contain essential fatty acids, which can help reduce pain and inflammation.

• Fruits and vegetables contain essential vitamins and minerals that help your body cope with stress (back pain).

• Herbal teas with ginger or green tea provide antioxidants that help reduce inflammation.

Foods to avoid:

• Fast foods and processed foods are typically high in saturated fats, sugar, and calories, which can affect your ability to manage your weight.

• While alcohol may temporarily make you feel better, it can worsen inflammation and lead to nutrient deficiencies that can negatively affect nerve, muscles, and bones.

SMOKING AND BACK PAIN

While many smokers feel that smoking lessens pain, it actually has the opposite effect. Studies have found that smoking can actually contribute to back pain and worsen the likelihood of developing a herniated disc. It is thought that smoking causes malnutrition of spinal discs, which in turn makes them more vulnerable to mechanical stress. Smokers also have diminished oxygen levels in their spinal tissues, which can hinder the healing process.

Lifestyle Suggestions

• Exercise regularly to strengthen your muscles and improve flexibility. Having strong abdominal and back muscles helps to reduce the risk of injuries and having good flexibility in your hips and legs will take the strain off your back. Walking, swimming, Pilates, yoga, and stretching are good choices.

• Don't smoke, as this can worsen pain and prevent healing.

• Wear a back support or brace if you are doing heavy lifting.

• Maintain a healthy body weight to reduce strain in your back muscles.

• Studies have shown that acupuncture, chiropractic, and massage are effective therapies for easing back pain.

• Apply cold and then heat to your back to soothe sore and inflamed muscles. If you have just strained your back, apply ice (wrapped in a towel) for 10–20 minutes several times a day. Use ice as long as spasms persist. Then you can apply heat using a heating pad or hot water bottle for 20 minutes.

• Use a topical cream that contains capsaicin, a hot pepper extract that reduces pain at the nerves. Four studies have found significant benefits for reducing lower-back pain. Look for a product that contains 0.025–0.075 percent capsaicin and apply three times daily. Do not apply to broken skin. Wash your hands after applying this cream as it can cause burning.

• When standing for long periods of time, alternate placing your feet on a low foot stool to take some pressure off your lower back.

• If your job involves sitting, use a chair with good lower back support and arm rests. Keep your knees and hips level and use a foot rest.

• Medium-firm mattresses are best for those with back pain. To recover from a backache, put a pillow under your knees when lying on your back or between your knees when on your side to ease the pressure on your back.

• Use proper form when lifting (see below).

•••

PROPER LIFTING TECHNIQUE

When lifting objects, keep your back straight, bend only at the knees, and let your legs do the work. Hold the object close to your body and avoid lifting and twisting at the same time. Have a partner help you when lifting heavy objects.

•••

Top Recommended Supplements

Devil's claw: Reduces inflammation and back pain, particularly due to osteoarthritis. Several studies have found benefits. Dosage: Look for a product that provides 60 mg of harpagoside (active constituent) and take twice daily. Avoid using if you have heartburn, ulcers, or gallstones.

Fish oil: Reduces pain and inflammation. Studies have found it helpful for reducing symptoms of arthritis, back pain, and neck pain. Dosage: 3–6 g daily of combined EPA and DHA.

S-adenosylmethionine (SAMe): Reduces inflammation and pain and improves joint mobility in those with arthritis and degenerative joint disease. Some studies have even shown SAMe to be as effective as anti-inflammatory drugs. Dosage: 400–1,200 mg daily.

Complementary Supplements

Boswellia: Reduces pain and inflammation due to arthritis. Dosage: 400–600 mg of a product that contains 40–60 percent boswellic acid three times daily.

Enzymes: Bromelain, chymotrypsin, papain, and trypsin have been shown in some studies to help reduce inflammation and pain caused by trauma, surgery, sports injuries, and arthritis. Follow product directions.

Glucosamine: Reduces pain and prevents the progression of osteoarthritis. Most studies have focused on its effects on hip and knee osteoarthritis, but it may offer benefits for the back as well. Dosage: 1,500 mg daily.

White willow: Reduces pain and inflammation. Studies have found it effective for treating low back pain. The active component is salicin, which is similar to aspirin, only it is better tolerated. Dosage: 60–240 mg salicin daily.

FINAL THOUGHTS

When dealing with back pain, remember the following:

1. For acute injuries, apply cold and then heat, and do light exercises.
2. To prevent injuries, exercise to increase strength and flexibility, use proper lifting techniques, and use proper form for sitting and standing.
3. Acupuncture, chiropractic, and massage can help relieve back pain.
4. For pain relief, use a cream containing 0.025–0.075 percent capsaicin and apply three times daily.
5. Supplements of devil's claw, fish oils, and SAMe offer benefits for reducing pain and inflammation. Boswellia, enzymes, glucosamine, and white willow may also offer benefits.

BAD BREATH (HALITOSIS)

Bad breath, known medically as halitosis, is a common condition that affects over 50 percent of the population. While it can be embarrassing and annoying, bad breath is not just a cosmetic problem—it can signify an underlying health problem.

Approximately 90 percent of cases of bad breath originate from problems in the mouth. Poor oral hygiene (not brushing or flossing regularly or properly) allows bacteria to grow and feed on food particles in the mouth. Bacteria emit sulphur gases, which not only cause bad breath, but also damage the tissues in the mouth, leading to inflammation of the gums (periodontitis). If left untreated, the bacteria continue to grow and cause gum recession, tooth decay, and even worse-smelling breath.

The ancient Greeks chewed tree resin and the Mayans chewed chicle (sap from sapodilla tree) to keep their breath fresh. Early American settlers made chewing gum from spruce sap and beeswax. In 1848, John B. Curtis made and sold the first commercial chewing gum called the State of Maine Pure Spruce Gum.

SIGNS & SYMPTOMS

- Unpleasant odour in the mouth and breath
- Unpleasant taste in the mouth

RISK FACTORS

- Constipation
- Diabetes
- Diet (garlic, onions, fish)
- Dieting and fasting
- Dry mouth (could be caused by medications, radiation therapy, or sleeping with your mouth open)
- Gum disease
- Infection in the mouth, throat, sinuses, or lungs
- Kidney or liver disease
- Poor oral hygiene (food caught between teeth)
- Smoking
- Tooth decay

"Morning breath"—we all have it, but did you know that this occurs because saliva flow is decreased when we sleep? Sleeping with your mouth open also causes dry mouth. Good saliva flow is important because the oxygen in saliva kills bacteria.

DOCTOR'S ORDERS

For bad breath caused by problems in the mouth, your dentist will advise you to improve oral hygiene: Brush at least twice daily, floss daily, or use an interdental cleaner to remove food between teeth, and have regular checkups. When brushing, don't forget to brush your tongue as it can trap large amounts of bacteria.

If the cause of bad breath is a lung, throat, or mouth infection, an antibiotic may be prescribed. If it is due to constipation and poor digestion, which can lead to the release of toxins into the breath, a laxative and/or fibre supplement may be recommended.

SHERRY'S NATURAL PRESCRIPTION

Dietary Recommendations

Foods to include:

- Fruits, vegetables, and whole grains are high in fibre, which aids digestive function and prevents constipation.

- Adding parsley to your foods or chewing on parsley after a meal is a natural way to deodorize your breath. Parsley contains chlorophyll, which neutralizes odour. Chlorophyll is also found in green vegetables, alfalfa, and watercress.

- Vitamin C is important for oral health; the best food sources are citrus, peppers, berries, spinach, cabbage, kale, and broccoli.

- Cranberries and cranberry juice contain powerful antioxidants that reduce bacterial adhesion to the gums.

Foods to avoid:

- Foods that move slowly through your digestive tract are more likely to cause constipation and bad breath, such as red meat, fried foods, and processed foods.

- Sulpher compounds found in meat, eggs, and dairy products interact with bacteria in your mouth, causing bad breath.

- Coffee and alcohol cause dry mouth and allow odour-causing bacteria to thrive.

- Minimize foods high in sugar (candy, pop, baked goods) as they promote tooth decay.

Note: Garlic, onions, and spicy food are commonly blamed for bad breath. However, food is only a temporary cause of the problem. The food we eat is digested and absorbed into the bloodstream. Odours are transferred to the lungs and expelled by our breath and continue until the food is eliminated.

Lifestyle Suggestions

- Brush your teeth after meals to remove food particles, especially after drinking coffee or eating sulphur-containing foods such as milk products, fish, eggs, and meat.

- Antibacterial mouthwash and toothpaste can help reduce bacteria in the mouth and teeth. Avoid those containing alcohol as it can dry out your mouth. Look for products that contain zinc (reduces sulphur compounds in the mouth), or tea tree or eucalyptus oil, which have antibacterial and antiseptic properties.

- If you wear removable dentures, take them out at night and clean them thoroughly before replacing the next morning.

- Drink lots of water to prevent dry mouth and flush food particles out of your teeth and mouth.

- Smoking—tobacco is a major cause of bad breath, teeth stains, and gum disease. It also negatively affects the taste of food and irritates the gums.

- Chewing gums and mints with xylitol help reduce bacteria and prevent dry mouth by stimulating saliva. Make sure there is no added sugar in the gum.

- Peppermint tea, mints, and gum also help to freshen breath and reduce bacteria in the mouth after meals.

Top Recommended Supplements

Chlorophyll: A component of green plants, chlorophyll helps neutralize odour. Dosage: 1 tsp of liquid or one or two capsules after meals.

Coenzyme Q10: A deficiency of coenzyme Q10, an antioxidant that is important for gum health, has been linked to gum disease, and studies have found that it can help promote healing of the gums. Dosage: 50–200 mg daily.

Probiotics: Friendly bacteria that help to reduce formation of bad bacteria that cause bad breath. Dosage: One or two capsules daily.

Complementary Supplement

Vitamin C: Essential for healthy gums and teeth; levels may be deficient in those with gum disease and in smokers. Dosage: 250–500 mg daily.

FINAL THOUGHTS

To prevent bad breath and maintain good oral hygiene:

1. Brush and floss daily and have regular dental visits.
2. Use mouthwash and toothpastes containing zinc, tea tree oil, or eucalyptus.
3. Drink lots of water and eat parsley and cranberry.
4. Don't smoke.
5. Chew gum with xylitol and/or peppermint and take supplements of chlorophyll, coenzyme Q10, and probiotics for gum health.

BLADDER INFECTION

Bladder infections, also known as urinary tract infections, are a common problem, especially among women. Normally the urine is sterile and does not contain any bacteria, viruses, or fungi. However, an infection can develop when these bugs enter the urethra (the tube that carries urine out of the body) and travel up into the bladder. This leads to inflammation of the bladder (cystitis) and unpleasant urinary symptoms. Over 90 percent of UTIs are caused by Escherichia coli (E. coli), a bacteria present in high amounts in the colon and rectal area.

If a bladder infection is not treated properly, it can spread to the kidneys and become very serious. Some people get recurrent bladder infections. This is often due to a structural abnormality in the urethra or bladder affecting the flow of urine.

DID YOU KNOW?

Infections of the bladder are the second most common infection in women and the most common complication of pregnancy.

SIGNS & SYMPTOMS

- Blood in the urine

- Cloudy or strong-smelling urine

- Fever

- Frequent urge to urinate

- Pain and burning upon urination

- Pain or discomfort in abdomen or lower back

- Passing small amounts of urine

RISK FACTORS

UTIs are much more common in women because of the following:

- Anatomy: The female urethra (tube that carries urine out of the body) is shorter and closer to the rectal area, making it easier for bacteria to enter during sex or after elimination.

- Pregnancy: The growing baby presses on the bladder, preventing it from completely emptying. When urine is left to stagnate in the bladder, the risk of developing infection increases.

- Menopause: A decline in estrogen leads to thinning of urinary tract, making it easier for bacteria to enter.

Other risk factors include:

- Dehydration: The urine becomes more concentrated.

- Catheter use: Insertion and removal can allow bacteria to enter.

- Enlargement of the prostate gland in men: Puts pressure on the urethra and prevents the bladder from completely emptying.

- Weak immune system: Conditions such as diabetes, AIDS, cancer, and stress can weaken the immune system, affecting its ability to fight off infection.

DOCTOR'S ORDERS

Treatment of a bladder infection often requires antibiotics, such as Bactrim or Noroxin. While necessary, there are various drawbacks to the use of antibiotics, including side effects such as diarrhea, stomach upset, and yeast overgrowth. Overuse of antibiotics causes resistance—the bugs become stronger than the drugs, leaving people vulnerable to attack by bacteria. Antibiotic therapy can also be expensive. Therefore, these drugs should be used only when absolutely necessary.

To relieve the pain and burning, a drug called phenazopyridine (Pyridium) may be prescribed. This is given for two to three days; it contains a dye and will cause discolouration of the urine and feces.

SHERRY'S NATURAL PRESCRIPTION

For those at risk of bladder infections, or those who suffer recurrent infections, preventative measures, including lifestyle changes and supplements, can be very helpful.

Dietary Recommendations

Foods to include:

- Drink eight or more glasses of water daily to help flush bacteria out of your bladder. Eat foods high in water such as watermelon and celery.

- Cranberry juice contains antioxidants called condensed tannins or proanthocyanidins, which prevent bacteria from adhering to the bladder walls. Many studies have shown that cranberry juice prevents bladder infections. Pure cranberry juice is best, but it is quite tart. You can sweeten it with stevia, which is a natural, low-calorie plant-based sweetener. Drink three 8 oz. glasses daily. Juice cocktails are an alternative that offer better taste and tolerability, but contain less juice and have added sugar; drink three 16 oz. glasses daily.

- Blueberries contain the same beneficial antioxidants as cranberries and may offer bladder benefits.

- Garlic strengthens the immune system response and helps fight infection.

- Pineapple contains the enzyme bromelain, which may enhance the action of antibiotics used to fight bladder infections.

Foods to avoid:

- Caffeine has diuretic properties, which promote fluid loss, making the urine more concentrated. Minimize or avoid consumption of coffee, soda pop, and caffeinated beverages.

- Alcohol is dehydrating and reduces immune function.

- Refined sugar and flour reduce immune function.

Lifestyle Suggestions

- Drink at least eight glasses of water daily or more if you are exercising or spending time in the sun. Dehydration concentrates the urine and increases the risk of infection.

- Urinate regularly as you feel the need. Holding in urine concentrates bacteria.

- Ladies, after going to the bathroom, wipe from front to back to prevent bacteria around the rectum from entering the urethra.

- Cleanse your genital area before and after sex and keep genital area dry. Wear cotton underwear, which allows the skin to breathe; change clothing promptly after swimming.

- Support immune function by exercising regularly, getting adequate sleep, and minimizing stress.

Top Recommended Supplements

Cran-Max: Studies show that it prevents bladder infections and may also be effective in treating early bladder infections if taken at the first sign of symptoms. Dosage: 500 mg daily for prevention, and twice daily for treatment.

Vitamin C: Acidifies urine, making it more difficult for bacteria to grow; inhibits the growth of E. Coli; and supports the immune system. Dosage: 500–2,000 mg daily.

Complementary Supplements

Oil of oregano: Has antibacterial properties, and is available in capsules or liquid. Dosage varies.

Probiotics: Support immune function, help fight off infections, and are essential for those on antibiotics because they restore the friendly bacteria destroyed by antibiotics. Dosage: One to three capsules daily.

FINAL THOUGHTS

A bladder infection is an uncomfortable problem that requires immediate treatment. To reduce the likelihood of a bladder infection:

1. Drink plenty of water and void regularly.
2. Eat cranberries, blueberries, and their juices.
3. Keep the genital area clean and dry.
4. Get regular exercise and adequate sleep.
5. For prevention, consider Cran-Max and vitamin C.

BRONCHITIS

Bronchitis occurs when the lining of the bronchial tubes (airways that lead to the lungs) become infected and inflamed. Acute bronchitis most commonly occurs following a respiratory infection, such as a cold or flu. It can also develop due to exposure to cigarette smoke or pollution, or in those who have gastroesophageal reflux disease due to backflow of acids into the lungs. Acute bronchitis caused by a viral infection often clears up on its own in a week or two without lasting effects.

Long-term exposure to lung irritants (particularly cigarette smoke) can lead to continual inflammation and thickening of the lining of your bronchial tubes, which is called chronic bronchitis. People with chronic bronchitis have a persistent productive cough and shortness of breath. It is an ongoing, serious disease that typically worsens over time. One of the best ways to improve this condition is to quit smoking.

If you have a cold or flu and symptoms persist beyond a few weeks, consult with your doctor.

SIGNS & SYMPTOMS

Acute bronchitis:

- Chest and sinus congestion (due to respiratory tract infection)

- Cough with yellowish-grey or green phlegm

- Fatigue

- Shortness of breath

- Sore throat

Chronic bronchitis:

- Chronic shortness of breath

- Continual need to clear your throat

- Persistent coughing: You're generally considered to have chronic bronchitis if you cough most days for at least three months a year in two consecutive years.

- Wheezing

If left untreated, bronchitis can lead to pneumonia in those at risk (elderly, smokers, and those with respiratory disease, such as asthma). Those with chronic bronchitis who smoke are at increased risk of lung cancer above and beyond the normal risk that a smoker faces.

RISK FACTORS

- Compromised immune function (the elderly, infants, and young children)

- Gastroesophageal reflux disease: Stomach acids that persistently back up into your esophagus may cause a chronic cough and bronchial irritation.

- Pollution and occupational exposure to chemicals that irritate the lungs, such as fumes from ammonia, strong acids, chlorine, hydrogen sulphide, sulphur dioxide, or bromine

- Smokers and those in contact with second-hand smoke

DOCTOR'S ORDERS

If you have acute bronchitis, your doctor will advise you to rest, drink fluids, and allow your body to recover. Since most cases of acute bronchitis are caused by a viral infection, antibiotics offer little benefit unless your doctor suspects a bacterial infection or you are at risk of this. Taking an antibiotic when not necessary can lead to resistance and secondary infections, such as thrush, yeast, and urinary tract infections, so it is important to ask your doctor if antibiotics are necessary if one is prescribed.

Cough suppressants are not recommended because coughing helps the lungs remove irritants. However, if your cough disrupts your sleep, then you may want to take a cough medicine at bedtime.

For severe cases of bronchitis, your doctor may prescribe an inhaler to reduce inflammation and help you breathe.

SHERRY'S NATURAL PRESCRIPTION

Dietary Recommendations

Foods to include:

- Drink lots of fluids (water, juice, and tea). Herbal teas, such as Throat Coat, which contains marshmallow and licorice, can help relieve sore throat.

- Essential fatty acids—which are found in fish, flaxseed, and olive oil—may help to reduce inflammation.

- Fruits and vegetables are rich in antioxidants and nutrients that can help support immune function and reduce free radical damage. Studies have shown that increasing fruit and vegetable consumption may reduce the risk of developing bronchitis.

- If you take antibiotics, increase your consumption of yogurt and cultured dairy products (kefir), which contain beneficial probiotics (friendly bacteria).

- Onions, garlic, and ginger have anti-inflammatory properties and immune benefits.

RESEARCH HIGHLIGHT

Eat your fruit and fish. Researchers at Harvard did a study of 2,112 teenagers and found an association between good lung function and levels of dietary intake of fruit and fish rich in omega-3 fatty acids. Teens who ate less of these foods (two servings of fruit per week and less than 22 mg of omega-3 fatty acids per day) had higher rates of asthma, wheezing, and symptoms of chronic bronchitis such as cough and phlegm (*Chest*, 2007: 132; 238–245).

Foods to avoid:

- Cow's milk allergy has been linked to bronchitis in children. Some practitioners feel that dairy products can increase mucus formation, and that people with bronchitis should minimize these foods.

- Sugar can hamper immune function. Avoid adding sugar to foods and minimize high-sugar foods (candy, soft drinks, and sweets).

Lifestyle Suggestions

- To prevent contracting or spreading a virus, avoid rubbing your eyes, nose, or mouth and wash your hands frequently.

- Avoid smoking and exposure to second-hand smoke. Tobacco is damaging to the lungs and increases your risk of chronic bronchitis and emphysema.

- For a sore throat, gargle with warm salt water and try lozenges that contain one or more of the following ingredients: slippery elm, marshmallow, vitamin C, zinc, eucalyptus, or menthol.

- For dry nose, try a nasal lubricant, such as Secaris or a saline nasal spray.

- Use an air purifier and humidifier in your room. Air purifiers remove bacteria, viruses, and dust from the air, cleaning the air you breathe. A humidifier adds moisture to the air, and warm, moist air helps relieve coughs and loosens mucus in your airways. But be sure to clean the humidifier according to the manufacturer's recommendations to avoid the growth of bacteria and fungi in the water container.

- Have a hot bath or use a vaporizer with essential oils of eucalyptus, peppermint, tea tree, or pine. These aromatic oils can help to clear congestion and improve breathing.

- Massage therapy to the back and chest can help to break up phlegm.

Top Recommended Supplements

Echinacea: Helps support immune function and studies show that it can reduce the severity and frequency of cold symptoms. It may also help prevent a cold from developing into bronchitis. Look for Echinacea purpurea. Dosage: 300–600 mg capsules twice daily or 2–4 mL tincture four to six times daily at the first sign of a cold for seven to 10 days. Some products combine echinacea with astragalus, which also has antiviral and antibacterial properties.

N-acetylcysteine (NAC): An amino acid derivative that helps break up mucus and reduce cough. Numerous clinical trials have found it beneficial for reducing symptoms in both acute and chronic bronchitis. Dosage: 300–600 mg daily.

Vitamin C: Supports immune function and helps prevent oxidative damage to the lungs. Studies have shown that it can reduce the severity and duration of the common cold, which may reduce the likelihood of complications, such as bronchitis. Dosage: 500 mg daily.

Complementary Supplements

Aged garlic extract: Contains antioxidant compounds that help support immune function. When taken regularly, it may help prevent colds and bacterial infections. Dosage: 600 mg daily.

American ginseng: Helps to prevent and relieve colds and flu, so it may help reduce these respiratory infections from leading to bronchitis. Look for COLD-fX, a patented extract of polysaccharides derived from North American ginseng that has been clinically studied. See package for directions.

Fish oils: Contain essential fatty acids that help reduce inflammation. One study in children found that daily fish oil supplements reduced the risk of recurrent respiratory tract infections. Dosage: Children should take 15 mg EPA plus DHA per pound of body weight per day; adults should take 1–3 g EPA plus DHA daily.

Vitamin E: An antioxidant that helps prevent oxidative damage to the lungs caused by environmental pollution and cigarette smoke exposure. Dosage: 400 IU daily.

FINAL THOUGHTS

To improve healing of bronchitis and prevent it from occurring, consider the following:

1. Eat more fruits, vegetables, fish, onions, garlic, and ginger.
2. Drink lots of fluids, especially water and herbal teas.
3. Avoid smoking and being around smoke and other irritants.
4. Use an air purifier and humidifier in your home.
5. Consider supplements of echinacea, NAC, and vitamin C.

BURNS

Whether they are the result of sunburn or a scalding pan, skin burns can be frightening and painful. They also may lead to serious complications, so proper treatment is critical.

Your skin is made up of three layers—the epidermis (outer layer of the skin), the dermis (under the epidermis, containing blood vessels, hair follicles, and connective tissue), and the subcutis (the final layer of skin containing adipose tissue and storage of nutrients). The skin provides a first line of defence against all forms of external toxins and bacteria, but this protective barrier may be burned at temperatures higher than 120°F. Skin burns occur from exposure to extreme heat such as the sun, fire, boiling water, hot beverages, or cooking heat, and hot objects such as an iron or steam. Other causes of burns include chemicals, electricity, lightning, or radioactive material.

Depending on the cause and length of exposure, burns can range from mild to severe and potentially fatal. Burns are classified according to their degree of severity and the amount of skin affected:

- **First-degree burns** damage the epidermis. These burns may be painful, but can usually be self-treated. They heal quickly and rarely cause scars.
- **Second-degree burns** damage the epidermis and dermis, and can cause acute pain, blisters, and scarring. Depending on the extent of the burn and subsequent tissue damage, second-degree burns may be self-treated, but must be diligently watched and treated to avoid infection.
- **Third-degree burns** severely damage the epidermis, dermis, and subcutis. They may affect muscles, bones, nerves, and blood vessels, requiring extensive treatment, skin grafts, and therapy. Because of the risk of shock and infection, third-degree burns are always considered a life-threatening medical emergency.

There are a variety of lifestyle recommendations and also natural products that can help relieve the pain and promote skin healing for first-degree and minor second-degree burns. Third-degree burns need to be managed by your doctor to reduce the risk of infection and serious complications.

SIGNS & SYMPTOMS

- First-degree burns: Mild pain where contact occurred for 24–48 hours, inflammation, redness, soreness

- Second-degree burns: Lingering pain, inflammation, redness, and blistering

- Third-degree burns: Skin may become white, brown, red, or black and quite swollen; unlike first- or second-degree burns, damage to the subcutis may mean there is no immediate pain; other symptoms include shock, dizziness, nausea, vomiting, fever, cold, and stiffness.

- Some burns may not leave visibly physical symptoms; exposure to smoke may burn the lungs; electrical burns may cause more internal than external damage; these are also considered medical emergencies because the extent of the damage is unseen by the naked eye and must be assessed.

RISK FACTORS

- Age: Children and the elderly have thinner skin, putting them at higher risk of burns.

- Chemicals, electrical wiring, lightning

- Lifestyle: Certain high-risk jobs or habits (such as drug or alcohol consumption) will increase the risk of burns.

- Most burns are caused by accidents in the home: boiling water, hot objects, hot oil, or grease, etc.

- Sun exposure or tanning beds

BURNS A LEADING CAUSE OF DEATH

Burns are the fifth leading cause of injury-related death of Canadian children. Three percent of burns reported are caused by hot-water scalding, most often in the bathtub. If you have children, make sure your hot-water heater is set no higher than 120°F. Most hot-water heaters are set at 140°F, which can instantly burn the thin skin of a child. At 120°F, it would take 10 minutes to cause a burn.

DOCTOR'S ORDERS

You should call a doctor if your burn is larger than the size of your palm or if it is painful; if your burn is on your face, hands, or genitals; if you have symptoms of infection, including fever, vomiting, chills, swelling, and stiffness; or if your burn is not healing. Third-degree burns always demand immediate medical attention.

The goals of burn treatment are to speed wound healing, prevent infection and scars, relieve pain, and restore the patient to normal health. As such, doctors may employ a variety of antimicrobial and antibiotic agents, as well as pain relievers, to achieve these goals. For extensive burns, extensive treatment is needed, which may include lengthy hospital stays to ensure that infection does not occur, and outpatient appointments for therapy.

SHERRY'S NATURAL PRESCRIPTION

For minor burns, there are natural ways to promote and support wound healing.

Dietary Recommendations

A healthy diet is critical for effective burn treatment to replace vital nutrients, promote wound healing, and reduce the risk of infection and scars. Also, for more serious burns, the healing process consumes many calories and a healthy diet can help keep your body strong during this process.

Foods to include:

- Drink plenty of water and electrolyte drinks to replace lost fluids. Caffeine-free herbal teas are also fine.

- Eat brightly coloured fruits and vegetables for vitamins A, C, and E and other bioflavonoids, which promote healthy skin and reduce inflammation.

- Ensure adequate protein intake to aid in skin repair. Eat lean poultry, fish, beans, nuts, and seeds.

- Essential fatty acids, which are found in fish and flaxseed, help reduce inflammation.

Note: Those with severe burns need to increase total caloric intake because as the body tries to repair, it burns calories at a faster rate.

Foods to avoid:

- Salty foods promote dehydration. Minimize eating chips, snack foods, deli meats, and other high-salt foods.

- Saturated fat can worsen inflammation and depress the body's immune system, delaying recovery.

- Sugar impairs immune function and slows skin and tissue regeneration. Minimize sweets, soft drinks, candy, and other high-sugar foods.

Lifestyle Suggestions

To prevent the risk of burns:

- Wear sunscreen everyday with a minimum of SPF 15; wear wide-brim hats to shield your face.

- Be mindful at all times about burn hazards in the home and your environment.

- Reduce the hot-water tank temperature to 120°F.

- Turn the handles of cooking pots and pans inward to avoid bumping.

- Get an automatic shut-off iron; unplug curling irons when not in use.

- Teach your children burn safety and first-aid treatment.

- Keep a first-aid and burn kit in your home that contains fresh gauze and antibacterial agents.

- Follow all precautions for electrical equipment.

To manage a minor burn:

- Gently cool and clean the area with cold water or cold wet compresses for at least 15 minutes. Do not apply ice.

- Cool compresses soaked in chamomile tea can help promote healing.

- Apply a topical anaesthetic cream, such as Polysporin Burn Cream or Calendula. Honey can also promote healing and reduce infection (see top of next page). Do not cover with any type of petroleum-based cream or butter, as they retain heat, slow healing, and increase risk of infection.

- Cover with a dry, sterile dressing. Do not wrap tightly.

- Do not break blisters or pick skin. Blisters keep infections out of the wound.

- Cleanse the wound daily with antiseptic solution or gauze soaked in green tea and change the dressing.

- Avoid exposing the burned area to hot water until it has healed.

RESEARCH HIGHLIGHT: HONEY SWEET FOR BURNS

Honey is hygroscopic—it attracts and absorbs moisture—which has proven helpful in the treatment of wounds because it retains the plasma released by a wound, allowing for reabsorption. In one study, 104 patients with first-degree burns were treated either with gauze soaked in silver sulfadiazine (SS), which is a conventional treatment, or honey. After seven days, 91 percent of honey-treated burns were infection-free compared with 7 percent of those treated with SS. After 15 days, 87 percent of honey-treated burns were healed compared with 10 percent of the SS-treated burns. Other studies have also found benefits. Honey products are also available in a spray, salve, or tincture (*The British Journal of Surgery,* 1991: 78; 497–498).

Top Recommended Treatments

Aloe vera gel: Cooling, helps relieve pain and inflammation, and also has anti-inflammatory properties. It is commonly used to manage burns and has a long history of use to promote wound healing, although the scientific research is lacking. Use aloe vera from a plant (split open a leaf) or get pure aloe gel at a health food store or pharmacy. Dosage: Apply two or three times daily.

Antioxidants: Studies have shown that oral supplements of vitamins A, C, E, zinc, and selenium can help to protect the skin from sunburn due to free radical-producing ultraviolet rays. These vitamins also help to promote skin healing. Dosage: Take a broad-spectrum antioxidant daily. Topical vitamin E cream or oil is commonly used to promote skin healing and may reduce scarring.

Complementary Treatments

Calendula cream: Soothing, has anti-inflammatory properties, and may help promote tissue repair. Dosage: Apply three times per day.

Ornithine alpha-ketoglutarate (OKG): Manufactured from two amino acids, ornithine and glutamine. It is used to stimulate the body to build muscle and tissue. Studies have shown that it can speed recovery. Dosage: 5–25 g daily as advised by your health care provider.

RESEARCH HIGHLIGHT: ORNITHINE ALPHA-KETOGLUTARATE

In one study, 60 severely burned subjects were randomly given either a placebo or 20 g of OKG daily for 21 days, starting an average of four days after the burn. The patients taking OKG showed significant improvement in wound healing compared to the placebo group. Previous studies of OKG-treated burn patients have reported shorter hospitalizations and fewer fatalities (*Clinical Nutrition,* 1999: 18; 307–311).

FINAL THOUGHTS

First-degree burns may be self-treated, but a doctor should see second- and third-degree burns immediately.

1. Take precautions to prevent burns. Keep a first-aid kit in the home.
2. Follow burn treatment protocol. After a burn has cooled, cleanse with chamomile tea and apply fresh aloe vera gel.
3. Antioxidants can help to protect against sunburn and help promote wound healing.
4. Eat a healthy diet packed with lots of fresh fruits and vegetables, whole grains, and fish. Increase total calorie intake during the healing process and drink lots of liquids.
5. Consider OKG supplements to speed healing.

CANCER

Cancer is one of the most feared diseases and rightfully so. It is the leading cause of premature death in Canada—about 1,006,000 potential years were lost in 2003 as a result of cancer. Cancer has become an age-related phenomenon: 44 percent of new cancer cases and 60 percent of cancer deaths will occur among those who are at least 70 years old. However, aging does not cause cancer. Rather, in many cases it is generally thought that our lifetime exposure to factors that increase our risk, such as smoking or eating a poor diet, leads to the development of cancer.

Cancer is a disease that starts in our cells. Our bodies are made up of millions of cells grouped together to form tissues or organs, such as muscles, skin, bones, and organs. Cancer occurs when there is an abnormal growth of cells, which can form lumps or tumours, or can spread through the bloodstream and lymphatic system to other parts of the body. Tumours can be either benign (non-cancerous) or malignant (cancerous). Benign tumour cells stay in one place in the body and are not usually life-threatening.

Malignant tumour cells are able to spread to invade nearby tissues and other parts of the body, which is a process called metastasis. When a malignant tumour spreads, it often causes swelling of nearby lymph nodes. Finding cancer early and getting treatment before it spreads can greatly help improve your chances of survival.

While we think of cancer as one disease, it is actually a group of more than 100 different diseases. It can involve any tissue of the body and have many different forms in each body area. Most cancers are named for the type of cell or organ in which they start. For example, if it starts in the liver it is called liver cancer. The four most common types of cancer in Canada are breast, prostate, lung, and colon.

A great deal of research has focused on the underlying causes of abnormal cell growth. We do know that certain factors, such as free radical damage, genetics, diet, and lifestyle, are involved. While many of us may blame our family history, only about 5–10 percent of cancers are attributed to faulty genes. Having a family history may increase your risk of certain cancers, but researchers feel that whether or not those genes are "switched on" may depend largely on lifestyle and environment. These critical yet often overlooked factors play a role not only in prevention but also in the treatment and recovery from cancer.

STARTLING CANCER STATISTICS

According to the Canadian Cancer Society, an estimated 159,900 new cases of cancer and 72,700 cancer deaths will occur in Canada in 2007. Based on current incidence rates, 39 percent of Canadian women will develop cancer during their lifetimes. Among men, 44 percent will develop cancer during their lifetimes.

Cancer is a very broad subject and it is beyond the scope of this chapter to discuss each type and make individualized recommendations. The goal here is to provide you with information on known risk factors for the most common forms of cancer, how to reduce your risk of getting cancer, and how to improve your chances of survival if you have cancer. If you have been diagnosed with cancer, it is critical that you consult with your health care provider to create an individualized program. In many cases, dietary and lifestyle strategies and supplements can be taken along with your other treatments. Certain supplements, however, could interact with chemotherapy or other medical treatments, so it is important to work with your health care provider.

Research shows that overall 30–35 percent of all cancers can be prevented by being active, eating well, and maintaining a healthy body weight.

SIGNS & SYMPTOMS

Cancer does not happen overnight. It may take months or years before there are any signs or symptoms, and these symptoms can vary greatly depending on the location of the cancer. Here are some key things to look for:

- A lump or area of swelling under the skin or bloating in pelvic area
- A mole that is asymmetrical, has an irregular border, is dark in colour, or grows in size or thickness
- Change in bowel or bladder habits
- Difficulty swallowing, upset stomach, nausea, or vomiting
- Persistent cough, hoarseness, or a cough that brings up blood
- Persistent low-grade fever
- Rectal bleeding or blood in the urine or stool
- Recurrent infections or wounds that do not heal
- Unexplained pain, especially in the bones, breasts, or pelvic area
- Unexplained vaginal discharge or bleeding
- Unexplained weight loss and loss of appetite
- Unusual fatigue, headaches

RISK FACTORS

- Becoming sexually active at a young age or having multiple partners increases the risk of cervical cancer.
- Exposure to environmental toxins such as tobacco, pollution, asbestos, heavy metals (arsenic, lead, nickel), and radiation (X-rays), and handling of petroleum products. Smoking is responsible for 30 percent of all cancer deaths. Chlorinated drinking water increases the risk of bladder cancer. Some substances used in pesticides are classified as known, probable, or possible carcinogens.
- Excessive sun exposure or sunburn during childhood increases the risk of skin cancer.
- Genetics: Family history of cancer increases risk.
- Heavy alcohol consumption increases risk.
- High insulin levels (hyperinsulinemia) and insulin resistance increase risk.

- High intake of saturated fat, trans fats, and high-glycemic foods (refined starches and sugar); low intake of fibre; consumption of pesticides, food additives; nutritional deficiencies (lack of antioxidants) increase risk.

- Lack of exercise increases your risk of several types of cancer.

- Obesity increases risk of breast, endometrial, cervical, ovarian, and gallbladder cancer for women and colon and prostate cancer for men.

- Poor liver function can increase risk. The liver plays a key role in removing toxins.

- Stress hampers immune function and may increase the risk of cancer (particularly breast cancer). Stress may also worsen recovery in those with cancer.

- Use of the hormones estrogen and progestin (HRT) increase the risk of breast cancer; risk is greatest with higher dosages for long periods of time (longer than five years).

- Weakened immune function, exposure to viruses and fungal infections increase risk.

Exposure to many different risk factors may increase a person's risk more than the risk associated with each individual toxin or chemical, so it is important to avoid as many known risk factors as possible. As you see from this list, many of the known risk factors are within our control.

GENETICS AND CANCER

There is evidence to show genetic inheritance has very little to do with who gets cancer. Researchers looked at a group of 44,778 pairs of twins from Finland, Sweden, and Denmark, in order to assess the risks of cancer for the twins of people with cancer. The researchers concluded that inherited genetic factors make only a minor contribution to the susceptibility of breast, prostate, and colorectal cancer. More importantly, they concluded that environmental factors make a major contribution to all of the 28 anatomical sites of cancer studied (*New England Journal of Medicine,* 2000: 343; 78–85).

DOCTOR'S ORDERS

The treatment of cancer depends on the location, stage of cancer, your existing health status, and many other factors. Today there are numerous options for medical treatment including chemotherapy, radiation, surgery, and hormone therapy.

There are a variety of important screening tests that can help in the early detection of cancer, such as:

- Breast self-exams, mammograms, and thermography scans
- Digital rectal exams
- Pap test (for cervical cancer) and pelvic exam
- Prostate exam and PSA test
- Skin exam
- Testicular exams

See your doctor yearly for a thorough health examination and bloodwork, and discuss any changes in your health or unexplained new symptoms.

SHERRY'S NATURAL PRESCRIPTION

Numerous studies have shown that good nutrition and various lifestyle measures can significantly reduce the risk of cancer. For those who have cancer, a good nutritional program can help prevent weight loss, aid digestion, support immune function, and boost energy levels. Supplements can also play an important supportive role.

Dietary Recommendations

Foods to include:

- Boost fibre intake: aim for 25–30 g daily of soluble and insoluble fibre. Eat 2 tbsps of milled flaxseed every day: it provides fibre and contains compounds that help in the prevention of cancer. Recent research found that it can also slow the growth of prostate cancer.

- Choose free-range poultry and wild (not farmed) fish, beans, and legumes.

- Choose healthy fats such as olive oil and flaxseed oil.

- Drink green tea, which is a potent antioxidant, and studies have linked drinking green tea to a lower risk of several cancers.

- Drink lots of purified water.

- Eat cancer-fighting foods such as broccoli, cabbage, cauliflower, Brussels sprouts, kale, tomatoes, garlic, onions, and carrots.

- Eat cancer-fighting herbs and spices like ginger, cayenne, rosemary, oregano, and curcumin.

- Eat lots of vegetables and fruit (10 servings daily). Choose organic produce as much as possible to avoid ingestion of pesticides. Foods that contain the highest amounts of pesticide residue include peaches, strawberries, apples, spinach, nectarines, celery, pears, cherries, potatoes, peppers, and raspberries. If organics are not available or cost-prohibitive, wash your produce with lots of water and scrub the skins. This will also help eliminate harmful bacteria.

- Eat small, frequent meals, which are easier on digestion and also help improve blood sugar control.

- Fermented soy products (tofu, tempeh and miso) appear to have cancer-fighting properties.

- Ginger tea may be helpful for managing nausea caused by chemotherapy.

- Yogurt and fermented dairy can aid digestion and intestinal function.

Consider doing a detoxification program, such as a juice cleanse. See Appendix C for more information.

EAT YOUR FRUITS AND VEGGIES

Overwhelming evidence from numerous clinical trials indicates that a plant-based diet can reduce the risk of cancer. In 1992, a review of 200 studies showed that cancer risk in people consuming diets high in fruits and vegetables was only one-half that in those consuming few of these foods. It is clear that there are components in a plant-based diet that can reduce cancer risk, but few Canadians get the recommended intake of these foods (Nutrition and Cancer, 1992; 18 (1): 1–29).

Foods to avoid:

- Reduce intake of saturated fat to less than 10 percent of total calories by limiting animal and dairy products. Avoid trans fats (found in many processed/snack foods and fried foods) completely. Read labels carefully.

- Avoid preservatives (nitrates and sulphites) and chemical food additives.

- Deli meats (bologna, salami) and hot dogs are full of nitrates and other chemicals that are associated with cancer and poor health.

- Eating charred meat (BBQ) and well-done meat has been associated with increased risk of breast cancer (see below).

- Minimize alcohol, as it is hard on liver and immune function. Heavy drinking increases the risk of cancers of the mouth, esophagus, breast, colorectal, and stomach. If you drink, limit yourself to one or two drinks daily and choose red wine as it contains antioxidants that may offer cancer-protecting properties.

- Minimize eating sugar and refined starches, which quickly raise blood sugar and insulin levels, increasing the risk of insulin resistance, which is associated with increased risk of certain cancers.

BBQ MEAT AND CANCER

Women who consistently eat well-done steak, hamburgers, and bacon have a 4.62 times increased risk of breast cancer. This conclusion was drawn from 41,836 women who took part in the Iowa Women's Health Study (*Journal of the National Cancer Institute,* 1998; 90 (22): 1724–1729). Marinating meat helps prevent the formation of these carcinogens. Marinades that contain olive oil, vinegar, garlic, mustard, lemon juice, rosemary, oregano, and curcumin have been to shown to be ideal. Meat should be marinated for at least two hours.

Lifestyle Suggestions

- Get regular exercise. Aim for one hour of moderate-intensity activity each day, such as walking, cycling, or swimming.

- Don't smoke, and avoid second-hand smoke and highly polluted areas.

- Manage your stress. Try yoga, meditation, and breathing techniques.

- Drink purified water. Several long-term studies have found that drinking chlorinated tap water increases the risk of cancer, particularly bladder cancer.

- Avoid storing food in soft plastic containers. Use glass or hard plastic (which contains high-density polyethylene).

- Minimize exposure to dangerous phthalates (see next page). Ask manufacturers about non-vinyl hard flooring alternatives, and consider other types of materials such as natural flooring and fabric shower curtains.

- Use stainless steel cookware. All non-stick cookware is made up of a chemical called PTFE (polytetrafluoroethylene). When heated to high temperatures (greater than 572°F), they can create fumes that contain a suspected cancer-causing chemical, tetrafluoroethene-TFE.

- Don't spray pesticides on your lawn. Look into natural methods of weed control. Don't let your children or pets on lawns that have recently been sprayed with pesticides as they can inhale the fumes and absorb the chemicals through their skin. Signs are posted when lawns are sprayed.

- Be sun smart. Wear sunscreen with at least SPF 15, and don't forget to apply it to your ears and the back of your neck. Wear a wide-brim hat and sunglasses when outdoors.

- Massage and acupuncture may be helpful for reducing stress and nausea associated with chemotherapy.

PHTHALATES: CANCER-CAUSING PLASTICS

Phthalates (pronounced THA-lates) are a group of chemicals often called "plasticizers," which are used in a variety of products, including polyvinyl chloride (PVC) products. Phthalates are added to PVC products to make them soft and flexible. Phthalates are associated with a number of health problems, including liver abnormalities, cancer, and fertility problems. There are many different types of phthalates. The most widely used is DEHP, which is found mostly in PVC plastics (vinyl flooring and medical plastics such as IV bags and tubes). DINP is another phthalate, which is also used in PVC plastics, including children's toys. Canadian guidelines suggest that DEHP and DINP shouldn't be used in items that are likely to be placed in children's mouths, but manufacturers aren't legally bound by these guidelines. Many suppliers of baby bottles use phthalate-free substances such as polypropylene (recycling code 5), but be sure to check with the manufacturer or use glass bottles. For nipples and pacifiers, choose those made of silicone or latex. In cosmetics, DBP, DEP, and DMP are the phthalates most often used.

Top Recommended Supplements

It is critical that you consult with a qualified natural health care practitioner for advice on supplements for cancer. There aren't any known cancer cures, but certain supplements can help to improve energy and well-being, support immune function, and may help the treatment of cancer. This section outlines some products that have shown benefits.

Coriolus versicolor: A traditional Chinese medicine that has been shown in many studies to enhance the effectiveness of various forms of standard cancer therapy. The two main active components are polysaccharide-K (PSK) and polysaccharopeptide (PSP), which are thought to work by stimulating the body's own cancer-fighting cells. This product may also be helpful in cancer prevention. Dosage: The typical dosage for use as an adjunct to standard cancer treatment is 2–6 g daily.

Ginseng: Studies have shown benefits for reducing fatigue, nausea and vomiting, and improving well-being in those undergoing cancer treatment. American ginseng has been shown to reduce fatigue in those with breast, lung, colon, and other forms of cancer. It may also increase the effectiveness of treatment for breast cancer. Panax ginseng has been shown to improve energy and well-being in those with cancer. Regular use of Korean ginseng was found to lower overall cancer risk. Dosage: Varies depending on product used; follow label instructions or the advice of your health care provider.

IP6 (inositol hexaphosphate): A supplement derived from rice bran. Animal research and preliminary human studies have shown that it has significant anti-cancer effects. It can help in the prevention of cancer and has growth-regulating effects on various cells and tissues, including those of the colon, breast, and prostate. Dosage: 4–8 g daily.

Multivitamin/mineral complex: Ensures that your body gets essential nutrients to support immune function and overall health. Look for a product that provides a full range of nutrients and is free of dyes and artificial chemicals. Dosage: Take daily. Consider extra antioxidants as it is difficult to obtain therapeutic dosages from a multivitamin. Dosages: 200–400 mcg selenium, 400–800 IU vitamin E (natural mixed tocopherols), and 500–2,000 mg vitamin C. Antioxidants may offer benefits for those undergoing chemotherapy, but it is important to consult with your health care provider.

GINSENG AND CANCER

According to research at Vanderbilt University in Nashville, TN, "Ginseng use after cancer diagnosis, particularly current use, was positively associated with quality of life scores, with the strongest effect in the psychological and social well-being domains. Additionally, quality of life improved as cumulative ginseng use increased" (*American Journal of Epidemiology,* 2006: 163 (7); 645–653).

Complementary Supplements

Aged garlic extract: Supports immune function and detoxification and has antioxidant properties. Dosage: 600 mg once or twice daily.

Green drinks: Contain barley and wheat grass, chlorella, spirulina, and other plants that support detoxification and overall health. Dosage: Take daily.

Probiotics: Replenish friendly bacteria that are depleted by treatment with chemotherapy and antibiotics. Probiotics aid digestion, support immune function and detoxification, and assist in nutrient absorption. They may also help to minimize diarrhea and upset stomach caused by chemotherapy and radiation. Dosage: One billion live cells twice daily.

FINAL THOUGHTS

To improve the management of cancer, consider the following:

1. Eat lots of vegetables (broccoli, cabbage, tomatoes, garlic, and onions), whole grains, milled flaxseed, and yogurt. Choose free-range poultry and wild fish. Drink green tea.
2. Reduce saturated fat, sugar and alcohol. Avoid trans fats and chemical food additives.
3. Get regular exercise, reduce stress, and don't smoke.
4. Avoid exposure to pesticides, phthalates, and other carcinogens.
5. Take a multivitamin/mineral complex and consider supplements of Coriolus versicolor, ginseng, and IP6.

CARPAL TUNNEL SYNDROME

Carpal tunnel syndrome (CTS) is a condition marked by pain, inflammation, and numbness in a small opening in the wrist that protects the main nerve and tendons that run to your hand. This nerve is sensitive to pressure. Repetitive wrist movements that cause inflammation or anything that narrows the space of the carpal tunnel and puts pressure on the nerve can lead to CTS. This condition is becoming increasingly common in recent years due to the types of jobs that people do today, particularly computer work, which leads to strain and pressure on the wrist. Bone spurs and arthritis can also cause swelling of the carpal tunnel and narrowing of this space, which place pressure on the nerve.

SIGNS & SYMPTOMS

The symptoms of CTS often start gradually and worsen over time, causing:

- Aching and pain in the wrist that may extend up your arm and your palm or fingers
- Numbness and tingling in your fingers or hand, which may be temporarily relieved by shaking your hand
- Weakness in your hands

RISK FACTORS

- Arthritis or bone spurs
- Gender (women are three times more likely to develop CTS)
- Genetics (being born with a narrow carpal tunnel)
- Injury (stress or force placed on the wrist area)
- Pregnancy or hormonal changes that cause fluid retention
- Repetitive use (working on computers, machinery, assembly line, or with power tools), particularly when done for an extended period without rest
- Smokers often have worse symptoms and slower recovery

DOCTOR'S ORDERS

Depending on the severity of the condition, there are a variety of options your doctor may recommend, such as wearing a wrist splint to provide support to the area and protect against further damage and injury. Non-steroidal anti-inflammatory drugs, such as ibuprofen, may be prescribed to reduce pain and inflammation. Stronger drugs called corticosteroids may be injected into the area to reduce inflammation. Neither of these drugs promote healing nor are they beneficial unless CTS is caused by underlying inflammation. For more severe forms of CTS, surgery may be done to cut the ligaments pressing on the nerve. This usually results in significant improvement, but there may still be some residual numbness, pain, stiffness, or weakness.

SHERRY'S NATURAL PRESCRIPTION

Dietary Recommendations

Foods to include:

- Beans, brewer's yeast, and whole grains (wheat germ) contain vitamin B6, which is important for nerve function.

- Vegetables and fruits contain vital antioxidants and nutrients that can help reduce inflammation and speed healing.

Foods to avoid:

- Minimize salt (processed foods and salt shaker), as it can cause fluid retention, which can worsen CTS.

- Saturated fat can impair circulation.

Lifestyle Suggestions

- Give your hands and wrists a break. When working on your computer or doing repetitive movements, take a break every 20 minutes and do some gentle stretches. Wear a wrist splint at night.

- Use proper form. For example, your keyboard should be at elbow height or slightly lower. Incorrect posture can cause strain on the neck and shoulders, which can worsen CTS. An occupational therapist can help by assessing your needs and making recommendations.

- Avoid using force with your hands. When working on a cash register or computer, hit the keys softly. Use a wide pen with a soft grip so that you don't have to squeeze the pen tightly.

- Warm paraffin wax treatments and hydrotherapy can help ease the symptoms.

- Massage, chiropractic, acupuncture, and physiotherapy are very beneficial.

- Yoga and stretching can help improve posture and strength and promote relaxation.

ACUPUNCTURE AND CARPAL TUNNEL SYNDROME

The National Institutes of Health released a consensus statement, after reviewing the scientific literature, and stated that acupuncture may be a useful treatment for treating the symptoms of carpal tunnel syndrome.

Top Recommended Supplements

Arnica: An herb that reduces pain and inflammation. One study found it particularly helpful in relieving pain after surgery. It is available in homeopathic tablets and topical creams and ointments.

Vitamin B6: Several studies have found that B6 can reduce the pain and symptoms of CTS. It may be particularly helpful in those with a B6 deficiency. Dosage: 100 mg three times daily. B6 is usually safe up to 500 mg daily; higher dosages can damage sensory nerves and cause numbness in the hands and feet.

Complementary Supplements

Boswellia: An herb with anti-inflammatory properties. Dosage: 1,000–1,500 mg two to three times daily.

Bromelain: An enzyme that may help to reduce inflammation. Dosage: 500 mg three time daily between meals.

Calcium and magnesium: These are important minerals for nerve and muscle function. Dosages: 500 mg calcium and 250 mg magnesium two to three times daily.

FINAL THOUGHTS

To prevent CTS or reduce the symptoms if you already have it, consider the following:

1. If you work on a computer or do repetitive wrist and arm movements, use proper form, take frequent breaks, wear a support, and avoid strong force.
2. Be gentle on your wrists.
3. Consider vitamin B6 and bromelain supplements.
4. Use topical products with arnica to reduce pain and inflammation.
5. Acupuncture, massage, and chiropractic are helpful.

CATARACTS

Cataracts are cloudy spots that develop on the normally clear lens of the eye. Initially they might not be noticeable; however, as they progress, cataracts cause gradual clouding and loss of vision.

Cataracts are the leading cause of blindness in North America. They are most common among older adults. In fact, about half of Canadians over 65 years have visual impairment due to cataracts. This can affect normal daily activities, making it difficult to read, drive a car, and walk safely.

In most people cataracts occur due to age-related changes in the lens. The lens is comprised mainly of protein fibres and water. With age, the lens undergoes changes; it becomes thicker, less flexible, and less transparent. The protein fibres break down and begin to clump together, creating cloudy spots on the lens, which become progressively worse. Cataracts tend to develop slowly in both eyes at the same time unless they are caused by an injury that affects only one eye. Cataracts that become completely white, known as overripe (hypermature) cataracts, can cause inflammation, pain, and headache.

Cataracts are not considered a "normal" part of aging, yet they do primarily affect older adults, likely due to lifetime exposure to free radicals from smoking, chemicals, UV light, and other factors that damage the lens.

There are other potential causes of cataracts. Infants may be born with cataracts if their mother contracted German measles (rubella) during pregnancy. They can also develop secondary to diabetes, injury, heavy metal poisoning, use of certain medications, and other factors as listed below.

For the majority of people, it is possible to delay and even prevent cataracts with lifestyle modifications and supplements. However, once a cataract has developed, it cannot be reversed; at this point surgery is the only option to restore vision.

SIGNS & SYMPTOMS

- Cloudy and blurred vision
- Fading or yellowing of colours
- Halos around lights
- Poor night vision
- Sensitivity to light and glare

RISK FACTORS

- Advanced age
- Diabetes and obesity
- Exposure to radiation
- Family history
- Heavy metal poisoning

- Injury, trauma, or surgery to the eye

- Poor diet (a deficiency of antioxidants such as vitamins C and E, beta carotene, and selenium)

- Smoking

- Use of corticosteroids (cortisone, prednisone)

- UV light exposure

DOCTOR'S ORDERS

Once a cataract is fully developed, the only way to remove it is through surgery. An ophthalmologist replaces the clouded lens with a clear lens implant. In some cases the cataract is removed and vision is corrected with glasses or contact lenses rather than with an implant.

SHERRY'S NATURAL PRESCRIPTION

Dietary Recommendations

Foods to include:

- Research shows that a diet high in fruits and vegetables can help prevent cataract development because these foods provide excellent sources of antioxidants, which help reduce free radical damage.

- Foods high in antioxidants include berries (acai, blueberry, and cranberry), cherries, tomatoes, peppers, carrots, grapes, mangos, and citrus fruits.

- Kale, collard greens, spinach, and broccoli are great sources of the carotenoids lutein and zeaxanthin, which lower the risk of cataracts and macular degeneration.

Foods to avoid:

- Fast food and processed foods contain hydrogenated (trans fats) and saturated fats, which generate free radicals.

- Limit alcohol, as it impairs the liver's ability to detoxify harmful chemicals from the diet and environment.

Lifestyle Suggestions

- Get regular eye exams at least every other year. While this won't prevent cataracts, early detection gives you a chance to take steps to slow or prevent their development.

- Don't smoke, as smoking is a known risk factor because it generates damaging free radicals. Avoid smoky environments and people who smoke, as second-hand exposure can be just as damaging.

- Wear proper-fitting sunglasses with UV protection and wide-brim hats to shield your eyes from the sun's damaging rays.

- Maintain a healthy body weight. Obesity is associated with increased risk of cataracts.

Top Recommended Supplements

Carotenoids: Beta-carotene and lutein are important antioxidants in the eye; numerous studies have shown that they protect against cataracts by shielding the eye against light damage. Dosages: 25,000 IU of beta-carotene; 6 mg of lutein.

Vitamin C: A major antioxidant in the lens; essential for healthy vision and to protect the eye against free radicals. Levels in the eye decrease with age. Research has shown that supplements of vitamin C can lower the risk of cataracts. Dosage: 500–1,000 mg daily.

Vitamin E: Activates glutathione, which is an important antioxidant in the eye. Low blood levels of vitamin E have been linked to increased risk of cataracts and some research shows protective benefits with supplements. Dosage: 400 IU daily.

HOW TO AVOID CATARACTS

The majority of the research evaluating the effect of antioxidant supplements has found protective benefits with long-term use lasting five to 10 years. Cataracts develop slowly over time. Consistent and long-term use of antioxidants, along with lifestyle changes, are your best defence. In one study, people who took multivitamins or supplements containing vitamins C or E for more than 10 years had a 60 percent lower risk of developing cataracts (*Archives of Ophthalmology*, 2000: 118;1556–1563).

Complementary Supplements

B-complex: Vitamins B2 and B3 protect glutathione in the eye, and some evidence shows protective benefits with supplements. Dosage: 50–100 mg of B-vitamins.

Bilberry: Rich in antioxidant flavonoids, which are protective to the lens. Dosage: 240–480 mg daily.

FINAL THOUGHTS

To delay the onset of cataracts and preserve your vision, consider the following:

1. Get regular eye exams.
2. Boost antioxidant and carotenoid intake by eating lots of berries, carrots, peppers, kale, collard greens, spinach, and broccoli.
3. Wear sunglasses with UV protection and wide-brim hats when outdoors or driving.
4. Don't smoke and avoid exposure to second-hand smoke.
5. Protect your eyes with supplements of vitamin C, E, and carotenoids.

CELIAC DISEASE (GLUTEN INTOLERANCE)

Celiac disease is a digestive disorder caused by an abnormal immune reaction to the consumption of gluten, a protein found primarily in wheat, barley, rye, and triticale. Celiac disease is much more common than previously thought. It is estimated to affect one in 133 Canadians. However, only about 3 percent of these have been diagnosed.

When a person with celiac disease eats gluten-containing food, the immune system reacts by producing antibodies, which attack the villi in the small intestine, reducing their ability to absorb nutrients. Over time, the reduced absorption of nutrients leads to malnutrition and vitamin, mineral, and essential fatty acid deficiencies. This can damage the health of every organ and body system and increase the risk of many diseases, such as osteoporosis and depression.

The cause of celiac is not known; however, three factors are typically present in those who develop the disease: genetic predisposition, a diet containing gluten, and a triggering event. Possible triggers include: introduction of grains into a baby's diet, puberty, pregnancy, menopause, stress, viral or bacterial infection, and trauma (accident, surgery).

There is no cure for celiac disease, but the condition can be managed by following a gluten-free diet for life. Supplements can play an important role in restoring health.

SIGNS & SYMPTOMS

Symptoms of celiac vary greatly and may include:

- Abdominal cramps and bloating
- Anemia
- Chronic diarrhea or constipation
- Dental and bone disorders
- Fatigue
- Irritability and depression
- Joint pain
- Skin rash or mouth sores
- Stunted growth in children
- Tingling in the legs and feet
- Weight loss

Note: Dermatitis herpetiformis is an itchy, blistering skin disease that also results from gluten intolerance. It typically affects the elbows, knees, and buttocks.

Those who do not adhere to a gluten-free diet are at greater risk of developing osteoporosis; cancer of the intestines, mouth, esophagus, or bowel; and neurological diseases (seizures and nerve damage).

- Existing autoimmune disease such as Lupus erythematosus, type 1 diabetes, rheumatoid arthritis, or thyroid disease

- Family history: Having a family member with celiac increases your risk by 10–20 percent.

DOCTOR'S ORDERS

Your doctor will recommend a strict gluten-free diet and a consultation with a dietitian to learn what this entails. Once gluten is removed from the diet, the villi start to heal and intestinal inflammation subsides. Complete healing and regrowth of the villi may take several months in younger people and as long as two to three years in older people. For severe cases that don't respond to dietary changes, medications such as prednisone are temporarily used to suppress the immune response.

SHERRY'S NATURAL PRESCRIPTION

A strict gluten-free diet is crucial for those with celiac disease. Vitamin, mineral, and essential fatty acid supplements are recommended to correct deficiencies and restore health.

Dietary Recommendations

Read labels carefully; look for products labelled gluten-free. If in doubt, contact the manufacturer. When eating out, ask to speak directly to the chef as service staff may not be familiar with gluten and the many possible hidden sources. Cross-contamination can occur if gluten-free foods are prepared in unwashed bowls previously containing gluten, or cooked in the same pots or deep-fryer.

Foods to include:

- Lean meats, fish and poultry, fruits, vegetables, corn, potato, rice, quinoa, and soy. Healthy fats (fish, nuts, and seeds) are very important to help restore essential fatty acids, which are depleted in those with celiac disease.

- Flours made from amaranth, buckwheat, rice, soy, corn, potato, and tapioca are allowed and can be substituted in recipes.

Foods to avoid:

- Foods containing wheat, barley, rye, bulgur, Kamut, spelt, and triticale, such as breads, pasta, cereals, baked goods, crackers, and pies.

- Watch for hidden sources of gluten—prepared and processed foods, such as sauces, dressings, and coating agents.

Note: Dairy should be limited initially as damage to the intestines reduces the ability to digest lactose (dairy sugar). After the intestines have healed, dairy consumption can resume.

• •

The safety of oats in those with celiac is controversial. Several small studies investigated this matter. These studies used pure oats, free of gluten contamination, and the amount per day was limited. The Canadian Celiac Association has stated that consumption of pure, uncontaminated oats is safe in the amount of 50–70 g per day (1/2–3/4 cup of dry rolled oats) by adults and 20–25 g per day (1/4 cup of dry rolled oats) by children with celiac disease. Note: Some individuals may not tolerate even pure oats, in which case they should be completely avoided.

Lifestyle Suggestions

To promote healing and support immune function, it is important to get adequate rest, reduce stress, and strictly adhere to the gluten-free diet.

Top Recommended Supplements

Digestive enzymes: May be depleted in those with celiac; they aid proper digestion of food and are particularly important in newly diagnosed individuals. Once the intestines have healed, enzymes may not be necessary. Look for a broad-spectrum product containing lipase, amylase, and protease. Take as directed before meals.

Essential fatty acids: Are highly recommended to correct deficiencies, reduce inflammation, and promote healing of intestinal cells. Look for a product that provides both omega-3 (fish) and omega-6 (borage, primrose) fatty acids.

Multivitamin and mineral complex: This is absolutely essential to correct deficiencies and promote healing. The most common deficiencies include calcium, magnesium, iron, zinc, vitamins D and K, and folic acid. Even those who are stable on a gluten-free diet and in remission may still have nutrient deficiencies and would benefit from a supplement. Those with severe malnutrition and deficiencies may require higher than typical amounts. Consult with a health care provider for recommendations.

Complementary Supplements

Fibre: Often deficient in a gluten-free diet due to the elimination of many grains, so supplements can help improve bowel function and prevent constipation. Look for a product that contains a combination of soluble and insoluble fibres.

Green Food supplement: Provides vitamins, minerals, and fibre; improves energy and recovery. Ensure that the product is gluten-free.

Probiotics: Support intestinal health, restore normal flora, and improve bowel function. Look for a product that is non-dairy, stable at room temperature and provides at least 1 billion live cells. Take one to three capsules daily.

FINAL THOUGHTS

To improve health and reduce complications from celiac disease, consider the following:

1. Adhere to a strict gluten-free diet.
2. Eat a healthy diet, including fruits, vegetables, lean protein, healthy fats, and gluten-free grains.
3. To promote healing, get adequate rest and reduce stress.
4. Take a quality multivitamin/mineral complex, essential fatty acids, and enzymes.
5. Consider fibre, probiotics, and green food supplements.

CERVICAL DYSPLASIA

Cervical dysplasia is a condition in which cells on the surface of the cervix become pre-cancerous or cancerous. There are various grades of cervical dysplasia, which are classified upon the extent of the abnormal cell growth. Low-grade cervical dysplasia progresses very slowly and typically resolves on its own. High-grade cervical dysplasia tends to progress quickly and usually leads to cervical cancer.

The primary cause of cervical dysplasia is infection with human papilloma virus (HPV), but additional factors are involved in causing the cervical cells to change and become pre-cancerous, such as smoking, long-term use of birth control pills, and nutritional deficiencies. Risk factors are discussed below.

An estimated 66 percent of cervical dysplasia cases progress to cancer within 10 years. Cervical cancer constitutes more than 10 percent of cancers worldwide and is the second leading cause of death in women between the ages of 15 and 34. This is unfortunate because cervical cancer is largely preventable. With early identification, treatment, and consistent follow-up, nearly all cases of cervical dysplasia can be cured and cervical cancer can be prevented. Most cervical cancer deaths occur in women who have not had a Pap smear.

SIGNS & SYMPTOMS

There are usually no symptoms of cervical dysplasia and it is detected only during a Pap smear. In some cases woman may notice:

• Abnormal bleeding

• Genital warts

• Low back pain

• Spotting after intercourse

• Vaginal discharge

Note: These symptoms are not unique to cervical dysplasia and may indicate a different problem.

RISK FACTORS

• Being born to a mother who took diethylstilbestrol (DES) to become pregnant or to sustain pregnancy

• Genital warts

• Having a sexual partner whose former partner had cervical cancer

• History of a sexually transmitted disease (such as herpes)

• Human papilloma virus (HPV) infection

• Long-term use (five years or more) of birth control pills, which contain estrogen

• Multiple sexual partners

- Nutritional deficiencies in folate, vitamin A, beta carotene, selenium, vitamin E, and vitamin C

- Sexual activity at a young age (less than 18 years)

- Smoking

- Suppressed immune function (HIV or use of chemotherapeutic medications)

DOCTOR'S ORDERS

Regular Pap tests are essential to detect changes in cervical cells and prevent cervical cancer. Every woman should have an annual Pap test beginning at age 18 and continuing on past menopause. Many women stop having this done later in life, which is dangerous since the highest incidence of cervical cancer is among those over age 65.

Cervical dysplasia is curable, although the lifetime recurrence rate is 20 percent. For early stages of cervical dysplasia doctors may simply recommend frequent monitoring, as pre-cancerous changes may disappear on their own. Treatment of more advanced stages involves surgical removal of abnormal tissue. The most commonly used procedures include laser therapy, cryocauterization (use of extreme cold to destroy abnormal tissue), and loop excision (using a wire loop to remove tissue).

THE PAP TEST

The Pap test, named after Dr. Georgios Papanicolaou, the inventor, screens for cervical dysplasia and cancer. Your doctor takes a little scraping of cells in the cervical area for analysis by a laboratory. All women age 18 and over should have this test done annually. It takes only a few minutes, is almost painless, and could save your life.

SHERRY'S NATURAL PRESCRIPTION

As there are various lifestyle and nutritional factors implicated in cervical dysplasia, it is possible to make adjustments and improve the health of your cervical cells and reduce your risk of dysplasia and cancer. These natural therapies do not replace the need for regular medical examinations and doctor's supervision.

Dietary Recommendations

Foods to include:

- Increase intake of whole grains, fresh vegetables, and fruits. These foods are high in antioxidants, which fight free radical damage. They also contain vitamin C, folate, and beta-carotene, which have been found to be deficient in those who develop cervical dysplasia. Choose organic as much as possible.

- Eat liver-supporting foods such as beets, carrots, onions, garlic, leafy greens, artichokes, apples, and lemons, to support detoxification.

- Broccoli, cauliflower, Brussels sprouts, and cabbage contain indole-3-carbinol, which helps the liver break down estrogen.

- Flaxseed, soy, beans, and legumes contain phytoestrogens, which may help reduce the impact of other hormones.
- Green tea contains polyphenols, which have been found to inhibit growth of cancer cells and reduce cervical dysplasia.

Foods to avoid:

- Alcohol, caffeine, refined foods, food additives, sugar, and saturated fats may affect hormone balance, impair immune function, and worsen symptoms.
- Red meat and dairy products may contain dioxins and chemicals that act as estrogen-mimickers.

•••

EAT YOUR FRUITS AND VEGGIES

Several population-based studies have suggested that eating a diet rich in nutrients from fruits and vegetables may protect against the development of cervical cancer.

•••

Lifestyle Suggestions

- Minimize exposure to environmental estrogens or xenoestrogens (phthalates, parabens, and dioxins), which are present in pesticides, plastics, and certain skin care products. Read labels and check with manufacturers.
- Don't smoke, and avoid second-hand smoke.
- Sexually active women should use a barrier method, such as condoms or a diaphragm, for protection against sexually transmitted diseases.
- Get regular exercise. This is a natural way to enhance immune function and prevent disease. Try walking, cycling, or aerobics.
- Reduce stress. Try yoga, Pilates, stretching, acupuncture, and massage.

Top Recommended Supplements

Green tea: Helps prevent cancer growth. One study also found that daily supplements of green tea providing 200 mg of EGCG (antioxidant component) significantly reduced or eliminated abnormal cells in those with cervical dysplasia. Look for a supplement providing 200 mg EGCG.

Indole-3-carbinol: A compound found naturally in cruciferous vegetables that aids in detoxification of estrogen, protects liver function, and may protect against hormonal cancers. In one study supplements were found to improve lesions in those with cervical dysplasia. Dosage: 400 mg daily.

Complementary Supplements

B-vitamins: Some research has shown that women with low dietary intakes of vitamins B1, B2, B12, and folic acid are at greater risk of developing cervical dysplasia and those with higher intakes of these nutrients from food and supplements are at lower risk. These vitamins may protect against cellular changes that lead to dysplasia. Look for a broad-spectrum B-complex and take daily for prevention.

Calcium D-glucarate: Helps the liver detoxify and eliminate excess hormones, particularly estrogen. Not specifically studied for cervical dysplasia, but may help by reducing the harmful effects of estrogen. Dosage: 300–500 mg daily.

Vitamin C: Deficiencies have been associated with cervical dysplasia. It is not known whether supplements can reverse this condition. However, it is known that vitamin C supports immune function and is an antioxidant that protects against cellular damage. Dosage: 500 mg daily.

Beta-carotene: Some research suggests that a deficiency in beta-carotene increases the risk of cervical dysplasia and cancer, and that supplements may promote a regression or decline in the signs of cervical dysplasia. Dosage: 25,000 to 50,000 units (15 to 30 mg) daily.

FINAL THOUGHTS

To improve cervical health and reduce your risk of cervical dysplasia and cancer, consider the following:

1. Have an annual Pap test and discuss the results with your doctor.
2. Eat organic vegetables, fruits, whole grains, legumes, and flaxseed.
3. Minimize red meat, dairy, alcohol, caffeine, and refined foods.
4. Avoid exposure to smoke and environmental estrogens; practice safe sex.
5. Top recommended supplements are beta-carotene, indole-3-carbinol, and green tea. Consider B-vitamins, calcium D-glucarate, and vitamin C.

CHRONIC FATIGUE SYNDROME

Chronic fatigue syndrome (CFS) is a condition marked by profound fatigue, weakness, and flu-like symptoms that may last from months to years.

CFS has become known only in the past few decades and is a mysterious condition as there is no obvious cause, no clear tests to make a diagnosis, and there are few (if any) medical treatment options available. This condition is not very common. It is estimated to affect about 60,000 Canadians.

The exact cause of CFS is not known, but there are several possible causes that have been suggested, including:

- Chemical sensitivities or toxic exposure
- Chronic inflammation
- Chronic low blood pressure
- Hormonal imbalance—low cortisol, DHEA, or thyroid levels
- Hypoglycemia—low blood sugar
- Immune system dysfunction
- Infection with a cold, virus (Epstein-Barr virus or Human Herpes Virus 6), or yeast (*Candida albicans*)
- Iron-deficiency anemia
- Stress

While there are many mysteries surrounding CFS, there are various lifestyle approaches and nutritional supplements that can help improve quality of life in those suffering with this condition.

DIAGNOSIS FOR CFS

According to the International Chronic Fatigue Syndrome Study Group—a group of doctors and researchers who determined a standard method for defining CFS—a person meets the diagnostic criteria of CFS when unexplained persistent fatigue occurs for six months or more with at least four of the eight primary signs and symptoms listed below.

SIGNS & SYMPTOMS

Primary signs and symptoms:
- Extreme exhaustion after normal exercise or exertion
- Headache of a new type, pattern, or severity
- Loss of memory or concentration
- Pain that moves from one joint to another without swelling or redness
- Painful and mildly enlarged lymph nodes in your neck or armpits
- Sleep disturbance
- Sore throat
- Unexplained muscle soreness

Other signs and symptoms:
- Abdominal pain
- Alcohol intolerance
- Bloating
- Chest pain
- Chronic cough
- Diarrhea
- Dizziness
- Dry eyes and mouth
- Earache
- Irregular heartbeat
- Jaw pain
- Morning stiffness
- Nausea
- Night sweats
- Psychological problems, such as depression, irritability, anxiety disorders, and panic attacks
- Shortness of breath
- Tingling sensations
- Weight loss

RISK FACTORS

CFS is more common among women, but sex is not a proven risk factor for this condition. It is thought that women are more likely to report the symptoms to their doctors than men.

DOCTOR'S ORDERS

There is no specific drug treatment for chronic fatigue syndrome. Lifestyle measures are often tried first. Doctors may prescribe medications to address certain symptoms. However, these drugs can cause side effects that may actually be worse than the symptoms of the condition. These medications include antidepressants (Paxil, Zoloft, and Wellbutrin), anti-anxiety drugs (Xanax and Ativan), anti-inflammatory drugs (Motrin), and allergy drugs (antihistamines and decongestants).

SHERRY'S NATURAL PRESCRIPTION

Dietary Recommendations

Foods to include:

- Fish provides omega-3 fatty acids that reduce inflammation.

- Vegetables, fruits, and whole grains are rich in essential nutrients for immune function and optimal health. Choose organic produce to avoid harmful pesticides.

- Yogurt contains beneficial bacteria that support immune function and digestion.

Food to avoid:

- Processed and fast foods contain chemicals that may trigger allergic reactions and stress the body, worsening symptoms.

- Caffeine can affect sleep quality and cause irritability and anxiety.

- Refined flour and sugar can affect immune function and cause blood sugar imbalances, which may worsen hypoglycemia.

Lifestyle Suggestions

- Reduce stress—promote relaxation with meditation, yoga, stretching, and breathing exercises.

- Get adequate sleep, which is essential to help the body recover from illness and to help cope with stress.

- Exercise—light to moderate activity can help improve both physical and emotional symptoms. Try to get a combination of both aerobic activities (walking, biking, and swimming) along with resistance training (working out with weights or machines) and stretching. Some people with CFS are sensitive to exercise and overexertion can worsen fatigue. It is important to start slowly and gradually increase intensity and duration.

- Don't smoke—smoking causes damage to the nervous system and can worsen CFS symptoms.

- Acupuncture and massage are helpful for relieving pain, promoting relaxation, and improving sleep.

- Change the air filters in your home. Pollution and germs can cause symptoms similar to CFS.

Top Recommended Supplements

B-complex vitamins: Some studies have shown that those with CFS have B-vitamin deficiencies (particularly B6 and B12). B-vitamins are required for energy production, enzyme reactions, and many other vital body processes. Look for a supplement that provides the range of B-vitamins and take daily.

L-carnitine: Required for energy production in cells. Those with CFS may be deficient and supplements have shown benefits for reducing fatigue and other symptoms. Dosage: 1–2 g three times daily.

Magnesium: Levels may be depleted in those with CFS and supplements may help improve energy and emotional symptoms. Dosage: 200 mg three times daily.

Complementary Supplements

Coenzyme Q10: Essential for energy production in the cells. Dosage: 100 mg twice daily.

Fish oils: Help reduce inflammation and support brain function. Preliminary research shows benefits for reducing CFS symptoms. Dosage: 1–3 g daily. Look for a product that provides at least 400 mg EPA and 200 mg DHA per gram of fish oil.

NADH: Supports energy production in the body. Preliminary research shows reduction in fatigue and other symptoms. Dosage: 10 mg daily on an empty stomach.

FINAL THOUGHTS

To reduce symptoms of CFS and improve quality of life, consider the following:

1. Eat more organic fruits, vegetables, whole grains, fish, and yogurt.
2. Reduce stress and get adequate sleep.
3. Exercise regularly.
4. Try acupuncture and massage.
5. Consider supplements of B-complex vitamins, magnesium, and L-carnitine.

CHRONIC VENOUS INSUFFICIENCY

Chronic venous insufficiency (CVI) is a common condition of poor circulation that affects an estimated 2–5 percent of Canadians. CVI occurs when there is damage to or an absence of the one-way valves in the veins. Without functioning valves to prevent the backflow of blood, the blood pools in the veins, causing them to enlarge.

CVI can be congenital (you are born with it) or it can result from a blood clot, which damages the vein walls and valves. It often starts with the failure of a single valve, which creates a high-pressure leak in the venous system. The vein dilates, leading to failure of other nearby valves. After a series of valves have failed, the affected veins can no longer direct blood upward toward the heart. Blood pools in the veins, causing them to enlarge. This scenario often continues as increasing numbers of valves fail under the strain and high pressure, and more and more veins become affected.

SIGNS & SYMPTOMS

The symptoms of CVI are worse during the day while you are upright and include:

- Burning and itching

- Enlarged veins (varicose veins)

- Heavy, aching legs

- Leg swelling

- Pain and pressure

- Restless legs

If the swelling is not controlled, inflammation occurs in the skin and tissues beneath the skin. The skin may develop reddish-brown spots called lipodermatosclerosis. Over time, the skin thickens and becomes hard, leathery, dry, and itchy. If a break in the skin occurs, a venous ulcer or chronic sore may develop.

RISK FACTORS

- Advanced age: Women over 40 and men over 70 years

- Chronic constipation: Increases venous pressure

- Gender: Women are at greater risk

- Lack of activity/movement: Minimizes the pump action of the calf muscles, causing higher venous pressure

- Obesity: Carrying excess weight increases venous pressure

- Occupation: Long periods of standing with little movement can increase venous pressure and weaken the vein walls and valves

- Pregnancy: Due to hormonal changes and carrying extra weight

- Previous vein problems: A history of deep vein thrombosis (DVT), which damages the valves, causing backflow and increased venous pressure

- Smoking: Causes damage to the valves and veins

DOCTOR'S ORDERS

Medical treatment is aimed at improving blood flow and preventing pooling of blood and further damage to the valves and veins. Options include:

Ablation/sclerotherapy/laser: Procedures that destroy the damaged vein; blood is rerouted through other veins, and the damaged vein is absorbed by the body.

Bypass: An artificial or transplanted vein is connected to the damaged vein to help improve blood flow.

Compression stockings: They provide firm support to improve blood flow back to the heart and prevent leg swelling; available for both men and women; custom ordered to size.

Hospitalization and antibiotic therapy: For severe venous ulcers.

Stripping: A surgical procedure to remove the damaged vein.

Valve repair: A surgical procedure to shorten the valves and improve valve function.

SHERRY'S NATURAL PRESCRIPTION

Dietary Recommendations

Foods to include:

- A high-fibre diet is essential to prevent constipation and straining. Eat plenty of fruits, vegetables, whole grains, legumes, nuts, and seeds. These foods are also high in antioxidants and good fats, both of which are helpful for circulation.

Foods to avoid:

- Saturated fats (animal fats) and trans fats (fast food and processed food) impede circulation, cause free radical damage, and trigger inflammation.
- Reduce sodium intake (soda pop, chips, crackers, and deli meats) as it can increase fluid retention and swelling.

Lifestyle Suggestions

- Exercise regularly: Activities that involve the calf muscle will help pump blood back to the heart. Try walking, cycling, and swimming.
- Elevate your legs above the thighs when resting.
- Avoid standing or sitting in the same spot for a long time. Move around, flex your ankles, circle your foot, do calf raises, and shift your body weight.
- Lose excess weight, which will reduce pressure on your legs.
- Avoid excessive heat on your legs (sunbathing and hot baths), which causes the veins to dilate, thus worsening the problem.
- Don't cross your legs, as it hampers circulation and worsens symptoms.
- Avoid wearing high heels and tight shoes or clothing, as they impair circulation.
- Avoid constipation and straining on the toilet, as this can increase vein pressure.
- Don't smoke, as smoking damages the veins and blood vessels, increases blood pressure, and impairs circulation.

Top Recommended Supplements

Diosmin: Improves the tone and strength of the veins, reduces swelling, fights free-radical damage, and stimulates lymphatic flow. It has a quick onset of action (one to two weeks) and is not associated with any side effects or drug interactions. Dosage: 600 mg once daily of a product standardized to provide 95 percent diosmin and 5 percent hesperidin.

••

Over 30 clinical studies have found diosmin safe and effective for improving vein disorders, including chronic venous insufficiency and varicose veins.

••

Horse chestnut seed extract: Promotes circulation, improves vein wall tone, and relieves swelling. It offers modest benefits and may take six to eight weeks. It may cause nausea and upset stomach and can enhance the effect of blood-thinning medications. Avoid it if you have kidney or liver disease. Dosage: 300 mg twice daily; standardized to 50 mg of aescin.

Pine bark extract: A flavonoid that offers antioxidant activity, strengthens capillaries, improves circulation, and supports vein health. A few small studies have shown benefits. Dosage: 100–300 mg daily. There are no known side effects or drug interactions.

Complementary Supplements

Antioxidants: Help improve circulation and vein health. In addition to diosmin and pine bark, other antioxidants to consider include vitamins C and E, bilberry, and grape seed extract. Follow label instructions.

Butcher's broom: Improves the strength and tone of the veins, acts as a mild diuretic, and has mild anti-inflammatory effects. Dosage: 100 mg three times daily.

Gotu kola: Is a plant extract shown in preliminary research to reduce swelling, pain, fatigue, sensation of heaviness, and fluid leakage from the veins. Dosage: 60–120 mg daily.

FINAL THOUGHTS

To prevent and improve CVI, consider the following:

1. Boost intake of fibre and antioxidant-rich foods; reduce your intake of saturated fats, processed foods, and sodium.
2. Don't smoke.
3. Exercise regularly, elevate your feet when resting, and avoid standing or sitting in the same spot.
4. Wear compression stockings.
5. Consider supplements of diosmin and pine bark.

COLD SORES

Cold sores, also known as fever blisters, are small lesions that appear on the lips or surrounding skin. They are primarily caused by infection with the herpes simplex type 1 virus (HSV-1), although they can result from herpes simplex type 2 virus (HSV-2), which is the virus that causes genital herpes. Approximately 80 percent of people carry the HSV-1 virus, and of those 20–40 percent experience recurrent cold sores (two or more outbreaks per year).

Most people contract cold sores during childhood, although some people get them later in life.

After infection with the virus, it can remain dormant for long periods of time and then periodically cause outbreaks, particularly when the immune system is weakened. There is no cure for the virus. However, there are a number of methods to reduce the risk of recurrence.

SIGNS & SYMPTOMS

The initial infection may cause flu-like symptoms (fever and fatigue). An outbreak of cold sores causes:

• Clusters of tiny, red, fluid-filled blisters

• Crusting once they burst

• Pain

Cold sores typically last for seven to 10 days. However, they can become infected if picked, which delays healing.

WARNING SIGNS: Those who get recurrent cold sores typically experience prodromal symptoms before an outbreak—tingling, itching, or burning around the lips. These symptoms usually occur 24–48 hours prior to the eruption of a lesion.

RISK FACTORS

The virus is spread through contact with the fluid from the cold sore blisters or the saliva of an infected individual. The lesions remain contagious until they have healed completely. Once you carry the virus, risk factors for an outbreak include:

• Drying of the lips (exposure to sun and wind)

• Fatigue

• Fever

• Hormonal changes in women (menstruation or pregnancy)

• Illness

• Stress

• Trauma

Those with a weakened immune system (having cancer, AIDS, or an organ transplant) are prone to more frequent and severe bouts of cold sores. In these individuals, cold sores can become a serious health risk.

DOCTOR'S ORDERS

Cold sores generally clear up without treatment. Contact your doctor if: the sores do not heal within two weeks; the symptoms are severe; you get frequent recurrences; you experience pain or irritation in your eyes.

Prescription antiviral drugs such as Valtrex and Zovirax may shorten the duration and severity of the infection, but are not approved for prevention. These drugs are expensive, associated with side effects (nausea, vomiting, and headache), and are not recommended for children, pregnant women, or those with impaired kidney or liver function.

Over-the-counter products that may be recommended include:

Aspirin, acetaminophen (Tylenol) or ibuprofen: Oral medications that help reduce pain.

Abreva: A cream that may help to shorten the duration of the outbreak.

Lipactin: A gel that helps to soothe the skin but does not shorten the duration.

SHERRY'S NATURAL PRESCRIPTION

There are several natural methods to speed healing of cold sores and prevent outbreaks.

Dietary Recommendations

Foods to include:

• Foods high in the amino acid lysine (legumes, fish, meat, and dairy) may help to reduce levels of arginine.

• Fruits, vegetables, and whole grains provide essential nutrients to support immune heath.

Foods to avoid:

• Foods that contain high amounts of arginine (chocolate, nuts, whole grains, and gelatin) allow the cold sore virus to thrive.

Lifestyle Suggestions

To avoid contracting or spreading the virus, don't share personal items such as drinking glasses, toothbrushes, razors, lipstick, or towels. If you have a cold sore, wash your hands before touching another person.

Those who suffer from recurrent cold sores can benefit from the following:

• intercept CS Cold Sore Prevention System: A device approved by Health Canada for the prevention of cold sores. It provides thermal therapy to enhance the immune system response and stop the virus. Clinical studies have shown that it can prevent outbreaks when used during the prodromal phase. There are no side effects; it can be used by children over six years and pregnant women; available without a prescription in most pharmacies.

- Sunscreen: Apply to lips and face before going out in the sun. Use a minimum of SPF 30.

- Moisturize: Use lip balm regularly to prevent the lips from becoming dry, chapped, or cracked.

- Relax: Work on reducing stress, which is a common trigger for cold sores. Try yoga, meditation, tai chi, and breathing exercises to promote relaxation.

- Sleep: Get adequate rest, which is essential for the immune system.

Once the blisters have appeared, try the following:

- Apply an ice pack, wrapped in a washcloth, for five minutes several times a day to ease pain and help dry out the sores.

- Dab the cold sore with a witch hazel on a cotton ball. Witch hazel has antiviral activity against HSV-1 and can reduce inflammation and spreading of the virus. Pharmacies keep this behind the counter, so you will have to ask for it.

Do not pick or squeeze a cold sore blister or scab. This may cause it to spread, delay the healing process, and lead to infection.

Top Recommended Supplements

Lemon balm: An herb, also known as *Melissa officinalis*, lemon balm has antiviral properties that can help speed healing and shorten the duration of an outbreak. Look for a cream containing 1 percent lemon balm extract. Apply two to four times daily for a week.

Lysine: An amino acid that inhibits growth of the cold sore virus and may reduce recurrence; take at the first sign of a cold sore. Dosage: 1–3 g daily. Creams containing lysine can help promote healing, but do not prevent outbreaks.

Complementary Supplement

Antioxidants: The antioxidants vitamins C and E may help to promote healing and strengthen the immune system's response to the virus. Vitamin E oil can also be applied directly to the affected area. In some studies this was found to reduce pain and accelerate healing.

FINAL THOUGHTS

Cold sores are an unpleasant, but largely preventable health concern. Here are the main points to keep in mind:

1. To cut your risk of an outbreak, get adequate rest, reduce stress, avoid sharing utensils or personal items, and wear sunscreen and lip balm.
2. Eat a healthy diet, including lysine-rich legumes and fish.
3. Never pick or squeeze cold sores.
4. Use a cold pack and witch hazel to relieve pain and prevent spreading, and a cream with lemon balm to promote healing.
5. To prevent outbreaks, use intercept CS and lysine supplements.

COMMON COLD

The common cold is an infection of the upper respiratory tract caused by a virus. There are over 200 viruses that cause colds; the most common is the rhinovirus. Colds are a major cause of doctor's appointments and lost work and school days. Children are most susceptible to contracting the virus and may experience as many as 10 colds a year. As we get older, we develop immunity to many viruses and are less likely to get colds.

Colds are highly contagious. The virus enters your body through your nose or mouth. For example, if you are beside someone who has the virus and coughs or sneezes and you inhale those virus droplets, then you can catch a cold. It can also be spread by hand-to-hand contact or by touching an object that has been contaminated with the virus and then rubbing your eyes, nose, or mouth.

A healthy functioning immune system is your best defence against a cold. If you catch a cold, there are a variety of lifestyle measures and supplements that can help speed healing and improve symptoms.

SIGNS & SYMPTOMS

Since there are many viruses that cause colds, symptoms and intensity vary, and include:

• Cough

• Head and body ache

• Low-grade fever

• Nasal discharge (yellow/green)

• Sinus congestion and runny nose

• Sneezing

• Sore, scratchy throat

• Watery eyes

Note: Colds typically last for seven to 14 days and improve without treatment. In some cases, though, a cold can lead to an ear infection, sinusitis, strep throat, bronchitis, pneumonia, or a flare-up of asthma.

IS IT A COLD OR FLU?

These infections are caused by different types of viruses. However, they do share some common symptoms such as aching, weakness, sore throat, and congestion. Here is where they differ: The flu causes a sudden onset of severe aching, pain, headache, and high fever (39°–40°C). Colds develop more slowly, don't usually cause fever, and cause only mild aching and fatigue. The flu is a serious respiratory illness and can lead to bronchitis, pneumonia, and respiratory failure. Contact your doctor if you suspect you have the flu.

- Age: Children are more susceptible because they have not developed resistance to viruses, plus children play together closely and are not careful about washing their hands and covering their mouths when they cough or sneeze.

- Poor diet: Nutritional deficiencies and excessive alcohol intake have all been linked to increased susceptibility.

- Season: Colds occur more frequently during the fall and winter because people spend more time indoors and are close together, which increases transmission; viruses survive better in low humidity, and cold temperatures make your nose drier and more susceptible to contracting a virus.

- Smoking: Damages nasal passages and makes it easier for viruses to enter.

- Stress and lack of sleep: Weaken the immune system and increase susceptibility.

DOCTOR'S ORDERS

Colds are not caused by bacteria, so antibiotics should not be used to treat a cold unless you develop a secondary bacterial infection such as strep throat or bronchitis.

Over-the-counter remedies, such as antihistamines, decongestants, and cough suppressants, may provide some symptom relief, but these products do not prevent or speed healing. As well, most of these products cause side effects. Antihistamines cause dry eyes/nose/mouth and drowsiness, and decongestants can raise blood pressure and cause dizziness and insomnia.

Tylenol (acetaminophen) can help reduce fever, aches, and pains, but it should be avoided by those with liver or kidney disease. Aspirin can also help these symptoms, but it should not be taken by children or teenagers because of the risk of Reye's syndrome. Those with kidney disease, ulcers, or risk of bleeding (taking blood thinners) should also avoid aspirin.

It is not necessary to see your doctor for a cold unless you or your child have a fever greater than 38°C along with aching, fatigue, sweating, and chills, or if there is vomiting, ear pain, coloured phlegm, or if symptoms persist longer than 10 days.

SHERRY'S NATURAL PRESCRIPTION

Dietary Recommendations

Foods to include:

- Fruits and vegetables (especially garlic, onions, ginger, and horseradish) provide important nutrients and compounds that support immune function.

- Drink plenty of fluids (water, juice, herbal tea, and soup). Elderberry juice has antiviral activity.

- Herbal teas, such as Throat Coat, which contains marshmallow and licorice, has been shown in research to help relieve sore throat.

Foods to avoid:

- Sugar hampers immune function, so avoid eating candy and sweets.

- Milk and dairy can be mucus forming, and may worsen congestion.

Lifestyle Suggestions

- Get extra rest to allow your body to recover.

- Manage stress—try breathing techniques, exercise, and meditation.

- For a sore throat, gargle with warm salt water and try lozenges that contain one or more of the following ingredients: slippery elm, marshmallow, vitamin C, zinc, eucalyptus, or menthol.

- For dry nose, try a nasal lubricant, such as Secaris or a saline nasal spray. Use a cool mist humidifier or vaporizer to add moisture to the air. Adding eucalyptus oil will help relieve nasal and sinus congestion and cough.

To prevent acquiring or spreading a cold:

- Wash your hands frequently.

- Don't rub your eyes, nose, or mouth unless you have just washed your hands.

- Cover your mouth and nose when you sneeze or cough.

- Avoid exposure to those who have a cold.

- Don't share drinking glasses and utensils.

- Disinfect your kitchen, bathroom, and common living areas, especially when someone in the house has a cold.

- Exercise regularly, as exercise enhances immune function.

Top Recommended Supplements

American ginseng: One particular product, Cold-FX, a patented extract of polysaccharides derived from North American ginseng, has been shown in clinical studies to be effective in the prevention and relief of colds and flus, as it strengthens immune function. See package for directions.

Echinacea: Shown in several studies to reduce the severity and frequency of cold symptoms. Look for Echinacea purpurea. Dosage: 300–600 mg capsules twice daily or 2–4 mL tincture four to six times daily at the first sign of a cold for seven to 10 days. Studies have not found this herb effective in children or as a cold preventative.

Vitamin C: Several studies have shown that vitamin C can reduce the duration and severity of colds. Dosage: 1–3 g daily throughout the cold season.

Zinc lozenges: Help relieve symptoms (coughing, sore throat, and runny nose) and shorten the duration of a cold. Look for a product that provides 13–25 mg of zinc (gluconate or acetate). Take at the first sign of a cold. Dosage: One lozenge every few hours while awake, up to a maximum 4 to 6 lozenges daily.

Complementary Supplements

Aged garlic extract: Taken regularly, it may help prevent colds by supporting immune function. Dosage: One to two capsules twice daily.

Probiotics: Support immune function and may help to prevent colds. Look for a product that provides at least one billion live cells and includes Lactobacillus acidophilus and bifido-bacterium, such as Kyo-Dophilus. Dosage: Take two to three times daily with meals.

Propolis: A resin collected from trees. Some research suggests that it can help prevent and shorten the duration of a cold. Dosage: 500 mg twice daily.

FINAL THOUGHTS

To reduce your chances of catching a cold, and speed the healing process when you do get a cold:

1. Eat a diet rich in fruits and vegetables; drink plenty of fluids.
2. Exercise regularly and reduce stress.
3. Wash your hands frequently and don't rub your eyes, nose, or mouth.
4. For prevention, consider Cold-FX and vitamin C.
5. To shorten the duration of a cold, try echinacea and zinc lozenges.

CONGESTIVE HEART FAILURE

Congestive heart failure (CHF), known simply as heart failure, occurs when your heart can't pump enough blood to meet your body's needs. CHF often results from other heart conditions, such as coronary artery disease or high blood pressure, which over time can damage and weaken the heart. When the heart can no longer pump blood efficiently through your body, blood and fluids back up into the circulatory system, causing swelling in your lungs, legs, feet, and ankles and congestive symptoms such as shortness of breath.

Heart failure can develop suddenly due to damage caused by a heart attack, or it can develop gradually after years of having high blood pressure, coronary artery disease, or a defective heart valve. A number of lifestyle factors contribute to heart failure such as smoking, obesity, and diet. In some cases, though, the heart becomes weakened without explanation. This is called idiopathic dilated cardiomyopathy.

Heart failure is treatable with medication and lifestyle modifications. In many cases it is possible to prevent heart failure by controlling the risk factors that damage the heart. Maintaining a healthy diet, exercising regularly, not smoking, and reducing stress can help significantly. There are also a variety of supplements that can strengthen the function of the heart.

SIGNS & SYMPTOMS

- Difficulty in concentrating or decreased alertness

- Fatigue and weakness

- Irregular or rapid heartbeat

- Lack of appetite and nausea

- Persistent cough or wheezing

- Reduced ability to exercise

- Shortness of breath when you exert yourself or lie down

- Sudden weight gain from fluid retention

- Swelling in your legs, ankles, feet, or abdomen

ACUTE HEART FAILURE

Acute heart failure occurs when something suddenly affects your heart's ability to function, such as a heart attack, a virus that attacks the heart muscle, severe infections, an allergic reaction, or a blood clot in the lungs. Signs and symptoms are similar to those of chronic heart failure, but are more severe and start suddenly. Acute heart failure can trigger a rapid heartbeat and abnormal rhythm. This requires immediate medical attention.

C

- Alcohol weakens the heart muscle.

- Arrhythmia, an abnormal heartbeat, weakens the heart.

- Congenital heart defects.

- Coronary artery disease: Plaque buildup causes the arteries to narrow, which limits the heart's supply of oxygen-rich blood.

- Diabetes increases the risk of high blood pressure and coronary artery disease.

- Heart attack damages the heart muscle.

- High blood pressure forces the heart to work harder.

- Kidney disease can cause high blood pressure and fluid retention, which contributes to heart failure.

- Obesity.

- Sleep apnea, an inability to breathe properly at night, results in low blood oxygen levels and increased risk of abnormal heart rhythms.

- Viral infection can damage the heart muscle.

DOCTOR'S ORDERS

Heart failure is a serious disease that requires medical care. Your doctor will recommend a combination of lifestyle measures and medications to help improve the strength of the heart and reduce symptoms of heart failure.

Commonly used medications include:

Angiotensin-converting enzyme (ACE) inhibitors: Vasodilator drugs that widen or dilate blood vessels to lower blood pressure, improve blood flow, and decrease the workload on the heart. Examples include enalapril (Vasotec), lisinopril (Prinivil, Zestril), and ramipril (Altace). A major unpleasant side effect of these drugs is chronic cough.

Angiotensin II (A-II) receptor blockers (ARBs): Work the same as the drugs above, but do not cause coughing. Examples include losartan (Cozaar) and valsartan (Diovan).

Beta blockers: Slow your heart rate and reduce blood pressure. Examples include carvedilol (Coreg), metoprolol (Lopressor), and propranolol (Inderal).

Digoxin (Lanoxin): Increases the strength of your heart muscle contractions and slows the heartbeat.

Diuretics: Commonly called water pills, diuretics make you urinate more frequently and keep fluid from collecting in your body. Examples include furosemide (Lasix) and spironolactone (Aldactone).

In some cases, surgery can be done to correct the underlying problem, such as replacing a faulty heart valve, or doing bypass surgery on severely narrowed arteries. For those with severe heart failure that can't be helped by surgery or medications, a heart transplant may be necessary.

SHERRY'S NATURAL PRESCRIPTION

The key to managing or preventing heart failure is to get the risk factors under control, namely, high blood pressure and coronary artery disease. In this section I outline dietary, lifestyle, and supplement strategies that help improve heart function.

Dietary Recommendations

Foods to include:

- Cold-water fish contains beneficial fatty acids that can help reduce blood pressure and cholesterol.

- Drink green tea, which contains antioxidants that offer benefits for the heart.

- Eat small, frequent meals. Overeating is hard on the heart.

- Garlic and onions contain antioxidants that help lower blood pressure and cholesterol.

- Soy foods can help lower blood pressure. Incorporate soy milk, tofu, soy protein, and soy nuts into your diet.

- Whole grains, vegetables, fruits, beans, and legumes contain lots of fibre along with essential nutrients, which help lower blood pressure and cholesterol.

Foods to avoid:

- Alcohol can weaken heart function and interacts negatively with many heart medications. Avoid or limit alcohol to one drink per day.

- Caffeine can increase heart rate and affect heart rhythm.

- Saturated fat (red meat and dairy) and trans fats can increase cholesterol and the risk of coronary heart disease.

- Sodium (salt) can cause water retention and worsen heart failure. Limit sodium intake to 2,000 mg per day. Foods high in sodium include snack foods (chips, pretzels), deli meats, soft drinks, and fast foods. Don't add salt to your foods—season with herbs instead.

Note: Those with heart failure may need to limit fluid intake to prevent water retention. Speak with your doctor about this.

Lifestyle Suggestions

- Don't smoke, and avoid second-hand smoke. Tobacco damages blood vessels, reduces the oxygen in your blood, and makes your heart beat faster.

- Maintain a healthy body weight. Being overweight increases stress to the heart.

- Get regular, moderate-intensity exercise, such as walking or swimming. Studies have shown that exercise can improve quality of life and function in those with CHF.

- Manage your stress. Stress increases heart rate and blood pressure, straining the heart. Try yoga, acupuncture, and meditation.

- Get adequate sleep at night (seven to nine hours). If you have shortness of breath during the night, prop up your pillow.

Top Recommended Supplements

Coenzyme Q10: An antioxidant that naturally occurs in all cells and is involved in energy production. People with CHF have lower levels of Q10. Several studies have shown that supplements can significantly improve CHF symptoms and quality of life. Dosage: 100–300 mg daily.

Hawthorn: Improves the heart's pumping ability and improves blood flow. Numerous studies have found that it can reduce symptoms of CHF and improve exercise capacity. Some research suggests that it may also help to prevent arrhythmias. Dosage: 300–600 mg three times daily.

L-carnitine: An amino acid naturally found in all cells. It helps the heart contract and produce energy more efficiently. Studies show that it improves heart function and can reduce the symptoms of CHF. Dosage: 1,000 mg three times daily.

Complementary Supplements

Calcium and magnesium: Essential for proper muscle contractions and blood vessel health. Levels of calcium and magnesium are depleted by diuretics and digoxin, commonly used CHF drugs. Several studies have found that these minerals can promote modest reductions in blood pressure and improve CHF. Magnesium can also help prevent abnormal heart rhythm. Dosage: 1,500 mg calcium and 500 mg magnesium daily. Take in divided dosages with meals.

Fish oils: Over 30 studies have shown that the omega-3 fatty acids in fish oil can help lower blood pressure, reduce atherosclerosis, and protect against heart attack. Dosage: 3 g of EPA plus DHA three times daily.

Garlic: Helps lower blood pressure and cholesterol, reduces clotting, and prevents plaque formation in the arteries. Most of the research showing benefits has been done on aged garlic extract (Kyolic). Dosage: 600 mg twice daily.

L-taurine: An amino acid that helps increase the force and effectiveness of heart-muscle contractions. Research has shown that taurine can reduce the symptoms of CHF. Dosage: 2 g three times daily.

Natural relaxants: Hops, lemon balm, passionflower, and valerian are herbs that can help promote calming, which can help those under stress. Lactium (milk protein extract) and Suntheanine (green tea extract) are also effective in promoting calming, reducing stress, and improving sleep. Dosage: Follow product label instructions.

Vitamin B1: Required for energy production in the cells of the heart. Taking diuretics depletes levels of vitamin B1, and studies have shown that vitamin B1 supplements can improve heart function and symptoms of CHF. Dosage: 100 mg daily as part of a B-complex.

FINAL THOUGHTS

To improve the management of CHF, consider the following:

1. Boost intake of fibre, fish, flaxseed, soy, garlic, and green tea.
2. Minimize intake of sodium, alcohol, caffeine, and saturated fat. Speak with your doctor about guidelines for fluid intake.
3. Don't smoke.
4. Get regular exercise and reduce your stress.
5. Consider supplements of coenzyme Q10, hawthorn, and L-carnitine.

CONSTIPATION

Constipation is a disorder of the lower gastrointestinal tract marked by a decrease in the frequency of stools, difficulty defecating, and/or the passage of dry, hard stools. Most people experience an occasional change in bowel habits; when it is persistent, it is referred to as chronic constipation.

During the digestive process, food passes from the stomach to the intestine where nutrients and water are absorbed into the body. The waste products of digestion create a stool, which travels through the intestines with muscle contractions. It normally takes six to 24 hours to pass a stool. Anything that slows the passage of stools through the intestines or increases the amount of water absorbed by the body—such as a lack of fibre, fluids, or physical activity; medication; or ignoring the urge to defecate—can lead to constipation.

Chronic constipation affects 31 percent of people between 19 and 65 years, and approximately 45 percent of people over 65 years. This can be a debilitating and uncomfortable problem, but there are a number of lifestyle recommendations that can help.

SIGNS & SYMPTOMS

- Abdominal pain, bloating, and gas

- Bowel movements less than three times a week

- Passing hard stools

- Straining during a bowel movement

Chronic constipation can also cause bad breath, headache, fatigue, hemorrhoids (due to straining), and worsen varicose veins.

Severe constipation may cause fecal impaction, a mass of hardened stool. This can be dangerous and may require removal by a doctor.

Note: See your doctor if you notice blood in your stool or have black stools, as this could signify a serious problem.

RISK FACTORS

- Age (more common in older adults)

- Diet (lack of fibre and/or fluids)

- Health conditions (irritable bowel, celiac disease, colon cancer, liver disease, and low thyroid)

- Lack of activity (sedentary or bedridden)

- Medications (sedatives, narcotics [codeine], chemotherapy, blood pressure drugs, Parkinson's drugs, and iron supplements)

- Pregnancy (causes hormonal changes)

- Stress (reduces intestinal motility)

DOCTOR'S ORDERS

Lifestyle approaches, such as increasing fibre and water intake and regular exercise, should be tried first. If this is not successful, your doctor may recommend drug therapy.

Stimulant laxatives irritate the colon wall to stimulate a bowel movement. Examples include Dulcolax (bisacodyl), Senokot (senna), castor oil, and cascara. These drugs work quickly (overnight), but may cause abdominal cramping and are recommended for short-term (a few days) use only. When taken regularly, they can cause dependence and other problems (see below).

Bulk-forming laxatives add bulk and water to the stools, which improves passage through the intestines. They are taken daily with plenty of fluids, and it may take a week to notice benefits. Side effects include temporary gas and bloating. Examples include bran, Metamucil (psyllium), and Benefibre (guar gum).

Stool softeners, such as Colace (docusate) cause water and fats to penetrate the stool, easing movement through intestines. They may cause tolerance and become ineffective with prolonged use. Mineral oil makes the stool slippery to facilitate passage; however, it should not be used regularly, as it can reduce the absorption of fat-soluble vitamins (A, D, E, and K).

CAUTION: DO NOT OVERUSE LAXATIVES

Overuse of laxatives may cause dependence (lazy bowel syndrome), poor absorption of vitamins and nutrients (particularly potassium), dehydration, damage to the intestinal tract, and worsened constipation. Those who take laxatives for a long time may need to go off them slowly to allow the bowels to return to normal function.

SHERRY'S NATURAL PRESCRIPTION

Dietary Recommendations

Foods to include:

- High-fibre foods improve bowel regularity. Eat whole-grain breads and cereals (made with wheat bran, whole oats, rye, and flaxseed), fresh fruits (especially strawberries, apples, and rhubarb), dried fruits, vegetables, and legumes.

- Broccoli, spinach, and kale contain magnesium, which improves gut motility.

- Aim for 25–35 g of fibre daily.

- Drink plenty of fluids—water is best, but pure fruit and vegetable juices and herbal teas are also fine.

Foods to avoid:

- Refined and processed foods are high in sugar and contain little fibre.

- Mucus-forming foods (dairy) slow the transit time of waste and can be constipating.

- Caffeine and alcohol are dehydrating and should be minimized.

CONSTIPATION IN INFANTS

Several clinical studies have found that chronic constipation in infants can be triggered by intolerance to cow's milk. In one study, two-thirds of the infants had constipation that was relieved when cow's milk was removed from their diet. (*New England Journal of Medicine*, 1998: 339; 1100–1104).

Lifestyle Suggestions

• Increase physical activity, as exercise helps stimulate intestinal and bowel contractions. Try walking, biking, or swimming.

• Set aside time to have a bowel movement, such as after breakfast.

• Don't resist the urge. The longer you delay going to the toilet once you feel the urge, the more water that is absorbed from the stool and the harder it becomes.

• Acupuncture, massage, and reflexology may help by improving intestinal motility.

• Detoxification, a short-term cleanse or juice fast along with fibre supplements (psyllium, flaxseed), allows the body to focus on removal of waste. This is particularly helpful for chronic constipation.

Top Recommended Supplements

Fibre supplements: Products containing psyllium husks, flaxseed, oat bran, guar gum, glucommannan, and fenugreek are effective and can be taken regularly. Take with plenty of water. Start with a small amount (one tablespoonful daily) and gradually increase to allow your bowels to adjust.

Probiotics: Supplements containing these "friendly bacteria" help to restore the normal gut flora and have been shown in studies to relieve constipation. Look for Kyo-Dophilus. Take one to three capsules daily.

Complementary Supplements

Aloe vera juice: Aids bowel movements by working as a stimulant and improving intestinal contractions. For short-term use only. Dosage: 65 mL twice daily.

Magnesium: Aids intestinal function and helps stool retain water; may be deficient in those with constipation. Dosage: 200 mg twice daily.

FINAL THOUGHTS

To prevent constipation and optimize bowel function:

1. Consume 25–35 g of fibre daily. Best sources are whole grains, vegetables, fruits, and legumes.
2. Drink lots of fluids, especially after exercising.
3. Get regular physical activity to stimulate intestinal contractions.
4. Take a fibre supplement if your diet is lacking.
5. Probiotics can help restore intestinal function.

CROHN'S DISEASE AND COLITIS

Crohn's disease and colitis are categorized as inflammatory bowel diseases or IBD. These diseases affect the digestive system and cause the intestinal tissue to become inflamed, develop sores, and bleed. In Canada, an estimated 170,000 Canadian men and women suffer from IBD. These diseases can be painful and debilitating and may lead to life-threatening complications, especially if untreated.

Crohn's disease and ulcerative colitis are very similar in that they both inflame the lining of your digestive tract and can cause severe bouts of watery or bloody diarrhea and abdominal pain. Where they differ is that Crohn's disease can occur anywhere in your digestive tract, often spreading deep into the layers of affected tissues whereas ulcerative colitis usually affects only the innermost lining of your large intestine (colon) and rectum. Symptoms may come and go and those affected may also experience long periods of remission.

The actual cause of these diseases is unknown. Stress can aggravate symptoms, and was once considered to be the underlying cause, but that is no longer the case. Many practitioners, especially those with knowledge of nutrition and preventative medicine, feel that diet may be responsible for triggering these diseases. Both diseases are rare in developing countries and among cultures that eat whole, unprocessed foods. As well, it wasn't until the mid-1900s that these diseases became a problem in North America. Our diets have drastically changed over the decades. Consumption of fast foods and processed and refined foods and ingestion of chemical food additives is common. Food allergies may also play a part.

It is also possible that the inflammation may stem from the immune system's response to infection with a virus or bacterium. Since the diseases are more common among those with a family history, genetic mutations may also be to blame.

While there is no known medical cure for Crohn's disease or colitis, there are a variety of lifestyle approaches, supplements, and medications that can reduce the symptoms and even bring about long-term remission.

SIGNS & SYMPTOMS

The signs and symptoms of Crohn's disease and ulcerative colitis can vary widely, depending on the severity of inflammation and where it occurs, and include:

- Abdominal pain and cramping: Inflammation and ulceration causes the walls of the bowel to swell and develop scar tissue, which causes pain as food moves through your digestive tract.

- Blood in the stool: Caused by the inflammation and ulceration.

- Diarrhea and gas: The inflammation causes cells in the intestine to secrete large amounts of water and salt, leading to loose stools or diarrhea.

- Fatigue, nausea, and headache.

- Loss of appetite and weight loss: The pain and cramping can affect appetite, and the damage to the intestine can impair food and nutrient absorption.

• Sores, ulcers, fistulas, and perforation of the intestine.

Some people with these diseases experience inflammation in other areas of the body (joints, skin, and eyes).

RISK FACTORS

• Age: Those between the ages of 15 and 35 are at greatest risk.

• Diet: Eating a diet high in refined foods and low in fibre

• Family history: Having a parent or sibling with the condition greatly increases the risk.

• Race: Caucasians, Jewish people, and those of European descent are four to five times more likely to develop Crohn's disease and colitis.

DOCTOR'S ORDERS

The goal of medical treatment is to reduce inflammation and promote healing of the intestine. In some cases it is possible to achieve long-term remission. Dietary changes and supplements (as discussed below) can be very helpful. Depending on your situation and the severity of the symptoms and intestinal damage, your doctor may prescribe drug therapy to control the inflammation. Commonly used drugs include sulfasalazine, mesalamine (Asacol), and corticosteroids, such as prednisone. Some drugs work well for some people, but not for others. As well, these drugs have serious side effects, so it is important to discuss the benefits and risks with your doctor. Anti-diarrheal medications or laxatives may be necessary sometimes. Iron supplements are used for anemia, which occurs from chronic intestinal bleeding. For severe cases, surgery to remove the diseased portions of the bowel may be necessary, but this is always the last resort.

SHERRY'S NATURAL PRESCRIPTION

Dietary Recommendations

Foods to include:

• Aloe vera juice has anti-inflammatory activity. One study of people with colitis found that 100 mL of aloe vera juice twice daily resulted in a complete remission or an improvement in symptoms in 47 percent of cases, compared with 14 percent of those given a placebo.

• Barley and wheat grass juice can help reduce intestinal inflammation, and some research has shown a reduction in symptoms of IBD.

• Drink plenty of fluids (water, broth, and juice) to prevent dehydration from chronic diarrhea. Herbal teas made from chamomile, slippery elm, and marshmallow can be very soothing to an inflamed gastrointestinal tract. These herbs also help facilitate digestion.

• Eat small, frequent meals, which is easier on digestion.

• Ensure adequate protein intake as protein deficiency is common in those with IBD. Eat lean poultry, fish, beans, and legumes. Fish contains beneficial fatty acids (EPA and DHA), which can help reduce inflammation. The best sources of these fatty acids are salmon, herring, mackerel, albacore tuna, and sardines.

- Include healthy fats such as fish and olive oil. Nuts and seeds contain good fats, but they can irritate inflamed intestines.

- Whole grains (whole oats, brown rice, and quinoa), vegetables, and fruits as tolerated provide energy and essential nutrients. During flare-ups when the intestines are inflamed, raw vegetables and fruits can be irritating, so it is best to cook (steam) these foods.

WHEAT GRASS FOR ULCERATIVE COLITIS

A double-blind controlled study of 23 people with ulcerative colitis compared the effects of wheat grass juice (100 mL daily) to placebo for one month. There was a significant clinical improvement (reduction in symptoms) in 78 percent of people who were given wheat grass compared to 30 percent who were given placebo. Wheat grass contains vitamins A, C, E, B-vitamins, calcium, magnesium, potassium, iron, natural enzymes, and chlorophyll. (*Scandinavian Journal of Gastroenterology*, 2002: 37; 444–449).

Foods to avoid:

- Alcohol, caffeine, and spicy foods can irritate the intestines.

- Dairy and wheat are common triggers for those with IBD. Carrageenan, a compound used to stabilize milk proteins, has been shown to induce ulcerative colitis in animals. Cow's milk contains a bacterium that has been linked to Crohn's disease.

- Fast foods are typically high in saturated fat, refined starches, and preservatives, all of which can worsen symptoms. One study found that those who eat fast foods at least two times per week more than triple their risk of developing Crohn's disease.

- Refined flour (white bread and foods made with refined flour) is associated with worsening of symptoms.

- Saturated fats (e.g., butter, cream, cheese, meat) can worsen inflammation and irritate your intestine.

- Sugar has been shown in some research to worsen IBD, so limit intake from all sources (table sugar, candy, soft drinks).

Try an elimination diet to determine if food allergies are worsening your symptoms. See Appendix D for more information.

Lifestyle Suggestions

- Manage stress. Stress can trigger flare-ups.

- Don't smoke. Smoking can increase the risk of relapse.

- Get regular exercise to reduce stress and improve mood and energy levels.

Top Recommended Supplements

Fish oil: Contains omega-3 fatty acids, which have been shown in studies to reduce inflammation and improve symptoms of IBD. One study also found that fish oil supplements reduced the risk of relapse and flare-up. Dosage: Take a supplement that provides at least 6 g of EPA/DHA daily.

Multivitamin and mineral complex: Nutrient deficiencies are very common in those with IBD due to malabsorption, decreased appetite, drug depletion, and increased nutrient loss through the stool. Nutrients most commonly deficient in those with IBD include vitamins A, B12, C, D, E, K, folate, calcium, copper, magnesium, selenium, and zinc. Taking a quality multivitamin every day can help restore nutrient levels and improve overall health. Those with severe damage to the intestine may not be able to absorb B12 so injections can be taken.

Probiotics: IBD can cause the normal bacteria flora of the intestine to be depleted, which can lead to digestive and bowel problems. Replacing the flora with probiotic supplements can help improve digestion and nutrient absorption and relieve constipation and diarrhea. Dosage: Look for a product that provides at least one billion cells per capsule and take twice daily. Recommended product: Kyo-Dophilus.

Complementary Supplements

Boswellia: An herb with ant-inflammatory properties. Some research has shown that it can reduce symptoms of both Crohn's disease and colitis, similarly to prescription drugs. Dosage: 550 mg three times daily.

Curcumin (from the spice turmeric): Has been shown to help maintain remission in individuals with ulcerative colitis. Dosage: 1 g twice daily.

Digestive enzymes: People with IBD may be deficient in digestive enzymes, particularly those with severe intestinal damage. Supplements can help aid food digestion and nutrient absorption. Take one or two capsules with each meal.

Glutamine: An amino acid that helps repair the intestinal lining. Dosage: 1,000 mg three times daily on an empty stomach.

Greens supplements: Contain barley and wheat grass, which can help soothe an inflamed intestine and provide essential nutrients. Recommended products include greens+ or Kyo-Greens. Dosage: Powders should be mixed with water or juice and taken daily.

FINAL THOUGHTS

To manage the symptoms of Crohn's disease and colitis, consider the following:

1. Avoid processed/refined/fast food, sugar, and dairy.
2. Eat small, frequent meals of fish, brown rice, and vegetables (cooked).
3. Drink barley, wheat grass, aloe vera juice, and plenty of water.
4. Reduce stress, get regular exercise, and don't smoke.
5. Fish oil, multivitamins, and probiotics are highly recommended.

DEPRESSION

Depression is a disorder that affects your mood, thoughts, feelings, and behaviour. It is the most common psychiatric ailment in Western society, affects approximately 1.4 million Canadians at any given time, and is the second leading cause of long-term disability. It is much more than a case of the "blues." Depression can be serious and debilitating.

Depression is most often caused by a number of underlying factors, including:

Biological: Imbalance of neurotransmitters (chemical messengers in the brain—dopamine, serotonin, and norepinephrine), or hormone imbalance (low estrogen, progesterone, testosterone, thyroid) such as post-partum depression

Environmental: Exposure to chemicals that disrupt brain chemistry (cigarette smoking, heavy metals, prescription and recreational drugs)

Nutritional: Deficiency of vitamins (B12), minerals (magnesium), or essential fatty acids; food allergies

Situational: Stress, trauma, injury, divorce, job loss, death of a loved one

Anyone suffering with depression should seek professional help to determine the underlying cause and an appropriate treatment.

SIGNS & SYMPTOMS

Adults with four or more of these symptoms that last at least two weeks and children with at least four signs are considered to have clinical depression:

- Agitation or sluggishness in movement and thought
- Changes in appetite
- Difficulty concentrating, indecisiveness
- Fatigue or loss of energy
- Feelings of worthlessness or guilt
- Insomnia or increased sleep
- Loss of interest or pleasure in usual activities
- Recurrent thoughts of death or suicide
- Reduced sex drive
- Significant weight loss or weight gain

RISK FACTORS

- Family history (having a parent or grandparent with depression)
- Gender (twice as many women experience depression, likely due to hormonal changes—post-partum, menopause, and PMS)

- Insomnia (due to effect on hormones in the brain)

- Medical conditions (cancer, stroke, diabetes, headaches, anxiety, hypothyroidism and other hormonal imbalances)

- Medications (sedatives, narcotics, corticosteroids, blood pressure and cholesterol-lowering drugs)

- Personality characteristics (low self-esteem; pessimism; attention, conduct, or learning disorders)

- Stress (loss of loved one, financial or relationship problems, trauma)

There is a strong link between insomnia and depression. Studies estimate that 20 percent of people with insomnia suffer from major depression and 90 percent of people with depression have insomnia.

DOCTOR'S ORDERS

Medical treatment typically involves prescription drugs and counselling. The three main classes of antidepressant drugs are: tricyclic antidepressant drugs (TCAs), monoamine oxidase inhibitors (MAOIs) and selective serotonin re-uptake inhibitors (SSRIs). TCAs include amitriptyline, clomipramine, and imipramine. MAOIs include phenelzine and tranylcypromine. These two classes are less commonly used since the discovery of the SSRIs, which include fluoxetine, fluvoxamine, citalopram, paroxetine, and sertraline.

While antidepressant drugs help some people, they are often overprescribed. It may take six to eight weeks to notice improvement. Side effects include nausea, weight gain/loss, headaches, anxiety, nervousness, insomnia or drowsiness, diarrhea, sweating, tremor, and sexual dysfunction. There are numerous drug interactions; consult with your pharmacist before taking any other prescription or natural products.

SHERRY'S NATURAL PRESCRIPTION

Dietary Recommendations

A healthy diet helps balance mood. Follow dietary recommendations outlined in Chapter 1. Eat small frequent meals to maintain good energy and mood. Since food allergies can also trigger depression, refer to Appendix D for information on identifying possible allergies.

Foods to include:

- Vegetables, fruits, whole grains, nuts, and seeds are good sources of vitamins, minerals, and essential fatty acids, which may be depleted in those with depression.

- Turkey and salmon contain the amino acid tryptophan, which elevates serotonin production. Fish is also a good source of essential fatty acids.

Foods to avoid:

- Sugar, refined carbohydrates, and caffeine can cause mood swings and irritability.

- Processed and fast foods often contain chemicals and preservatives that may upset brain chemistry.

- Alcohol is a nervous system depressant and should be minimized or avoided completely, especially by those taking medication.

Note: If you are taking MAOI drugs, avoid soy sauce, bologna, canned meats, fermented sausage, salami, ripened cheese, red wine, and yeast concentrates.

Lifestyle Suggestions

- Acupuncture: Studies have found it beneficial for depression. It may work by stimulating the production of neurotransmitters.

- Counselling: Therapy with a psychologist or psychiatrist can be very beneficial. Some research has found cognitive therapy equally effective to drug therapy.

- Exercise: Research has shown that exercise offers powerful benefits for relieving depression and stress and improving mood, well-being, and sleep. Aim for 30 minutes of activity daily—walking, cycling, swimming, yoga, or any activity you enjoy.

- Massage and reflexology: Help to relieve stress and tension and promote relaxation.

....

A review of 28 clinical studies on SAMe for depression found it to be equally effective compared to conventional antidepressants. (Agency for Healthcare Research and Quality, Evidence Report/Technology Assessment, Number 64, AHRQ Publication No. 02-E033, August 2002.)

....

Top Recommended Supplements

Fish oil: Rich in omega-3 fatty acids, which are essential for the nervous system, and support neurotransmitter function. Levels may be depleted in those with depression. Studies show benefits for depression, especially for those not getting adequate response to antidepressant drugs. Dosage: 3–9 g daily.

S-adenosylmethionine (SAMe): Supports the production of serotonin, dopamine, and norepinephrine; improves communication between nerve cells; is an antioxidant (protects brain tissues against damage from free radicals); has been shown to be beneficial for depression in many studies. SAMe is well tolerated, has positive side effects (supports joint and liver health), and a quick onset of action (two weeks). Not recommended for those with bipolar disorder (manic-depression) as it can worsen the manic symptoms. Dosage: 400–1,600 mg daily on empty stomach; start with a low dose and gradually increase if needed.

St. John's wort: Increases neurotransmitter levels, and is effective for mild to moderate depression. May take two to four weeks to notice benefits; side effects are rare and include stomach upset, fatigue, itching, sleep disturbance, skin rash, and sun-sensitivity. St. John's wort interacts with many drugs, such as oral contraceptives, blood thinners and other antidepressants; check with your pharmacist. Dosage: 300 mg three times daily.

Suntheanine: A patented extract of theanine (an amino acid present in green tea), it reduces stress and anxiety without causing drowsiness or addiction, and also improves sleep quality. It works quickly to promote calming (30 minutes to one hour), and there are no known side effects. Dosage: 50–200 mg daily.

Complementary Supplements

B-Complex: B-vitamins (such as B12 and folic acid) may be deficient in those with depression. Folic acid works with SAMe to boost neurotransmitter levels. Several studies have found benefits. Take 400–1,000 mcg folic acid along with 50–100 mg of other B-vitamins daily to support brain function.

5-hydroxytryptophan (5-HTP): A substance used by the body to create serotonin. Preliminary research shows benefits for depression. Side effects are rare and minor (upset stomach). Avoid use with other products that affect serotonin levels. Dosage: 100 mg three times daily.

Ginkgo biloba: Improves blood flow to the brain; improves memory and cognitive function; may also improve serotonin response. Supplements may be particularly beneficial for the elderly. Dosage: 40–120 mg daily. Note: Ginkgo may enhance the effect of blood-thinning medications.

Tyrosine: An amino acid that helps depression. Dosage: 200–500 mg daily. Do not combine with prescription antidepressants.

D

Depression

FINAL THOUGHTS

If you or someone you know is suffering with depression, seek professional help and consider the following:

1. Eat a healthy diet and avoid sugar, refined/processed foods, caffeine, and alcohol.
2. Exercise regularly to reduce stress and improve mood and sleep.
3. Try acupuncture, massage, and professional counselling.
4. Consider a supplement of SAMe or St. John's wort.
5. Take fish oils daily for overall brain function and improved mood, and consider Suntheanine to reduce stress and anxiety.

DIABETES

Diabetes is a chronic disease where the body does not make enough insulin, or becomes insensitive (resistant) to the insulin that is produced. According to the Canadian Diabetes Association, over two million Canadians have diabetes, and this figure is expected to rise.

When we consume food, it is broken down into glucose, which causes a rise in blood glucose levels. Insulin is a hormone secreted by the pancreas in response to that rise in blood sugar. Insulin's role is to transport glucose from the bloodstream into the cells to be used for energy.

There are three main types of diabetes. Type 1 diabetes is responsible for approximately 10 percent of cases and occurs when the pancreas produces little or no insulin. The exact cause of type 1 diabetes is unknown, but it is thought that the immune system attacks and destroys the insulin-producing cells of the pancreas. Genetics may also play a role. Type 1 diabetes was previously known as juvenile diabetes or insulin-dependent diabetes because it typically appears during childhood or adolescence, and people who get this form require insulin injections to manage their blood sugar.

Type 2 diabetes is the most common form, accounting for about 90 percent of people with diabetes. This form occurs when the pancreas does not produce enough insulin or when your cells become resistant to the action of insulin. Obesity, inactivity, and poor diet (eating too many high-glycemic foods) are some of the causes of type 2 diabetes. Other risk factors are discussed below. In the past, type 2 diabetes affected primarily adults. However, a growing number of children and adolescents are being diagnosed today.

The third type of diabetes is gestational diabetes, a temporary condition that occurs during pregnancy. It affects approximately 3.5 percent of all pregnancies and involves an increased risk of developing diabetes for both mother and child.

All forms of diabetes can have serious consequences if left untreated. There is no cure for diabetes, but there is much that can be done from a lifestyle perspective to improve blood sugar control and prevent potentially life-threatening complications.

SIGNS & SYMPTOMS

- Blurred vision: High blood sugar causes fluid to be pulled from all tissues, including the lenses of the eyes, which can affect vision.

- Fatigue and irritability

- Hunger: Your muscles and organs become energy depleted because insulin is not able to move glucose into your cells, which can trigger persistent hunger.

- Impaired wound healing or frequent infections.

- Increased thirst and frequent urination; as excess sugar builds up in your bloodstream, fluid is pulled from your tissues, which can make you thirsty, so you may drink and urinate more than usual.

- Weight loss: Even though food intake may be increased, weight loss can occur because your muscles and fat stores may shrink because they are not getting the necessary glucose.

Some people with type 2 diabetes develop patches of dark, velvety skin in the folds and creases of their bodies, usually in the armpits and neck. This condition, called acanthosis nigricans, is a sign of insulin resistance. However, it is important to realize that many people who have type 2 diabetes have no symptoms until complications develop.

DIABETIC COMPLICATIONS

If left untreated, diabetes can lead to serious complications. Uncontrolled high blood sugar can cause damage to blood vessels throughout the body. Diabetes dramatically increases the risk of heart disease and stroke. In fact, about 75 percent of people who have diabetes die of some type of heart or blood vessel disease. Other complications include kidney and eye disease, nerve damage (diabetic foot and erectile dysfunction), and increased risk of infection.

RISK FACTORS

- Age: The risk of type 2 diabetes increases with age, especially after age 40. Aging does not cause diabetes, but people tend to exercise less and gain weight with age.

- Diet: Studies have shown that people who eat high-glycemic diets (lots of quick-release carbohydrates) are at increased risk of type 2 diabetes.

- Gestational diabetes: Developing diabetes during pregnancy increases the risk of developing type 2 diabetes later in life.

- Heredity: Having a parent or sibling with either type 1 or 2 diabetes increases the risk.

- Inactivity increases the risk of type 2 diabetes; conversely, physical activity improves insulin sensitivity and reduces the risk.

- Obesity greatly increases the risk of type 2 diabetes because carrying excess body fat reduces insulin sensitivity.

- Race: Those of Aboriginal, Hispanic, Asian, or African descent are at greater risk.

DOCTOR'S ORDERS

People with type 1 diabetes require insulin injections in order to manage blood sugar. In the past the only way to get insulin was through injection with a needle and syringe. Now there are insulin pen devices and pumps that are more convenient and less painful. There are also several types of insulin that vary in their onset and duration of action. Your doctor will help devise a plan based on your needs.

Some people with type 2 diabetes can manage their blood sugar with diet and exercise alone, but in some cases, medication or insulin is required. There are a variety of oral medications used for diabetes. These drugs work by stimulating the pancreas to produce and release more insulin, inhibiting the production and release of glucose from your liver (so that less insulin is needed to transport sugar into your cells) or increasing tissue sensitivity to insulin.

A number of factors can affect blood sugar levels such as diet, activity level, illness, medication, alcohol, and stress. Careful monitoring is essential to ensure that your blood sugar levels are within the recommended range. Depending on your situation, your doctor may advise you to check your blood sugar once a day or more often. Fasting blood glucose levels should be between 4 and 7 mmol/L. The recommended range two hours after meals is between 5 and 10 mmol/L.

In addition to daily blood sugar monitoring, your doctor may recommend an A1C test, which measures your average blood sugar level for the past 120 days. This test indicates how well your diabetes treatment plan is working overall. The recommended A1C level for diabetics is 7 percent or less.

HYPOGLYCEMIA

Hypoglycemia or low blood sugar occurs when your blood sugar drops to less than 4 mmol/L. Symptoms include shakiness, lightheadedness, irritability, confusion, racing heart, and sweating. Hypoglycemia can result from not eating at regular intervals, intense physical activity, taking too much medication, or drinking alcohol. Blood glucose levels can drop quickly, and in severe cases can lead to loss of consciousness and seizures, so it is important to act quickly and eat or drink a fast-acting carbohydrate such as glucose tablets, honey, juice, or candy to raise blood sugar levels.

SHERRY'S NATURAL PRESCRIPTION

Dietary Recommendations

Foods to include:

- Cinnamon contains compounds that work synergistically with insulin, helping to reduce blood sugar levels. One study found benefits with just ½ tsp daily. Add cinnamon to your cereal, oatmeal, or breakfast shakes.

- Chromium is essential for blood glucose regulation. It is found in brewer's yeast, whole grains (especially wheat germ), onions, and garlic.

- For a natural and healthy sugar substitute, try stevia or xylitol.

- High-fibre, low-glycemic (slow-release) carbohydrates such as whole grains (whole wheat, oats, brown rice, spelt), vegetables, fruits, and legumes help to balance blood sugar.

- Protein (lean poultry, meat, and fish) and healthy fats (nuts, seeds, olive oil, and flaxseed oil) in each meal will slow carbohydrate digestion and promote better blood sugar control.

Note: To promote steady blood sugar levels, eat small, frequent meals (every three hours).

Foods to avoid:

- Alcohol can cause either high or low blood sugar depending on how much you drink and if you are eating while drinking. Limit alcohol intake to no more than two drinks daily.

- High-glycemic (quick-release) carbohydrates such as white bread and baked goods, refined cereals, potatoes, white rice, and sugar (candy, cookies, soda) cause rapid and profound increases in blood sugar, creating a problem for diabetics. Studies have also found that those who eat high-glycemic diets are also at increased risk of developing type 2 diabetes.

- Saturated fat (animal products such as meat and dairy) can worsen blood glucose control.

Lifestyle Suggestions

- Lose excess weight. Being overweight can impair insulin sensitivity.

- Get regular physical activity. Aim for 30 minutes to one hour of moderate intensity activity each day, such as brisk walking, cycling, or swimming. Exercise helps with weight management and also improves blood glucose control and insulin sensitivity.

- Don't smoke. People with diabetes who smoke are at greater risk for heart, kidney and eye disease, and nerve damage.

- Manage your stress. Stress triggers the release of hormones that impair insulin sensitivity. Try yoga, meditation, and other relaxation techniques.

- Practise good oral hygiene. Brush your teeth at least twice a day and floss daily to reduce the risk of gum infection. Visit your dentist regularly for professional cleaning.

- Take care of your feet. Diabetics are prone to nerve damage, which can make sores on the feet unnoticeable and delay wound healing. Inspect your feet daily for blisters or cuts. Apply moisturizer particularly to your heels. See your doctor if you develop any sores that do not heal within a few days.

- Have regular physicals and eye exams to screen for potential complications.

Top Recommended Supplements

Alpha lipoic acid: A powerful antioxidant that can help improve insulin sensitivity and reduce the risk of diabetic complications such as neuropathy and nephropathy (kidney disease). Dosage: 600–1,200 mg daily.

Chromium: An essential trace mineral that plays a role in sugar metabolism. It helps improve insulin sensitivity and glucose tolerance. Some studies have found that diabetics are deficient in chromium, and that supplements can help improve blood sugar management. Look for chromium picolinate as this is the most widely studied form of chromium. Dosage: 400–1,000 mcg daily.

Fibre: Helps improve blood glucose control and weight management. Studies involving fibre supplements of psyllium, oat bran, and glucomannan have shown benefits for diabetics. Dosage: Varies with product and formulation. Follow instructions on label and take with plenty of water.

Complementary Supplements

B-vitamins: Essential for proper nerve function and energy metabolism. Take a B-complex or a multivitamin that contains at least 50 mg of the B-vitamins.

Fenugreek: Seeds and supplements containing this herb have been shown to lower blood sugar and improve insulin sensitivity. Dosage: 15 g of powdered seeds with a meal or 1 or 2 g of an extract daily.

Fish oil: Helps improve glucose tolerance, reduce triglycerides and cholesterol levels, and may help improve diabetic complications (neuropathy and nephropathy). Dosage: Look for a product that provides at least 400 mg EPA and 200 mg DHA per dosage, and take three times daily.

Gymnema: Preliminary research shows that this herb can help stimulate insulin secretion and improve blood glucose control in those with both Type 1 and Type 2 diabetes. Dosage: 400 mg once or twice daily of a product standardized to 25 percent gymnemic acid.

Magnesium: Required for energy metabolism and nerve function. People with diabetes tend to have low magnesium levels and a deficiency is associated with insulin resistance. Supplements can help improve insulin sensitivity and glucose control. Dosage: 200–600 mg daily.

Phase 2: White kidney bean extract that reduces starch digestion. Studies have shown that it can lower after-meal blood sugar levels. Dosage: 500–1,000 mg before starchy meals.

Vitamin E: Helps to improve glucose tolerance and reduce glycosylation (binding of sugar to proteins in blood vessels). Many studies have found that it can prevent and reverse nerve damage and help protect against retinopathy and nephropathy. Dosage: 800 IU daily.

FINAL THOUGHTS

To improve blood sugar control and reduce the risk of diabetic complications, consider the following:

1. Eat small, frequent meals with low-glycemic, high-fibre carbohydrates, protein, and healthy fats. Add cinnamon to your diet.
2. Avoid eating fast/processed/refined foods, alcohol, and saturated fat.
3. Reduce your stress and aim for at least 30 minutes of activity daily.
4. Maintain good oral and foot hygiene and see your doctor regularly for checkups and blood glucose testing.
5. Consider supplements of alpha lipoic acid, chromium, and fibre.

DIARRHEA

Diarrhea, which is loose, watery stools, is one of the most common digestive disorders. In fact, most people will experience diarrhea several times every year. Diarrhea is considered acute if it lasts just a few days or chronic if it persists for more than four weeks.

During digestion, the food we eat is broken down and nutrients are absorbed through the intestine. The waste material passes through the colon where most of the fluids are absorbed, creating a soft stool. The most common causes of acute diarrhea are dietary factors and infection. The body secretes extra fluid and intestinal contractions propel the toxins out of the body. When diarrhea occurs, the food and fluids you eat pass quickly through the colon so that the fluids are not adequately absorbed, causing soft, watery stools. Chronic diarrhea can occur due to digestive disorders or use of medications that affect bowel function.

Aside from being unpleasant and embarrassing, diarrhea can lead to serious complications such as dehydration and nutrient deficiencies. In some cases it will clear up on its own, and in other cases treatment is necessary to get it under control and prevent complications.

SIGNS & SYMPTOMS

- Abdominal pain or cramps
- Bloating and gas
- Fever
- Frequent, loose, watery stools

RISK FACTORS

- Antibiotics and other medications
- Diet: Fast foods, processed foods, preservatives, and artificial sweeteners, such as sorbitol and mannitol
- Digestive disorders (Crohn's disease, colitis, celiac disease, and irritable bowel syndrome)
- Infection with bacteria, viruses, or parasites
- Lactose intolerance

DOCTOR'S ORDERS

Acute diarrhea often clears up in a few days and rarely requires treatment. However, to prevent dehydration, your doctor will advise you to increase fluid intake. There are special rehydration solutions, such as Gastrolyte and Pedialyte, available in pharmacies, that contain electrolytes (salt, potassium, and other minerals) that are necessary for health and to prevent dehydration. If you become depleted in these nutrients, it can lead to heart problems and other consequences.

If you develop diarrhea while taking an antibiotic, contact your doctor and stop the medication. Antibiotics destroy both the good and bad bacteria, which can disturb the balance of your normal flora in your intestine, leading to overgrowth or potentially dangerous bacteria, such as *Clostridium difficile*, which can cause very serious diarrhea and requires medical treatment.

If lactose intolerance is causing the diarrhea, you will be advised to avoid dairy products or to take lactase (enzyme needed to digest lactose) when eating dairy.

There are over-the-counter anti-diarrheal medications, such as Imodium (loperamide), which can help to slow the diarrhea. However, these drugs should not be used if you have infectious diarrhea as they can prevent your body from eliminating the offending organism.

SHERRY'S NATURAL PRESCRIPTION

Dietary Recommendations

Foods to include:

- Carob contains tannins that have an astringent or binding effect on the mucous membranes of the intestinal tract. One study of 41 infants with diarrhea found that carob powder (at a dose of 1 g per kilogram per day) significantly improved resolution of diarrhea as compared to placebo. Carob can also be used for treating adult diarrhea. It is available in health food stores and some grocery stores.

- Drink plenty of fluids (water, vegetable juice, broth). Teas containing chamomile or blackberry, blueberry, or red raspberry leaves can be helpful in alleviating diarrhea because these herbs contain tannins, which have astringent properties. Ginger tea can help reduce intestinal inflammation.

- During an acute attack, avoid solid foods and consume liquids. As you start to feel better, eat foods that are nutritious and easy to digest, such as bananas, brown rice, and potatoes. When your bowel movements have normalized, add more fibre-rich foods back into your diet.

- Fermented milk products (yogurt and kefir) help to restore beneficial bacteria in the gut and suppress growth of pathogenic bacteria.

Foods to avoid:

- Caffeine, alcohol, and spicy foods (hot peppers) are too stimulating to the digestive tract.

- Dairy products (other than fermented dairy), fats, and oils can worsen symptoms and should be avoided until the diarrhea has cleared.

- Sugar should be avoided if you have a bacterial infection. Fruit juices (especially apple and pear) are high in sugar and should be minimized until you have recovered.

Lifestyle Suggestions

- Get plenty of rest to allow your body to recover.

- See your doctor if diarrhea persists beyond five days or if you or your child develops dehydration.

SIGNS OF DEHYDRATION

Diarrhea can lead to dehydration rapidly, especially in young children and requires immediate medical attention. Signs of dehydration include excessive thirst, dry mouth or skin, little urination, severe weakness, dizziness or lightheadedness, or dark urine. Signs of dehydration in infants include dry mouth, crying without tears, unusual sleepiness, sunken eyes or cheeks, and skin that doesn't flatten if pinched and released. If this occurs, see your doctor immediately.

Top Recommended Supplements

Multivitamin and mineral complex: Persistent diarrhea can lead to deficiencies of various vitamins and minerals, and taking a multivitamin can help prevent deficiencies. Certain nutrients (such as folic acid and zinc) can promote healing of the intestine. Speak to your pharmacist or health adviser for a recommendation as products vary depending on age, activity level, lifestyle, and gender.

Probiotics: Regular use of these beneficial bacteria can help prevent traveller's diarrhea and also help treat infectious diarrhea. Over 13 clinical studies have shown that probiotics can reduce the severity and duration of diarrhea and help prevent it from occurring. They can also help prevent and treat antibiotic-induced diarrhea. Dosage: One capsule three times daily with meals. Look for a product that provides at least one billion live cells per dosage and is stable at room temperature, such as Kyo-Dophilus. To prevent antibiotic-induced diarrhea, take your probiotic when you start your antibiotic and for at least two weeks after the antibiotic is finished.

CAUTION: If you have diarrhea, avoid taking large doses of vitamin C or magnesium (more than 500 mg or 100 mg respectively), as these nutrients can cause loose stools.

Complementary Supplements

Brewer's yeast: Some research has shown that this supplement can help relieve infectious diarrhea, particularly when caused by *Clostridium difficile* (associated with antibiotic use). Dosage: Three capsules three times daily.

Goldenseal: Has antibiotic properties and contains a chemical called berebine, which prevents infectious bacteria from attaching to the gut and blocks the action of toxins produced by bacteria. Dosage: 250–500 mg three times daily, or 1 mL of tincture three times daily.

PREVENTING TRAVELLER'S DIARRHEA

Travelling to developing countries and exposure to poor sanitation and contaminated food and water is a very common cause of diarrhea. To reduce your risk, avoid tap water and ice cubes and drink only bottled water and beverages; avoid raw fruits and vegetables unless you can peel them yourself; avoid raw or undercooked meats; use bottled water to brush your teeth; and keep your mouth closed while showering. Taking a probiotic (friendly bacteria) every day while away can also help reduce the risk of traveller's diarrhea. These beneficial bacteria (such as lactobacilli and bifidobacteria) normally live in the colon and inhibit the overgrowth of disease-causing bacteria. Look for a product that is stable at room temperature, such as Kyo-Dophilus.

FINAL THOUGHTS

To manage diarrhea, consider the following:

1. Drink lots of fluids (especially water and herbal teas).
2. Avoid dairy, fats, oils, spicy food, sugar, caffeine, and alcohol.
3. Get adequate rest.
4. Take a probiotic, multivitamin and mineral complex, and rehydration solution.
5. See your doctor if diarrhea persists beyond five days or if you develop dehydration.

DIVERTICULAR DISEASE

Diverticulosis is a common condition where small, bulging pouches (diverticula) develop in the gastrointestinal tract. Diverticula usually develop when weak places in your colon give way under pressure, causing the formation of pouches, which can protrude through the colon wall. These pouches rarely cause problems, so people often don't realize that they have them. However, if the diverticula become infected (diverticulitis), this can cause abdominal pain, fever, nausea, and change in bowel habits.

It is possible to prevent diverticular disease by eating a high-fibre diet and avoiding constipation.

SIGNS & SYMPTOMS

Most people with diverticulosis do not have any symptoms. If diverticulitis occurs, it can cause:

- Abdominal pain (severe and sudden onset)

- Constipation or diarrhea

- Fever, nausea, vomiting

- Rectal bleeding

Note: Complications of diverticulitis include blockage in the colon and abscess or fistula formation. If a pouch ruptures, the waste material can spill into the abdominal cavity, leading to peritonitis, which is a serious medical problem that needs immediate attention.

RISK FACTORS

- Age: Diverticular disease is most common in those over age 40. About 10 percent of those over age 40 and 50 percent of those over age 60 are affected

- Poor diet: Lack of fibre

- Lack of exercise

THE FIBRE FACTOR

Diverticular disease is very rare in countries where people eat a high-fibre diet, but it is very common in Canada, the United States, and Europe where people eat more refined carbohydrates and less fibre. Prior to the 1900s when refining of grains started, diverticular disease was rare in North America. A high-fibre diet can reduce your risk of diverticular disease and also help prevent flare-ups in those who already have it.

DOCTOR'S ORDERS

The treatment of diverticulitis depends on the severity of the symptoms. For those with mild symptoms, dietary changes and antibiotics for the infection may be all that is needed. During a flare-up, your doctor will advise a temporary low-fibre diet to allow the colon to heal. Once the symptoms subside, you can gradually increase the fibre in your diet.

Surgery is a last resort, but may be necessary for those with bowel obstruction or severely damaged intestine.

SHERRY'S NATURAL PRESCRIPTION

Dietary Recommendations

Foods to include:

- Drink plenty of fluids (water, juice, herbal tea) to aid the effect of fibre.

- Eat healthy fats (fish, olive oil, flaxseed), which can help reduce inflammation.

- Eat small, frequent meals to facilitate digestion and elimination.

- Fermented milk products (yogurt and kefir) can help reduce the risk of infection by supporting growth of beneficial bacteria in the gut.

- High-fibre foods, such as fresh fruits and vegetables and whole grains (oats, whole wheat, brown rice, and flaxseed), keep stools soft, reducing the pressure on your colon and preventing constipation. Aim for 25–30 g of fibre daily. Increase your intake gradually to avoid bloating and gas.

Foods to avoid:

- Fast foods and processed foods contain chemicals that can damage intestinal health.

- Minimize saturated fat (red meat).

- Refined grains (white flour/bread/rice/pasta) contain little to no fibre.

In the past, those with diverticular disease were told to avoid nuts or seeds, but there is no evidence that these foods trigger flare-ups, so they can be enjoyed as part of a healthy diet.

Lifestyle Suggestions

- Get regular physical activity. Aim for 30 minutes to one hour each day. Studies have found that jogging can help protect against diverticular disease.

- Respond to bowel urges. Avoid holding it in as that can create dry, hard stools that are hard to pass, increasing colon pressure.

Top Recommended Supplements

Fibre: Helps prevent constipation and improve bowel function. One study of glucomannan, a water-soluble dietary fibre derived from konjac root, found that it reduced symptoms of diverticular disease. Other good fibre supplements include psyllium, milled flaxseed, and oat bran. Dosage: Varies with the product. Aim for 25–30 g of fibre daily from foods and supplements.

Probiotics: Beneficial bacteria help to reduce the risk of gut infection and also aid digestion and nutrient absorption. Dosage: Take one to three capsules daily of a product that provides at least one billion live cells. A recommended product is Kyo-Dophilus.

Complementary Supplement

Aged garlic extract: Supports immune system function and helps to reduce the risk of infection. This form of garlic is odourless and has been widely researched. Dosage: 600 mg daily.

FINAL THOUGHTS

To prevent diverticular disease, consider the following:

1. Boost your fibre intake by eating whole grains and avoiding refined foods.
2. Include healthy fats (fish and flaxseed) and fermented milk products (yogurt and kefir) in your diet.
3. Drink plenty of fluids.
4. Get regular exercise.
5. Consider fibre supplements and probiotics to complement your diet.

EAR INFECTIONS

Ear infections are the most common childhood illness, and the reason for more children's visits to the doctor than any other illness. Ear infections, known medically as Otitis Media, are a non-contagious infection of the middle ear, just behind the eardrum.

Ear infections often develop from a viral infection, such as a cold. If the middle ear becomes inflamed from the infection, fluid builds up behind the eardrum, creating a breeding ground for infection. These infections can also occur when there is swelling or problems with the eustachian tubes (the tubes that connect the middle ear to inner nose). These tubes equalize pressure inside and outside the ear. In children, the eustachian tubes are narrower and shorter, making it easier for fluid to get trapped in the middle ear during an infection.

In most cases, ear infections will clear up without treatment. More serious infections, particularly in infants and toddlers, may require medical treatment. A healthy diet and lifestyle can help support proper immune function and reduce the risk of developing ear infections.

YOUNG CHILDREN MOST AFFECTED

Children under three years of age are most at risk for developing an ear infection. Statistics show that three out of four children younger than three have had at least one ear infection.

SIGNS & SYMPTOMS

Pain in the ear is the most common symptom of an ear infection. Children often don't recognize that their ears are the source of their discomfort, so it is important to look for other signs and symptoms such as:

- Balance difficulties
- Crying and irritability
- Ear drainage (look for a thick, yellow fluid, but do not be alarmed)
- Fatigue/malaise
- Fever
- Hearing problems
- Trouble sleeping
- Tugging at ears (though this is not a telltale sign)

RISK FACTORS

- Age: Young children are at greater risk because their eustachian tubes are not fully developed (they are shorter and more horizontal), making fluid drainage more difficult.
- Exposure to smoke and air pollution

- Group child care increases the spread of germs

- Season: More common during the fall and winter (cold and flu season)

- Swollen adenoids can block the eustachian tubes

- Teething and feeding position: Babies who drink from a bottle while lying down tend to get more ear infections than those who feed upright.

- Weakened immune system: Colds or flus can increase a child's risk of getting an ear infection.

SWIMMER'S EAR

Swimmers often suffer from painful plugged ears when water becomes trapped in the outer ear and ear canal. When this happens, the skin inside the ear becomes watery, reducing the natural acidity that fights incoming pathogens and infection may result. Swimmer's ear usually clears up on its own, but requires a trip to the doctor if there is pain.

DOCTOR'S ORDERS

About 80 percent of all ear infections clear up on their own without antibiotic treatment. For infants older than six months who are otherwise healthy and have mild symptoms, it is recommended to just keep an eye on your child for 72 hours. If symptoms persist beyond this period, a visit to the doctor is recommended. The doctor will use a tool to look inside the child's ear for inflammation or pus. Once symptoms are detected, the ear infection is treated with a course of antibiotics to avoid complications. Doctors may also recommend an analgesic to relieve pain.

For severe cases where a child has recurrent ear infections, surgery may be recommended to place small tubes inside the ears to drain fluid and relieve pressure. The concern is that hearing loss from chronic ear infections may delay language and speech development. (See below.) A specialist will place a small plastic tube in a surgical hole made in the eardrum. The tubes allow air to enter the middle ear and fluid to drain properly out of it. They are also thought to relieve pressure and pain. Children are under general anaesthesia during surgery, and usually recover quickly with little pain. There are maintenance issues and minor complications that may result from ear tubes, so it is important to discuss all factors with your doctor before proceeding with surgery.

RESEARCH HIGHLIGHT: EAR TUBES MAY NOT BE NECESSARY

In the January 2007 issue of *The New England Journal of Medicine*, a large research study found that early treatment with ear tubes did not affect developmental outcomes when comparing treated and untreated children. Children involved in this long-term study were followed from approximately age three to age 11. Some were treated with tubes and some were not. Over the years, the researchers tested the children for reading, writing, spelling, behavioural issues, social skills, and intelligence, and found that there was no significant difference between the two groups. As a result of this groundbreaking study, guidelines regarding the treatment of chronic ear infections with tubes were re-evaluated and changed to encourage a watchful, waiting approach to treatment.

SHERRY'S NATURAL PRESCRIPTION

Dietary Recommendations

Foods to include:

- Brightly coloured vegetables, fruits (especially berries), and whole grains contain essential vitamins and minerals that support the immune system.

- Chewing gum that contains xylitol (a natural sugar found in some fruits) can help reduce the risk of ear infections. Studies have shown that xylitol interferes with the growth of some bacteria that may cause ear infections.

- Fish and flaxseed contain essential fatty acids that help to reduce inflammation.

- Yogurt contains beneficial bacteria that help to reduce the risk of infections.

Foods to avoid:

- Dairy products may increase the risk of infection in those with sensitivities or allergies to cow's milk.

- Sugar suppresses immune function. Minimize soft drinks, candy, and sweets.

Lifestyle Suggestions

- Avoid second-hand smoke, as it weakens immunity.

- Breast-feeding supports lifelong healthy immunity: Always breast-feed with the baby slightly vertical and never put a child to sleep with a bottle.

- Discourage children from submerging their heads in water for prolonged periods, especially in lakes that are polluted.

- Healthy sleep patterns promote wellness.

- If your child exhibits signs of an ear infection, keep a close eye and check his or her temperature.

- Regular exercise boosts immune function.

- Use earplugs for swimming and bathing for children who are prone to infections.

- Wash hands regularly to avoid infections and encourage your children to wash their hands and avoid rubbing their eyes, nose, or mouth.

Top Recommended Supplements

Echinacea: Can help to reduce the severity and duration of cold symptoms, which may help to prevent ear infections from developing, although this has not been specifically studied. Dosage: 1–2 mL (depending on age) of echinacea tincture taken three times per day or more. Echinacea should be started as soon as symptoms appear and continued until a few days after they are gone.

Garlic: Contains potent sulphur compounds that boost immune function. Studies have shown that aged garlic extract can destroy the major bacteria that cause ear infections. Dosage: Adults should take two to six capsules daily; children should take one or two capsules daily.

Please refer to Chapter 9 for homeopathic recommendations for ear infections.

Complementary Supplements

Oil of oregano: Has antibacterial and antifungal properties. Consult with your health care provider for dosage guidelines.

Vitamin C: Helps support immune function and reduces the severity of cold symptoms. Dosage: Adults should take 1,000 mg; children should take 250–500 mg three times daily.

FINAL THOUGHTS

To help reduce the risk of ear infections, consider the following:

1. Encourage a healthy diet, including lots of vegetables, fruits, whole grains, fish, flaxseed, yogurt, and chewing gum with xylitol. Minimize sugar intake.
2. Keep children away from cigarette smoke.
3. Discourage children from submersing their heads underwater for prolonged periods.
4. Encourage regular handwashing, especially for children in daycare facilities.
5. Consider echinacea to shorten the severity and duration of a cold. Aged garlic extract can help support immune function and protect against infections.

ECZEMA

Also known as dermatitis, eczema is an inflammatory skin condition marked by extremely itchy, red, scaly, and irritated skin. Eczema affects about six million Canadians and is the most common skin problem in children under the age of 12. There are several forms of eczema, including:

Atopic dermatitis: Atopic dermatitis is the most common form of eczema, affecting about 10 percent of all Canadians. It usually begins in infancy and varies in severity during childhood and adolescence. It is thought to be due to a combination of dry, irritable skin and a malfunction in the body's immune system.

Contact dermatitis: This is caused by exposure to an irritant or allergen, such as laundry soap, dyes, cosmetics and skin products, cleaning products, or plants (poison ivy).

Neurodermatitis: This form develops in areas where something, such as tight clothing, rubs or scratches your skin and causes an irritation.

Seborrheic dermatitis: Seborrheic dermatitis is a red rash with yellowish and oily scales, which is known as cradle cap when it affects infants. It may also affect adults and can be triggered by stress or other health conditions such as Parkinson's disease.

Stasis dermatitis: This may be caused by varicose veins and chronic venous insufficiency, which cause a buildup of fluid beneath the skin of the legs. This fluid buildup interferes with your blood's ability to nourish your skin and places extra pressure against the skin.

While eczema can be uncomfortable to deal with, it is not contagious and can be managed well with a variety of conventional and natural methods.

SIGNS & SYMPTOMS

Eczema can appear on various parts of the body. Symptoms vary in severity and include:

• Dryness

• Itching

• Redness

• Skin lesions (crusty, scaly patches)

• Swelling

In severe cases, fluid-filled vesicles, ulcers, or cracks may occur. Open sores and ulcers can become infected if picked or scratched. If the skin becomes red and warm to the touch, it may be infected and require immediate medical attention.

RISK FACTORS

• Age: While eczema can occur at any age, it is most common in infants and young children.

• Diet (deficiency of essential fatty acids; exposure to food allergens)

- Digestive problems (leaky gut syndrome and celiac disease)

- Exposure to skin irritants (chemicals, detergents, latex, cosmetics)

- Genetics (it tends to run in families)

- Having hay fever, allergies, asthma or a family history of these conditions

- Stress (physical or emotional)

- Climate changes, stress and illness, or infections can trigger flare-ups.

FOOD ALLERGENS AND ECZEMA

Common food allergens associated with eczema include eggs, milk, peanuts, soy, and wheat. Eczema flare-ups can also be triggered by food additives (preservatives and dyes) and spices.

DOCTOR'S ORDERS

Doctors often prescribe steroid creams, such as hydrocortisone, clobetasol, or mometasone, to reduce the itching and inflammation. These products should not be used over the long term, as they may cause side effects such as burning, itching, blistering, easy bruising, and thinning of skin. Antihistamines are given for those with severe itching. Elidel (pimecrolimus) is a drug that affects the immune system and helps reduce flare-ups. This is also not recommended for long-term use.

SHERRY'S NATURAL PRESCRIPTION

Dietary Recommendations

Foods to include:

- Nuts, seeds (flaxseed, pumpkin, and hemp), coldwater fish, and olive oil contain essential fatty acids, which can help reduce inflammation. Pumpkin and sunflower seeds also contain zinc, which is important for skin health.

- Fruits and vegetables contain valuable antioxidants and fibre (which prevents constipation).

- Drink lots of purified water to help flush toxins out of the body.

Foods to avoid:

- Spices, dairy, caffeine, alcohol, and chemicals present in processed and fast foods may trigger flare-ups.

Note: Since food allergies can cause eczema, consider an elimination diet (see Appendix D) to determine if dairy, wheat, or other common allergens are the source of your skin problems.

Lifestyle Suggestions

If you have contact dermatitis, avoid exposure to known irritants. For all forms of eczema, the following tips can help reduce flare-ups:

- Use only hypoallergenic skin products, soaps, and detergents and rinse well with water.

- Take short baths or showers (five to 10 minutes) with warm (not hot) water. Bathing in oatmeal can help reduce itching. Gently pat your skin dry. Do not rub hard.

- Moisturize your skin after bathing and throughout the day. Look for creams that are thick and emollient and contain one or more of the following: chamomile; vitamins A, E, and C; calendula; licorice; and lavender. Avoid products containing perfumes, dyes, or chemical irritants.

- Wear soft, natural fabrics, such as cotton, hemp, or silk.

- Don't scratch or rub your skin. If you are itchy, apply moisturizer.

Top Recommended Supplements

Fish oils: Contain omega-3 fatty acids (EPA) that reduce inflammation. Several studies have shown significant benefits with high dosages (10 g per day). Lower dosages may also offer benefits.

Gamma-linoleic acid (GLA): An essential fatty acid that may be lacking in those with eczema. Studies have found benefits with GLA supplements (primrose, borage, and blackcurrent oil) to reduce itching and improve eczema. Dosage range: 3–6 g daily.

Complementary Supplements

Celadrin: A mixture of fatty acids that reduce inflammation. Available in creams and capsules. Dosage: 3–6 capsules daily.

Probiotics: Beneficial bacteria with immune-regulating properties; help improve digestion and reduce allergic reactions. Dosage: one to three capsules daily.

Witch hazel: An astringent that helps dry up weeping eczema and reduces itching and inflammation. Apply topically with gauze pads.

FINAL THOUGHTS

Eczema is a manageable condition. To reduce flare-ups:

1. Avoid exposure or ingestion of known allergens or triggers.
2. Use only hypoallergenic household and skin products.
3. Bathe briefly; moisturize regularly with products made for sensitive skin.
4. Consider supplements of fish oil, GLA, or Celadrin.
5. Probiotics may be helpful for those with digestive problems and to reduce allergic responses.

ENDOMETRIOSIS

Endometriosis is a condition where cells that make up the lining of the uterus grow outside the uterus, most commonly on the fallopian tubes, ovaries, or tissue lining the pelvis. This tissue behaves similarly to that within the uterus. It thickens, breaks down, and bleeds each month with the menstrual cycle. However, because there is nowhere for this blood to exit the body, it becomes trapped, irritates surrounding tissue, and may cause scar tissue to form, which is painful.

Endometriosis affects about 10–20 percent of women of child-bearing age. The actual cause is unknown; however, it is known that endometriosis is an estrogen-dependent condition and estrogen is necessary to induce or maintain endometriosis. One theory is that menstrual blood containing endometrial cells flows back through the fallopian tubes, and cells start to grow outside the uterus. Many women have some retrograde menstrual flow, yet the immune system is able to clear the debris and prevent implantation and growth of cells. In some women, though, this endometrial tissue implants and grows. It is thought that a compromised immune system or environmental toxins (xenoestrogens) may be at play. Since endometriosis often occurs in those with a family history, it is possible that there could be a genetic flaw. Another theory is that endometrial cells are carried via the bloodstream to other sites in the body.

While endometriosis can be painful, it doesn't increase the risk of uterine cancer or ovarian cancer, and there are a number of lifestyle approaches and natural remedies that can be very helpful.

SIGNS & SYMPTOMS

One-third of women with endometriosis have no symptoms. When symptoms do occur, they include:

- Heavy or irregular menstruation
- Infertility or miscarriage
- Pain with bladder or bowel function, or intestinal pain
- Painful intercourse
- Pelvic pain, especially during menstruation

ENDOMETRIOSIS AND PREGNANCY

Approximately 30–50 percent of women who have difficulty becoming pregnant have endometriosis. Endometriosis can produce adhesions that can trap the egg near the ovary and prevent it from travelling through the fallopian tube to the uterus. Despite this, many women with endometriosis are still able to conceive, but it often takes them longer. During pregnancy, most women have no signs or symptoms of endometriosis.

- Age: Women of child-bearing age are at greatest risk.

- Family history (having a mother or sister with the condition)

- Retrograde menstrual flow

- High estrogen levels (exposure to xenoestrogens)

- Immune system dysfunction

DOCTOR'S ORDERS

Doctors may prescribe anti-inflammatory medications such as ibuprofen (Advil and Motrin) to ease pain and swelling. Oral contraceptives are sometimes used to regulate hormone levels and control heavy bleeding. For women having difficulty conceiving, laparoscopic laser techniques can be done to shrink and remove lesions.

Hysterectomy should be considered only as a last resort for those with severe symptoms that have not benefited from other conventional and natural approaches. Having this radical surgery does not guarantee an end to the symptoms and is associated with various risks and complications.

SHERRY'S NATURAL PRESCRIPTION

The natural approach to endometriosis focuses on supporting liver function (the liver breaks down estrogen), optimizing intestinal health (normal flora also aid in estrogen metabolism), and balancing immune function.

Dietary Recommendations

Foods to include:

- Increase intake of whole grains, fresh vegetables, and fruits. These foods are high in fibre and help balance levels of friendly bacteria in the intestine. Choose organic as much as possible.

- Eat liver-supporting foods such as beets, carrots, onions, garlic, leafy greens, artichokes, apples, and lemons.

- Broccoli, cauliflower, Brussels sprouts, and cabbage contain indole-3-carbinol, which helps the liver break down estrogen.

- Flaxseed, soy, beans, and legumes contain phytoestrogens, which may help reduce the impact of other hormones.

- Yogurt increases the amount of friendly bacteria in the intestine.

Foods to avoid:

- Alcohol, caffeine, refined foods, food additives, sugar, and saturated fats may affect hormone balance, impair immune function, and worsen symptoms.

- Red meat and dairy products may contain dioxins and chemicals that act as estrogen-mimickers. To avoid these chemicals and hormones choose organic meat.

Lifestyle Suggestions

- Have regular pelvic examinations and report any changes in symptoms to your doctor.

- Get regular exercise. This is a natural pain reliever and boosts mood. Try walking, cycling, or aerobics. Kegel exercises (contracting and releasing the pelvic muscles) may help release pelvic tension.

- Reduce stress. Stress can trigger flare-ups and worsen symptoms. Try yoga, Pilates, stretching, and breathing techniques.

- Acupuncture and massage may help relieve pelvic congestion and pain.

- A castor oil pack may help with abdominal pain and swelling. Apply oil directly to abdomen, cover with a clean soft cloth and plastic wrap. Place a heating pad on top and let sit for 30–60 minutes.

- Do not use tampons. They block menstrual flow and may increase the likelihood of retrograde blood flow. Use unbleached, unscented cotton pads instead.

- Minimize exposure to environmental estrogens or xenoestrogens (phthalates, parabens, and dioxins), which are present in pesticides, plastics, and certain skin care products and cosmetics.

Top Recommended Supplements

Calcium D-glucarate: Helps the liver detoxify and eliminate excess hormones (particularly estrogen). Dosage: 300–500 mg daily.

Chasteberry: Balances the estrogen to progesterone ratio and may help normalize ovulation. Dosage: 150–300 mg daily.

Indole-3-carbinol: A compound found naturally in cruciferous vegetables that aids in detoxification of estrogen, protects liver function, and may protect against hormonal cancers. Dosage: 400 mg daily.

Milk thistle: Supports liver function and aids detoxification. Dosage: 50–100 mg daily.

Complementary Supplements

Calcium and magnesium: Aid in hormone metabolism and may help reduce menstrual pain. Dosages: 500 mg of calcium and 200 mg of magnesium three times daily.

Evening primrose oil: Helps reduce pain and inflammation. Dosage: 3,000 mg daily.

Fish oils: Contains omega-3 fatty acids that may help with pain and inflammation. Dosage: 1 g three times daily.

Iron: Required for those with heavy bleeding and anemia. Dosage varies. Take only under advice from your health care provider.

Vitamin C: Improves healing of tissues damaged by lesions and scarring; it also helps control heavy bleeding by strengthening capillary walls. Dosage: 1,000 mg daily.

E

Endometriosis

FINAL THOUGHTS

To improve endometriosis and prevent worsening, consider the following:

1. Eat organic vegetables, fruits, whole grains, legumes, flaxseed, and yogurt.
2. Minimize red meat, dairy, alcohol, caffeine, and refined foods.
3. Get regular exercise and reduce stress.
4. Avoid exposure to environmental estrogens.
5. Top recommended supplements are indole-3-carbinol, calcium D-glucarate, chasteberry, and milk thistle.

ERECTILE DYSFUNCTION (IMPOTENCE)

Erectile dysfunction (ED), also known as impotence, is the inability to achieve or maintain an erection that is adequate for sexual performance. This is the most common sexual problem among men—almost every man will experience an episode of ED at one point in his life. Persistent ED affects approximately 25 percent of men over age 50 and this figure rises with age.

A series of factors are involved in developing an erection. Sexual arousal causes nerves in the brain and spine to signal arteries in the penis to swell up with blood. The spongy tissues in the penis expand and it becomes erect. Any interference with this process, whether physical or psychological, can prevent an erection.

As men age, there are changes in erectile function. It may take longer to develop an erection and it may not be as rigid, and more direct stimulation may be required. Orgasm may become less intense and the volume of ejaculate reduced.

The majority of cases of ED are caused by physical factors such as diabetes and nerve damage. It can also be caused by psychological issues, or the use of certain drugs. In most cases it is not caused by low sexual desire.

While ED was once a sensitive subject to discuss, the advent of drugs such as Viagra has brought this topic into the limelight and more men are seeking treatment. Aside from drug therapy, there are many things that can be done to prevent ED and improve erectile function.

SIGNS & SYMPTOMS

- Inability to obtain a full erection
- Inability to maintain an erection for sexual performance

RISK FACTORS

- Diabetes: Elevated blood sugar damages blood vessels in the penis
- Diseases of the nerves, blood vessels, heart, prostate, and kidneys
- Hormonal imbalances: Low testosterone, growth hormone, or DHEA levels
- Surgery or trauma that causes nerve damage (spinal cord injury, prostate surgery)
- Drugs: Antidepressants, beta-blockers, antihistamines, tranquilizers, and anti-cancer drugs
- Alcohol, marijuana, cocaine, and other illicit drugs
- Smoking causes damage to blood vessels and nerves in the penis, affecting erectile function.
- Psychological factors: Stress, anxiety, depression, and lack of sleep

DIABETES AND ED

Diabetes is the leading cause of erectile dysfunction. Approximately 80 percent of men with diabetes develop erectile dysfunction, and it occurs at an earlier age.

DOCTOR'S ORDERS

Medications such as Viagra, Cialis, and Levitra have revolutionized the treatment of ED. These drugs work by enhancing the effects of nitric oxide, a chemical that relaxes muscles in the penis, leading to increased blood flow. Arousal and stimulation is still required for an erection, but the drug assists the physical aspect. Do not use these drugs if you have had a heart attack, stroke, or other serious heart problems, or if you are taking drugs for angina (nitroglycerine).

Yohimbe is a plant-based drug that dilates blood vessels and increases circulation. It has been shown in several studies to improve ED. Yohimbe was previously available over the counter, but is now available by prescription only due to numerous side effects such as nervousness, irritability, insomnia, and increased blood pressure. It should be avoided by those with heart or kidney disease.

Other medical options include injectable drugs, implants, hormone therapy, vacuum devices, surgery to repair blood vessels or nerves, and counselling.

SHERRY'S NATURAL PRESCRIPTION

Dietary Recommendations

Foods to include:

- Fibre-rich foods help promote blood sugar balance.

- Zinc helps support testosterone production; the best food sources are pumpkin seeds, soybeans, oysters, and wheat germ.

- Vitamin E dilates blood vessels and improves blood flow; the best food sources include nuts and seeds, whole grains, and leafy green vegetables.

Foods to avoid:

- Foods high in saturated and trans fats can be damaging to the blood vessels and reduce circulation (red meat, dairy, processed and fast foods).

- Minimize refined flour and sugar as these foods cause blood sugar fluctuations, which can be damaging to the blood vessels.

- Avoid alcohol before sex.

Lifestyle Suggestions

- Exercise: Regular activity is essential to improve blood flow and circulation, reduce stress, and increase energy levels. Activities such as walking, squats, and lunges are particularly good for increasing blood flow to the pelvic area.

- Don't smoke. Smoking has serious consequences, as it damages blood vessels and nerves.

- Maintain a healthy body weight. Obesity leads to diabetes and heart disease, both of which can impact sexual function.

- Get adequate sleep at night and be aware that a lack of sleep can affect performance.

- Reduce stress whether through exercise, breathing techniques, or visualization. Find what works to promote relaxation and practise it regularly.

- Communicate with your partner and your doctor.

Top Recommended Supplements

Arginine: An amino acid used to make nitrous oxide, a substance that dilates blood vessels and increases blood flow. Dosage: 1,000 mg three to five times daily.

Korean ginseng: Also called panax ginseng, Korean ginseng increases energy and the ability to maintain an erection; several studies have found it effective for improving erectile function. Dosage: 1,800–2,700 mg daily.

Complementary Supplements

Antioxidants: Vitamins C and E and flavonoids (grape seed and pine bark) help improve blood flow and reduce oxidative damage to the blood vessels. Follow label directions.

Ginkgo biloba: Opens blood vessels and increases blood flow to the penis; is particularly helpful for ED caused by antidepressant drugs or vascular problems (diabetics). Dosage: 120–200 mg daily.

Maca: Rich in the amino acid arginine, which increases blood flow to the penis and histidine, which helps support orgasm and ejaculation; preliminary research has found it helpful. Dosage: 500–1,000 mg three times daily.

FINAL THOUGHTS

To prevent or improve ED, consider the following:

1. Exercise regularly; eat a high-fibre diet with lots of whole grains, nuts, and seeds; and reduce stress.
2. Maintain a healthy body weight.
3. Don't smoke and minimize alcohol.
4. The best supplements for ED are Korean ginseng and arginine.
5. Ginkgo biloba may be helpful for ED caused by antidepressant use or those who have diabetes.

FIBROCYSTIC BREASTS

Fibrocystic breasts are described as benign (non-cancerous) changes that occur in the breast tissue, making them lumpy and fibrous. This condition is also known as cyclic mastalgia. It was once known as fibrocystic breast disease, but the term "disease" is no longer used because research has shown that this condition is a variation of normal breasts, not a disease, yet it can cause significant pain and discomfort.

Fibrocystic breasts affect as many as 60 percent of women typically between ages 30 and 50. During the menstruating years, fluctuating monthly hormonal cycles can lead to the accumulation of fluid, cells, and cellular debris within the breast. It is believed that excess levels of the hormones estrogen and prolactin cause breast cysts to become chronically inflamed and surrounded by fibrous tissue that can harden and thicken the cysts, creating the lumpy breasts. Other hormones, such as growth factor, insulin, and thyroid hormone, are also implicated.

While this condition can be painful, the lumps are benign and do not increase your risk of breast cancer. If you do discover a lump in your breast tissue, it is important to consult with your doctor.

There are a number of lifestyle modifications and natural treatments that can help reduce the symptoms of fibrocystic breasts and promote good breast health.

SIGNS & SYMPTOMS

- Breast pain and tenderness

- Changes in nipple sensation (itching)

- Dense and bumpy consistency in the breast tissue

- Feeling of fullness in the breasts

- Swelling in the breasts before the menstrual period

Note: Symptoms may range from mild to severe and typically peak just before each menstrual period, and improve immediately after the menstrual period.

FIBROCYSTIC BREASTS AND BREAST CANCER

Fibrocystic lumps are benign and don't increase your breast cancer risk, but they can make diagnosing breast cancer more difficult because of the dense, fibrous tissue and lumps. Fibrocystic lumps move freely when touched and they get worse with the menstrual cycle. In contrast, a cancerous growth in the breast is often not tender or freely movable when touched. See your doctor if you notice a lump in your breast. To rule out breast cancer, a needle aspiration of the cyst and/or mammogram can be done.

RISK FACTORS

- Age: Women between the ages of 30 and 50 are at greatest risk

- Diet: High intake of saturated fat and caffeine

- Family history of fibrocystic breasts or breast cancer

F

Fibrocystic Breasts

- Irregular menstrual cycles

- Hormones: Having an imbalance of estrogen to progesterone (estrogen dominance), which can be caused by exposure to xenoestrogens (estrogen-like chemicals in food and environment, such as pesticides and plastics) or taking estrogen replacement therapy

- Low thyroid function (hypothyroidism)

- Not having children

- Poor lymphatic drainage

SHERRY'S NATURAL PRESCRIPTION

Dietary Recommendations

Foods to include:

- Boost fibre intake (whole grains, vegetables, and fruits) as fibre helps the body eliminate excess hormones and toxins, which worsen fibrocystic breasts. Onions, garlic, beets, artichokes, and lemon help support liver function and the elimination of hormones.

- Choose organic foods as much as possible to avoid harmful chemicals.

- Cruciferous vegetables (broccoli, cauliflower, Brussels sprouts, and cabbage) contain substances that help the body detoxify estrogen.

- Drink plenty of water. Try dandelion tea, which may help reduce breast pain and supports detoxification.

- Fish and flaxseeds contain beneficial fatty acids that can help reduce inflammation. Flaxseed also contains lignans which act as a phytoestrogen and help to block the effects of estrogen.

- Sea vegetables (kelp and nori) contain iodine, which may be deficient in those with fibrocystic breasts. Iodine deficiency can increase tissue sensitivity to estrogen stimulation.

- Soy products contain phytoestrogens, which can help balance hormone levels and counter the effects of excess estrogen stimulation. Soy also contains amino acids which aid in detoxification.

- Use oils containing beneficial fats such as olive, flaxseed and sunflower oil.

Foods to avoid:

- Minimize caffeine as it can worsen symptoms. Aside from coffee, it is also in black tea (and, to a lesser extent, in green tea), cola, chocolate, and some over-the-counter medications.

- Reduce saturated fat (meat and dairy products) as studies have shown that it can worsen fibrocystic breasts.

Lifestyle Suggestions

- Examine your breasts monthly.

- Exercise regularly to improve circulation and help the body detoxify.

- Work on losing excess weight. Women who are obese have higher levels of estrogen because this hormone can be stored in fat tissue.

- Reduce stress, which can cause hormonal changes that may worsen symptoms. Try yoga, tai chi, and breathing techniques.

- Get your hormones checked. Ask your doctor to check your thyroid as low thyroid can worsen symptoms of fibrocystic breasts. Urine and saliva tests can be done to check for estrogen dominance. See Appendix E for more information.

- Massage can help improve circulation and lymphatic drainage.

- Wear a proper-fitting bra. If it is too tight, it can cut off circulation and worsen symptoms.

- Apply castor oil packs to the breasts. Soak flannel cloth in castor oil, wring out, and apply to breasts. Cover with a heating pad or hot water bottle and leave on for 30 minutes. This will help relieve pain and improve circulation.

Top Recommended Supplements

Chasteberry (vitex): Helps to balance hormone levels of estrogen, progesterone, and prolactin. Studies have shown that it can help reduce breast pain and swelling. Dosage: 150–300 mg daily of a product standardized to contain at least 0.5 percent agnuside. Do not take if you are on oral contraceptives or if you are pregnant.

Fish oils: Contain beneficial omega-3 fatty acids, which have anti-inflammatory effects, help reduce breast pain, and also help the body absorb iodine. Iodine deficiency is associated with fibrocystic breast changes. Dosage: 1 g three times daily.

GLA: Found in flaxseed, primrose, and borage oil, which contain beneficial fatty acids that may help reduce pain and inflammation associated with fibrocystic breasts. Dosage: 1 g three times daily.

Indole-3-carbinol: A compound found naturally in cruciferous vegetables that aids in detoxification of estrogen, protects liver function, and may protect against hormonal cancers. Dosage: 400 mg daily.

Complementary Supplements

Magnesium: Helps reduce pain and inflammation of fibrocystic breast changes, particularly symptoms associated with the menstrual cycle. Dosage: 100–200 mg twice daily with meals.

Vitamin B6: Helps the liver process estrogen. Studies have shown that it can reduce breast pain and swelling associated with the menstrual cycle. Dosage: 50–100 mg daily as part of a B-complex.

Vitamin E: Helps reduce pain, tenderness, and swelling. Some (but not all) studies have found benefits. Dosage: 400–800 IU daily.

FINAL THOUGHTS

To prevent and manage fibrocystic breasts naturally, consider the following:

1. Examine your breasts monthly and report any changes to your doctor.
2. Reduce exposure to xenoestrogens (plastics, pesticides, non-organic meat, and dairy). Eat more fibre, sea and cruciferous vegetables, and soy products.
3. Reduce stress and get regular exercise.
4. Try castor oil packs to relieve pain and promote better circulation.
5. Consider supplements of chasteberry, fish oils, GLA, and indole-3-carbinol.

FIBROIDS (UTERINE)

Uterine fibroids are non-cancerous tumours or growths of the uterus. They are also known as myomas, fibromyomas, or leiomyomas. Despite their name, fibroids are not fibrous; they are comprised of connective tissue and muscle. They can appear in groups and grow either inside or outside of the uterus. Approximately 50 percent of women have fibroids; however, many are unaware. They can be smaller than a pea, or grow as large as a football. In rare cases fibroids can develop into cancer; however, most often they are not harmful, but may cause pain and discomfort when they become large and put pressure on the abdomen and bladder.

Fibroids typically appear during the child-bearing years, particularly between the ages of 30 and 40 years, and then shrink in menopause. While the actual cause of fibroids is uncertain, it is known that their growth is stimulated by estrogen. Fibroids are becoming increasingly common today, which has been attributed to high amounts of xenoestrogens (estrogen-like compounds) in our food supply and environment.

ENVIRONMENTAL ESTROGENS

Xenoestrogens are substances that have estrogen-like activity in the body. They are present in foods (fish, meat, and dairy) and in the environment (plastics, pesticides, and skin care products). Research suggests that xenoestrogens may play a role in uterine fibroids, certain cancers, and premature sexual maturity in young girls.

SIGNS & SYMPTOMS

Many women do not realize they have fibroids until it is discovered as a result of a pelvic examination or prenatal ultrasound. For those who develop large fibroid tumours, signs and symptoms vary depending on location, and may include:

- Anemia (due to heavy bleeding)
- Backache or leg pains
- Constipation
- Heavy menstrual bleeding and prolonged periods
- Infertility and miscarriages
- Pelvic pressure or pain
- Urinary frequency or incontinence

RISK FACTORS

- Age: Most common between the ages of 30 and 40 years
- Estrogen excess (promotes growth of fibroids)
- Family history (fibroids contain genetic alterations)
- Insulin-like growth factor (may stimulate fibroid growth)
- Race (fibroids are more common among Black women)

Some studies have suggested that obese women are at increased risk for fibroids, while other studies have not found this link. Studies have also found a link between consumption of red meat and ham with the presence of fibroids. Pregnancy and childbirth may have a protective effect, but more research is needed.

DOCTOR'S ORDERS

In most cases, doctors recommend watchful waiting for fibroids. Since fibroids tend to grow slowly and then shrink after menopause, surgical procedures are recommended only if the fibroids are large and cause heavy bleeding and pain, or if they are impairing fertility. Surgical options include myomectomy (incision into abdomen and removal of fibroids), hysterectomy (removal of uterus), and uterine artery embolization (procedure that cuts off blood supply to the uterus to cause the fibroid to shrink). Medications are also used to reduce estrogen levels and shrink fibroids; however, there are many side effects with these drugs. Progesterone cream is popularly used for fibroid treatment; however, in some women it can cause fibroids to grow, so it should be used only under a physician's supervision.

SHERRY'S NATURAL PRESCRIPTION

A holistic approach to treating fibroids is aimed at reducing levels of circulating estrogens and supporting liver function (the liver detoxifies estrogen). This can be achieved through dietary, lifestyle, and supplemental approaches.

Dietary Recommendations

Foods to include:

- Fibre-rich foods such as fruits, vegetables, and whole grains will help extract excessive estrogen stores from the body.

- Cruciferous vegetables such as broccoli, cauliflower, and Brussels sprouts are particularly helpful, as they contain compounds that help the liver detoxify estrogen.

- Choose organic foods whenever possible to reduce ingestion of xenoestrogens from pesticides.

- Foods containing phytoestrogens (plant-based estrogens), such as soy foods and flaxseed, help balance estrogen levels.

- Artichokes, beets, carrots, dandelion greens, garlic, and onions contain compounds that support liver function and detoxification of hormones.

- Drink more green tea, as it contains polyphenols that block the negative effects of estrogen and help protect against estrogen-related cancers.

- Those with heavy bleeding may require additional iron to prevent anemia. The best food sources of iron include clams, oysters, organ meats, beef, pork, poultry, and fish. Iron is also present in eggs, dried beans, fortified cereals, and dark green leafy vegetables.

Foods to avoid:

- Meat, dairy, and fish (farmed salmon) may contain dioxins and other xenoestrogens that can stimulate fibroid growth and worsen symptoms.

- Minimize sugar and caffeine, which can trigger pain and inflammation.

Lifestyle Suggestions

• Reduce stress, as it can cause hormonal changes that may worsen fibroid symptoms. Try yoga, tai chi, and breathing techniques.

• Regular exercise of moderate-intensity activity for one hour daily reduces stress and will help to maintain a healthy body weight.

• Acupuncture helps relieve pelvic pain and swelling.

• Apply castor oil to your pelvic area, cover with plastic and a hot towel. Leave in place for one hour and do this three times per week.

Top Recommended Supplements

Calcium D-glucarate: Assists in the elimination of estrogen. Dosage: 400–500 mg daily.

Indole-3-carbinol: Helps with the detoxification or breakdown of estrogen. Dosage: 200–400 mg daily.

Chasteberry: Helps to normalize hormone levels. Dosage: 160–240 mg daily.

Complementary Supplements

Dandelion root and milk thistle: Help support liver detoxification. Dosage varies. Follow label directions or the advice of your health care provider.

Pancreatic enzymes: May help reduce unusual cell and tissue growths. Dosage: One capsule between meals three times daily.

Red raspberry tea: An astringent that helps reduce uterine inflammation and prevents fibroid growth. Dosage: 500–1,000 mL daily.

FINAL THOUGHTS

Fibroids are a common condition that affects women of child-bearing years. To prevent and manage fibroids naturally, consider the following:

1. Reduce exposure to xenoestrogens (plastics, pesticides, non-organic meat, and dairy).
2. Boost fibre intake; eat more cruciferous vegetables.
3. Reduce stress and get regular exercise.
4. Acupuncture can help relieve pain and promote relaxation.
5. Consider supplements of indole-3-carbinol, calcium D-glucarate, and chasteberry.

FIBROMYALGIA

Fibromyalgia (FM) is a common disorder that has only recently received recognition by the medical community. It is marked by widespread pain, fatigue, and tender points.

The exact cause of FM is unknown. However, researchers have identified several factors that contribute to the development of FM:

- Allergies or chemical sensitivities
- Alterations in muscle metabolism: Reduced blood flow to muscles can cause fatigue and pain
- Chemical imbalance in the brain: Alterations in the neurotransmitters serotonin and norepinephrine
- Elevated levels of a chemical called substance P, which is involved in our sensation of pain signals
- Infection: Viruses (Epstein-Barr, HHV-6, and cytomegalovirus) and fungal infections by *Candida albicans* have been implicated
- Nutritional deficiencies in magnesium and antioxidants
- Sleep disturbances: Disturbed sleep patterns may be a cause rather than just a symptom
- Trauma or injury, particularly in the upper spinal region

The word "fibromyalgia" comes from the Latin terms for fibrous tissue (fibro), muscle (myo), and pain (algia).

SIGNS & SYMPTOMS

Symptoms of FM vary among people and can be affected by weather, stress, and physical activity.

- Anxiety
- Chest pain
- Depression
- Difficulty concentrating
- Dizziness
- Dry eyes, skin, and mouth
- Fatigue and sleep disturbance
- Headaches
- Irritable bowel or bladder
- Numbness or tingling in the hands and feet
- Pain: Most commonly in the neck, shoulders, hips, lower back, and thighs
- Painful menstrual periods
- Swollen lymph nodes

F

Fibromyalgia

- Age: Early and middle adulthood
- Autoimmune disease: Those with arthritis, lupus, and other autoimmune diseases
- Disturbed sleep: Those with nighttime muscle cramps, restless legs, or sleep apnea
- Family history
- Gender: Women are at greater risk

According to a report in the Annals of Internal Medicine, 33 percent of FM patients also suffer from multiple chemical sensitivities. *Annals of Internal Medicine,* 1999: 130 (11); 910–921.

DOCTOR'S ORDERS

There is no cure for FM. Prescription drugs are given to reduce symptoms, with limited success. Those commonly prescribed include muscle relaxants (Flexeril), anti-inflammatory drugs (ibuprofen), and pain relievers (acetaminophen, codeine). In some people, antidepressants help to improve sleep, depression, and anxiety.

SHERRY'S NATURAL PRESCRIPTION

A comprehensive program that includes lifestyle strategies, nutrition, and supplements to reduce symptoms and improve well-being offers the greatest benefit for FM sufferers.

Dietary Recommendations

Foods to include:
- Focus on fresh fruits, vegetables, whole grains, lean protein, and healthy fats to ensure your body gets essential nutrients and energy.
- Eat plenty of magnesium-rich foods such as green vegetables, soybeans, almonds, and cashews.

Foods to avoid:
- Caffeine interferes with sleep, causes anxiety, and reduces mineral absorption.
- Sugar reduces immune function, interferes with sleep, causes mood swings, and encourages growth of yeast, which has been linked to FM.
- Minimize or avoid processed/fast/fried foods, which are high in saturated fats and can trigger inflammation.

Note: Since food allergies have been implicated in FM, it is important to identify possible allergens. Refer to Appendix D for more information.

Lifestyle Suggestions

- Reduce stress, which can trigger or aggravate the symptoms of FM. Try breathing exercises, meditation, yoga, and massage.

F

Fibromyalgia

- Exercise to improve mood, reduce pain, and improve overall well-being.

- Chiropractic improves spinal alignment and nerve flow; can reduce pain and improve sleep.

- Acupuncture can help reduce pain and promote relaxation.

- Sleep is essential; lack of sleep can intensify pain, anxiety, and responses to stress.

- Laughter improves mood and well-being; watch funny movies, read humorous books, and spend time with funny people.

Top Recommended Supplements

5-hydroxytryptophan (5-HTP): Elevates serotonin levels and alleviates depression; may also reduce tender points, anxiety, and improve sleep quality. Do not combine with prescription antidepressants or products that modify serotonin levels. Dosage: 100 mg three times daily. This is less expensive than SAMe (see below) and is a good second choice.

Melatonin: A hormone that regulates our sleep cycles. Supplements shorten the time needed to fall asleep, reduce night wakening, improve sleep quality, and reduce tender points. Dosage: 3 mg one hour before bed.

S-adenosylmethionine (SAMe): Supports production of neurotransmitters (serotonin), antioxidants, hormones, and joint compounds. Studies for FM have shown that it can reduce pain, fatigue, and stiffness, and improve mood. SAMe is very safe and better tolerated than antidepressant drugs. Dosage: 800 mg daily. Choose a product that is enteric coated. Take on an empty stomach.

Complementary Supplements

Vitamin E: Antioxidants may be depleted in those with FM; preliminary research found that vitamin E improved symptoms of FM. Dosage: 400 IU daily.

Capsaicin: A component of cayenne pepper that helps relieve pain, and works by depleting substance P, thus reducing the sensation of pain. Look for Zostrix or Menthacin, which are available without a prescription. Apply to painful areas; wash hands after application, as it can burn the eyes.

Celadrin: Reduces pain and swelling; improves joint mobility. Dosage: 1,500 mg daily. Celadrin is also available in a cream, which can be applied to sore joints and muscles.

Magnesium: Reduces inflammation; promotes muscle relaxation. Dosage: 200 mg three times daily; may provide additional benefits when taken with malic acid (1,200–2,400 mg), which reduces pain.

F

Fibromyalgia

FINAL THOUGHTS

FM is a chronic and painful condition that is not curable, but can be greatly improved with lifestyle strategies and supplements. Key points to keep in mind:

1. Nourish your body with a healthy diet and eliminate foods that trigger inflammation.
2. Exercise regularly to reduce stress and pain and improve sleep and mood.
3. Consider massage, chiropractic, and/or acupuncture to reduce symptoms.
4. Top supplements include SAMe or 5-HTP and melatonin.
5. Consider supportive supplements of Celadrin, magnesium, and antioxidants.

FLU

The flu, which is short for influenza, is a viral infection that affects the upper respiratory tract (nose, throat, bronchial tubes, and lungs). Every year, approximately 10–25 percent of Canadians are infected with the flu. While it can be unpleasant, most people recover within a week to 10 days. However, an estimated 4,000–8,000 Canadians, mostly seniors, die every year from pneumonia related to flu or from other serious complications of flu.

The flu is caused by three strains (types) of viruses: influenza A, B, and C. Type A is responsible for the deadly influenza pandemics (worldwide epidemics) that strike every 10–40 years. Type B can lead to smaller, more localized outbreaks that generally occur every three to 15 years. And either types A or B can cause the flu that circulates almost every winter. Type C is less common and causes only mild symptoms.

In Canada, flu season typically runs from November to April. During these months when the weather is colder outside, we spend more time indoors, closer to one another and sharing germs. This is how the flu is spread—by close contact with someone who has the virus. The virus travels through the air in droplets when someone with the infection coughs, sneezes, or talks. You can inhale the droplets directly, or you can pick up the germs from an object (doorknob, telephone, or keyboard) and then transfer them to your eyes, nose, or mouth.

There is no cure for the flu, but there are measures that can be taken to reduce your risk of infection and speed healing and reduce complications if you are infected.

IS IT THE FLU?

The flu is often confused with cold or stomach flu, but both are caused by other viruses. There is no such thing as stomach flu. A sudden onset of diarrhea, vomiting, and upset stomach is often caused by a virus (not influenza) that infects the digestive tract or by a change in diet. A cold is also caused by a virus (rhinovirus), but it differs from the flu in that it has a slower onset and is not usually associated with high fever or muscle or joint aching. Cold symptoms are also less severe than flu.

SIGNS & SYMPTOMS

Once you are in contact with the virus, it takes about 48 hours for symptoms to develop.

• Chills and sweats

• Headache

• Loss of appetite

• Nasal congestion

• Nausea and vomiting (more common in children)

• Sore throat, dry cough

• Sudden onset of fever, muscle and joint aching, weakness, and fatigue

In most cases, the symptoms resolve in a week to 10 days. However, young children, the elderly, and those with a weakened immune system are at risk of developing complications such as ear infections, acute sinusitis, bronchitis, and pneumonia.

RISK FACTORS

Anyone can get the flu, but the following are at greatest risk of infection and developing complications of the flu:

- Adults and children with chronic heart and lung disease

- Health care workers

- People living in a nursing home or chronic care facility

- People with chronic conditions such as diabetes, anemia, cancer, immune suppression, HIV, or kidney disease

- Those younger than two years or over age 65

DOCTOR'S ORDERS

For most people, the best way to manage the flu is to rest, drink fluids, and allow the infection to run its course. Those who are at risk of complications (infants, the elderly, and those listed above) should consult with their doctor. There are antiviral drugs (such as Tamiflu) that can be given within the first 48 hours to reduce the length of illness and help prevent complications.

Anyone with signs and symptoms of pneumonia should seek medical attention. These include a severe cough (with phlegm), a high fever, and a sharp pain in the lungs when you breathe deeply. If you have bacterial pneumonia, you'll need treatment with antibiotics.

Over-the-counter products such as Tylenol and Motrin can be used to help reduce pain and fever. While they may help ease the symptoms, they do not shorten the duration of infection and can cause side effects. Tylenol can be hard on the liver and Motrin can cause stomach pain, bleeding, and ulcers. Children under age 16 should not be given aspirin because of the risk of Reye's syndrome, a rare but potentially fatal disease.

Health Canada recommends yearly flu vaccination for those at risk. Vaccines don't offer 100 percent protection, but they do help reduce the risk of infection and complications if you get sick. Children under six months and those who are allergic to eggs should not receive the vaccine.

There is great debate about the long-term safety of vaccination and possible consequences, such as allergic reactions and increased risk of Guillain-Barré syndrome, an autoimmune disease that attacks the nervous system and results in weakness and abnormal sensations. There has also been ongoing concern about a possible link between thimerosal (a mercury-based preservative found in vaccines) and the risk of autism. At this point the Centers for Disease Control and Health Canada feel that there is not enough evidence to link the two, but there are numerous case reports linking autism to vaccinations. It is important to review the benefits and risks with your health care provider.

F

Flu

SHERRY'S NATURAL PRESCRIPTION

Dietary Recommendations

Foods to include:

- Citrus fruits and berries contain vitamin C, which helps support immune function.

- Drink plenty of fluids, especially during the first few days of infection, to prevent dehydration and weakness. Choose water, juice, herbal teas, and broth. Elderberry juice contains compounds that can speed healing.

- Eat light meals of nutritious foods such as soups and stews with vegetables and beans, brown rice, fish, and poultry.

- Garlic, ginger, and onions contain antioxidants that support immune function.

Foods to avoid:

- Dairy products can worsen mucus (phlegm).

- Minimize sugar (candy, soft drinks, and sweets) as it can hamper immune function.

Lifestyle Suggestions

- Get adequate rest as this is essential to help your body recover. Not getting enough rest on a regular basis can weaken your immune system and make you more susceptible to the flu and other infections.

- Minimize stress, which can hamper immune function. Try meditation, yoga, and breathing techniques.

- Get regular exercise to support proper immune function. Studies have shown that those who exercise regularly have less severe symptoms and recover quicker than those who don't exercise. During an episode of the flu you will not have the energy to exercise and should rest.

- Wash your hands frequently (especially after touching your eyes, nose, or mouth and after coughing or sneezing) to prevent spreading germs to others.

Top Recommended Supplements

Echinacea: Contains compounds that are thought to stimulate the immune system. Studies have shown that supplements can reduce flu symptoms and duration of infection. There are many forms of echinacea. A mixture containing all the parts of E. purpurea above the ground (flowers, leaves, stems) has the best supporting evidence for effectiveness in treating flu. Dosage: 3–5 mL of tincture or 300 mg of extract three times daily. Take at the first onset of symptoms and continue for seven to 14 days. There is no evidence that taking it all the time will reduce the risk of infection, so take it only when you need it.

Garlic: Has antiviral properties and enhances immune function. Studies of aged garlic extract (a special extract that contains potent sulphur compounds) found that regular use can reduce the risk of cold and flu. Dosage: 600 mg daily.

Complementary Supplements

Elderberry: Can stimulate the immune system and inhibit viral growth. Studies of a product containing elderberry, echinacea, and bee propolis found that it reduced symptoms and sped recovery from influenza. Dosage: Follow label instructions.

Panax ginseng: Strengthens immune function. A few studies have shown that it can reduce the risk of cold and flu. Dosage: 200 mg daily of an extract standardized to contain 4–7 percent ginsenosides.

• •

FLU PROTECTION

To reduce the risk of contracting the flu, wash your hands frequently and avoid touching your eyes, nose, or mouth; get adequate sleep; eat a healthy diet; exercise regularly; and limit exposure to crowded places during flu season. If you are at high risk of the flu, discuss the benefits and risks of having a vaccine with your doctor.

• •

FINAL THOUGHTS

To improve healing from the flu, consider the following:

1. Drink plenty of fluids, such as water, elderberry juice, and herbal teas.
2. Eat citrus, berries, garlic, onions, and ginger.
3. Minimize sugar and dairy products during an infection.
4. Get lots of sleep and rest to allow your body to recover.
5. Consider echinacea to speed recovery and aged garlic extract for prevention.

GALLSTONES

Gallstones are solid deposits of cholesterol or mineral salts that form in your gallbladder or nearby bile ducts. It is estimated that about 20 percent of Canadians have gallstones by age 60. In many cases they do not cause a problem or symptoms. However, some people with gallstones develop a gallbladder attack, which causes abdominal pain, bloating, and nausea.

The gallbladder is a pouch-shaped digestive organ that is located near the liver and is responsible for storing and concentrating bile, a greenish-brown fluid composed of bile salts, fatty compounds, cholesterol, and other chemicals produced by the liver. When you eat, food enters the small intestine and the gallbladder contracts and releases bile into the common bile duct. The common bile duct carries bile to the upper part of your small intestine (duodenum), where it helps break down fat from your food. Aside from aiding digestion, bile is also involved in the absorption of fat-soluble nutrients, the retention of water in the colon to promote bowel movements, the excretion of bilirubin (the residue from the breakdown of red blood cells), and the elimination of drugs and chemicals from the body. If the bile becomes chemically unbalanced, it can form into particles that eventually grow into stones, which can lead to inflammation and infection of the gallbladder, known as cholecystitis.

There are two main types of gallstones: cholesterol and pigment gallstones. Cholesterol gallstones, as the name implies, are comprised mainly of cholesterol. They are yellow in colour and may also contain calcium and bilirubin. About 90 percent of gallstones are cholesterol stones. They can be caused by too much cholesterol in the bile (which is not related to high blood cholesterol) or infrequent or incomplete emptying of the gallbladder (which causes the bile to become more concentrated). Pigment gallstones are dark brown or black stones that form when your bile contains too much bilirubin. This may result from having cirrhosis, biliary tract infection, or sickle cell anemia.

Problematic gallstones are treatable with medications and/or surgery. Lifestyle measures can go a long way to help prevent gallstones and also to help eliminate them.

CHOLESTEROL AND GALLSTONES

About 90 percent of gallstones are comprised of cholesterol. Normally, your bile contains enough bile salts and lecithin to dissolve the cholesterol excreted by your liver. However, if your bile contains high amounts of cholesterol, it may form into crystals, which can develop into stones over time. Diets high in saturated fat can increase the risk of gallstones threefold. Don't cut out fat completely as some is necessary for proper function of the gallbladder. Just choose healthy, polyunsaturated fats, such as olive oil, fish, nuts, and seeds.

SIGNS & SYMPTOMS

Gallstones vary greatly in shape and size. They can be as small as a grain of salt or as large as a golf ball. They can be smooth and round or irregular with jagged edges. Some people get just one, and others have several or even hundreds of them. About 90 percent of people have no symptoms. Others may experience:

- Fever when the stones get trapped in the neck of the gallbladder

- Indigestion (gas and bloating)

- Nausea and vomiting

- Upper abdominal pain and aching

Untreated gallstones can lead to serious, even fatal, complications, such as the following:

- Blockage of the bile duct: Occurs when a small stone escapes the gallbladder and enter the ducts leading from your gallbladder, liver, or pancreas to your small intestine (common bile duct). Symptoms include yellowing of the whites of the eyes and skin (jaundice), dark urine, and pain in the upper abdomen. If the pancreas becomes inflamed, it can cause intense, constant pain in your upper abdomen that may radiate to your back or chest. The pain is usually worse when you lie down and better when you sit up. You may also have nausea, vomiting, and fever.

- Gallbladder cancer: Gallstones may cause your gallbladder to release bile more slowly, which increases inflammation and the amount of time cells are exposed to cancer-causing substances in the bile. This type of cancer is quite rare.

G

Gallstones

RISK FACTORS

- Age: Risk increases with age. About 25–30 percent of women and 10–15 percent of men develop gallstones by age 70.

- Ethnicity: The incidence of gallstones is higher in certain racial groups. For example, in Canada 70–80 percent of the Native population is affected by this disease.

- Gender: Women between the ages of 20 and 60 are three times more likely to have gallstones than men. This is attributed to estrogen, which causes more cholesterol to be excreted in the bile.

- Medical conditions such as cirrhosis, biliary tract infection, and sickle cell anemia increase the risk of pigment gallstones.

- Obesity raises cholesterol levels in the bile and also reduces the frequency of gallbladder emptying.

- Pregnancy and use of oral contraceptives or estrogen therapy increase the risk.

- Yo-yo dieting: Rapid weight loss can upset bile chemistry and skipping meals or eating too little fat can reduce gallbladder contractions.

DIETING AND GALLSTONES

Rapid weight loss from fad dieting can increase your risk of gallstones. In fact, losing more than 3 lbs a week may increase your risk of developing gallstones when compared with losing weight more gradually. Skipping meals or cutting fat out of your diet reduces gallbladder emptying and this also increases your risk of gallstones.

DOCTOR'S ORDERS

Most gallstones do not cause any symptoms. Treatment is required only if you are experiencing serious symptoms. The most common treatment for gallstones causing symptoms is removal of the gallbladder (cholecystectomy). This can be done by laparascopic surgery where a small tube is inserted into the abdomen and tiny instruments are used to remove the gallbladder. This is preferred as the incisions are small and recovery is quick (a few days). For severe cases, open surgery through a large abdominal incision is necessary. Recovery from this procedure can take weeks.

For those with small stones, sound wave therapy can help break up stones. Medications, such as ursodiol, are then used to dissolve the stone fragments.

SHERRY'S NATURAL PRESCRIPTION

Dietary changes, exercise, and supplements can be helpful in preventing gallstones and to prevent them from growing and causing inflammation and infection. However, if you are experiencing severe pain, fever, or any of the above listed symptoms of a blockage of the bile duct, it is critical to see your doctor.

Dietary Recommendations

Foods to include:

• Beets, artichokes, and dandelion greens help to improve the flow of bile.

• Coffee is actually protective. Caffeine increases bile flow and stimulates gallbladder contractions. In one study of 46,000 men, those drinking 2 or 3 cups of regular coffee per day had a 40 percent lower risk of gallstones compared with men who did not drink coffee.

• Eat small, frequent meals.

• Diets high in fibre are associated with a lower risk of gallstones. Eat more wheat and oat bran, milled flaxseed, legumes, vegetables, and fruits.

• Include lean protein (fish and poultry) and healthy fats (olive and flaxseed oil).

Foods to avoid:

• Diets high in sugar are linked to increased risk of gallstones. Minimize high-sugar foods such as candy, soft drinks, pastries, and other sweets.

• Eating lots of saturated fat and cholesterol increases the risk of gallstones. Minimize red meat, high-fat dairy, eggs, deep-fried and processed foods.

Lifestyle Suggestions

• Maintain a healthy body weight. If you are overweight, follow a healthy diet (not fad diet) and boost activity levels to promote slow, gradual weight loss. Rapid weight loss can actually increase your risk of gallstones.

• Get regular physical activity every day.

Top Recommended Supplements

Milk thistle: May help prevent gallstones from occurring. The active component, silymarin, helps to reduce cholesterol levels in bile and improve bile flow. Dosage: 420 mg daily.

Peppermint oil: Aids digestion; some research has shown that it can help dissolve gall-stones. Dosage: One capsule three times daily. Choose an enteric-coated capsule to prevent upset stomach.

Complementary Supplements

Lecithin: Contains phosphatidylcholine (PC), which helps to protect against gallstone formation. Some preliminary studies suggest that 300–2,000 mg per day of PC may help dissolve gallstones.

Vitamin C: Needed to convert cholesterol to bile acids. A low intake of vitamin C is associated with increased risk of gallstones. Dosage: 500 mg daily.

The herbs artichoke leaf, dandelion root, and turmeric are often used to treat gallstones. It is thought that they work by improving bile flow and stimulating the gallbladder to contract and expel the stone. The research to support the benefits of these herbs is weak and there are certain side effects, so it is important to consult with your health care provider.

FINAL THOUGHTS

To reduce the risk of gallstones, consider the following:

1. Eat small frequent meals with high-fibre grains, vegetables, and fruits along with lean protein and healthy fats.
2. Coffee in moderation (2 or 3 cups per day) is helpful for prevention.
3. Get regular physical activity.
4. Maintain a healthy body weight, but avoid fad diets and rapid weight loss.
5. Consider supplements of peppermint oil and milk thistle.

GLAUCOMA

Glaucoma refers to a group of eye diseases that cause damage to the optic nerve and elevated pressure inside the eye, or intraocular pressure (IOP). One of the most common causes of blindness, glaucoma affects one in 100 Canadians over the age of 40.

The optic nerve is a bundle of nerve fibres at the back of the eye that carries images from the back of the eyeball (retina) to the brain. As the optic nerve deteriorates, blind spots develop in the visual field, usually starting with the peripheral (side) vision. If left untreated, glaucoma may lead to blindness in both eyes.

Elevated IOP is one of the primary causes of optic nerve damage; however, not everyone with elevated IOP develops glaucoma and glaucoma can develop in those with normal IOP. IOP is regulated by the production and drainage of eye fluids. In a healthy eye, fluid is produced and drained at equal rates. If too much fluid is produced, or not enough is drained, then IOP increases.

The two main types of glaucoma are open-angle and angle-closure. Open-angle glaucoma is the most common form and occurs when the eye fluids drain too slowly, causing a fluid backup and increased IOP. Damage to the optic nerve occurs slowly and is painless, so visual loss may occur without symptoms. Angle-closure glaucoma develops when the drainage canals within the eye become blocked and IOP increases. This can result from a narrow drainage angle that you are born with, or as a result of aging. If you have a narrow drainage angle and your pupils dilate, this can cause a sudden increase in IOP, along with severe pain and headache. Vision loss can occur rapidly and requires immediate medical attention.

Other forms of glaucoma include low-tension glaucoma in which IOP is normal, yet the optic nerve becomes damaged. The cause of this is unknown. Childhood glaucoma is an inherited form of the disease that is similar to open-angle glaucoma. There may not be any symptoms initially, but it leads to blindness if left untreated. Congenital glaucoma appears soon after birth and causes noticeable signs, including tearing, light sensitivity, and cloudiness of the cornea. With secondary glaucoma IOP increases due to a structural problem within the eye, such as eye injury or other medical conditions.

SIGNS & SYMPTOMS

Many people with glaucoma are unaware of it until a serious loss of vision occurs. Signs and symptoms vary depending on the type of glaucoma.

Open-angle glaucoma:
- Loss of peripheral vision
- Progressive visual loss
- Tunnel vision

Acute angle-closure glaucoma:
- Blurred vision, halos around lights
- Headache
- Intense eye pain
- Nausea and vomiting
- Red, watery eyes

- Age: Caucasians over 60 years and Blacks over age 40 are at increased risk.

- Family history (genetic defects may be inherited)

- Increased intraocular (internal eye) pressure

- Injuries (trauma to the eye, eye tumours, or inflammatory eye disease)

- Medical conditions: Having diabetes, high blood pressure, heart disease, hypothyroidism, or nearsightedness increases your risk.

- Medications (chronic use of corticosteroids)

- Race: Blacks are at much greater risk; Mexicans and Asians are also at increased risk.

DOCTOR'S ORDERS

There is no cure for glaucoma and the damage to the optic nerve cannot be reversed. In the early stages, if there is no damage to the optic nerve, your doctor may just recommend more frequent exams to monitor any changes. Those with elevated IOP and nerve damage often require treatment for life. There are a number of therapies that lower IOP and prevent further damage, such as eyedrops, oral medications, laser therapy, and surgery. Since the disease can progress without symptoms, regular checkups are critical.

SHERRY'S NATURAL PRESCRIPTION

Dietary Recommendations

Foods to include:

- Vegetables that contain vitamin C and carotenoids (antioxidants)—such as carrots, bell peppers, broccoli, kale, collard greens, and tomatoes—are important for eye health.

- Berries and cherries contain plant pigments (anthocyanidins) that prevent free radical damage to the eye and protect blood vessels.

- Fish contain omega-3 fatty acids that may reduce the risk of glaucoma.

Foods to avoid:

- Regular coffee consumption can increase IOP.

- Food allergies may be implicated in glaucoma. Refer to Appendix D.

- Alcohol impairs liver function, which can affect the removal of toxins.

CAFFEINE AND GLAUCOMA

Caffeine has been shown in studies to elevate intraocular pressure. If you have glaucoma, minimize coffee, pop, tea, and other caffeinated beverages.

Lifestyle Suggestions

- Drink fluids in small amounts over the course of a day. Drinking a lot in a short time may increase eye pressure.

- Exercising at least three times per week has been found to reduce IOP in those with open-angle glaucoma. Avoid exercises that require you to lower your head (in certain yoga poses, for example), as this can increase IOP.

- Reduce stress, which can trigger an attack in those with angle-closure glaucoma. Try breathing exercises, acupuncture, massage, and meditation.

- Wear sunglasses when outdoors and safety glasses or goggles for sports or when using tools or working with chemicals.

- Get frequent eye examinations as advised by your doctor.

Top Recommended Supplements

Note: Supplements may be used in conjunction with prescribed therapies under doctor's supervision. Do not stop taking any prescribed medication unless advised by your doctor.

Ginkgo biloba: One study found that ginkgo can improve vision in those with glaucoma. It may work by enhancing circulation. Dosage: 40 mg three times daily.

Vitamin C: Studies have shown that it can help to lower IOP. Dosage: 2 g or more daily.

Complementary Supplements

Alpha lipoic acid: May help improve vision. Dosage: 150 mg daily.

Bilberry: Helps improve blood flow and blood vessel health. Dosage: 160 mg twice daily.

Magnesium: Preliminary research suggests it may improve vision in those with glaucoma. Dosage: 250 mg twice daily.

FINAL THOUGHTS

To prevent worsening of glaucoma and preserve your vision:

1. Get regular eye exams and follow your doctor's orders.
2. Exercise regularly and reduce stress.
3. Wear appropriate eye protection.
4. Eat more vegetables, berries, and fish; avoid caffeine and alcohol.
5. Consider supplements of vitamin C and ginkgo biloba.

GOUT

Gout is a form of arthritis that occurs when uric acid accumulates in a joint, leading to a sudden onset of intense pain and inflammation. While this problem is not life threatening, it can be debilitating.

Uric acid is a substance created by the breakdown of foods containing high amounts of purines, a component of protein found in organ meat, seafood, and fish. Uric acid is normally eliminated in the urine. However, some people produce high amounts or are not able to eliminate it properly, leading to a buildup in the blood and the formation of uric acid crystals in the joints.

DID YOU KNOW?

Gout was once known as the "disease of kings" due to its association with consumption of rich foods and alcohol.

SIGNS & SYMPTOMS

Gout attacks often occur suddenly, affecting the big toe, heel, or ankle and then later progressing to the knees, wrists, elbows, and fingers. Symptoms include:

• Back pain

• Fever

• Intense pain

• Joint swelling

• Red and warm joints

• Upset stomach

RISK FACTORS

• Age: Those over 40 are at greater risk

• Alcohol consumption (rye, beer, and wine)

• Carrying excess weight

• Eating foods high in purines (see below)

• Elevated triglycerides

• Family history

• Gender: Men are affected more frequently

• High blood pressure

• Kidney disease

• Lead exposure

• Medications (antibiotics, aspirin, chemotherapy, diuretics, niacin)

• Stress (trauma, surgery, emotional stress)

DOCTOR'S ORDERS

For an acute attack, non-steroidal anti-inflammatory drugs (NSAIDs) such as ibuprofen, naproxen, and indomethacin are often prescribed. They reduce pain and inflammation and work within 12–24 hours, but may cause side effects, including upset stomach, bleeding stomach, and ringing in the ears. They can be hard on the liver and kidneys. Use only when absolutely necessary—the lowest dose for the shortest period of time.

One of the oldest remedies for a gout attack is colchicine, which is derived from the herb autumn crocus. It can also be used for prevention, but is limited by unpleasant side effects, such as severe diarrhea and upset stomach.

The primary drug used for prevention is allopurinol. It reduces the production of uric acid and is generally well tolerated. Skin rash is the most common side effect. There are a number of drug interactions with allopurinol, so check with your pharmacist before taking new medications.

SHERRY'S NATURAL PRESCRIPTION

An acute gout attack will most likely require medical treatment. However, certain lifestyle changes and nutritional supplements may help ease symptoms of an attack and prevent recurrences.

Dietary Recommendations

Foods to include:

- Cherries (fresh, canned, or juice) help to reduce uric acid levels. Strawberries, blueberries, and celery also seem to help.

- Flaxseed provides essential fatty acids, which help reduce inflammation.

- Foods high in vitamin C (red peppers, tangerines, mandarins, oranges, and red cabbage) reduce uric acid.

- Pineapple is high in bromelain, a digestive enzyme that may help reduce inflammation.

- Whole grains and flaxseed are high in fibre and help with elimination of uric acid.

Foods to avoid:

- Organ meats (heart), sardines, herring, mackerel, mussels, and sweetbreads contain very high amounts of purines, which can substantially increase uric acid levels.

- Minimize (once weekly) anchovies, veal, bacon, liver, kidneys, goose, scallops, salmon, crab, lobster, turkey, and haddock, which contain high amounts of purines.

- Limit consumption (four times weekly) of legumes (dried beans, peas, and soybeans), asparagus, gravy, mushrooms, oysters, tongue, spinach, and tuna.

- Refined flour (white bread, pasta) and sugar should be minimized as these foods can raise uric acid levels and are also unhealthy.

- Reduce consumption of alcohol, especially beer, as it interferes with uric acid elimination.

- Drink plenty of water (2–3 L per day) to help flush uric acid through the kidneys. However, if you have heart or kidney disease and are on fluid restriction, consult your doctor before changing fluid intake.

Note: Purines are found in all protein foods, and should not be eliminated completely. Avoid foods highest in purines during an acute attack, and gradually resume eating these foods once symptoms disappear.

Lifestyle Suggestions

- Acupuncture helps to relieve pain and inflammation and promote relaxation.

- Exercise: Activities such as swimming, cycling, and stretching can help improve blood flow, reduce pain, and promote relaxation. Avoid high-impact activities, such as running, which are hard on the joints.

- Go easy on the joints—be careful not to bruise or hurt your joints as this can bring on an attack.

- Massage: Gentle massage helps promote relaxation and encourage removal of toxins. Avoid rubbing the joints affected by gout.

- Reduce stress through massage, meditation, or breathing exercises, which can help prevent a recurrence of gout.

- Weight loss: Slow, gradual weight loss may reduce attacks. Avoid rapid weight loss or fasting as this can raise uric acid levels and aggravate gout.

Top Recommended Supplements

Celadrin: Reduces joint pain and inflammation and also helps improve joint mobility. Dosage: 1,500 mg daily.

Vitamin C: Reduces uric acid levels. Take 500 mg daily for prevention. Higher amounts (4 g and higher) have been used to relieve an attack, but this should be done only under the supervision of a health care professional.

Complementary Supplements

Bromelain: An enzyme that helps reduce inflammation during an attack. Dosage varies by product potency; check label directions.

Fish oil: Omega-3 fatty acids help reduce inflammation and improve joint health. Dosage: 1 g three times daily.

Quercetin: A flavonoid that in preliminary studies was found to help prevent gout attacks. Dosage: 150–250 mg three times daily.

FINAL THOUGHTS

Gout is a painful condition that can often be prevented and certainly improved by dietary and lifestyle modifications. To reduce your risk of an attack:

1. Minimize intake of high-purine foods and alcohol.
2. Eat gout-fighting foods such as cherries, berries, and pineapple; drink plenty of water.
3. Try acupuncture and massage to reduce stress and pain.
4. Engage in regular, light exercise such swimming, cycling, and stretching.
5. Top supplements for gout include vitamin C and Celadrin.

G

Gout

GUM DISEASE

Gum disease, also known as gingivitis, is a very serious, yet often overlooked health problem. Initially it causes red, swollen, and bleeding gums. If left untreated, gum disease can lead to periodontitis, a very serious infection that destroys the soft tissue and bone that support your teeth, leading to tooth loss. Chronic periodontitis is very serious as it can lead to other health problems such as high blood sugar and increased risk of heart attack and stroke. In pregnant women it can affect the health of the un-born child and lead to premature babies.

There are many factors that affect gum health such as smoking, heredity, and immune function. However, the most common cause of gum disease is poor oral hygiene. The disease starts with the formation of plaque on the teeth when starches and sugars in food interact with bacteria in the mouth, creating a sticky film on the teeth. Brushing and flossing help to reduce plaque formation, but it reforms quickly and any that is missed and stays on the teeth longer than two or three days can harden under the gum line into tartar. Tartar acts as a reservoir for bacteria. It cannot be eliminated by brushing or flossing; only professional cleaning can eliminate this substance.

Plaque and tartar irritate the gums, causing inflammation. In time this inflammation causes pockets to develop between the gums and teeth that fill with more plaque, tartar, and bacteria. Over time the pockets become deeper and more bacteria accumulate under the gum tissue, leading to loss of bone and tissue, and even tooth loss.

With proper oral hygiene, regular dental cleaning, and a healthy diet and lifestyle, gum disease can be prevented.

CHECK YOUR GUMS

Healthy gums are firm and pale pink. If your gums are puffy, red, and bleed easily, see your dentist. The sooner you seek care, the better your chances of reversing damage and preventing more serious problems.

SIGNS & SYMPTOMS

- Breath odour or bad taste in mouth
- Gum recession
- Loose teeth or a change in how the teeth fit together
- New spaces between teeth
- Pus between teeth and gums
- Swollen, red gums
- Tenderness and bleeding of the gums

- Diabetes increases the risk of gum infection, and gum disease impairs the body's ability to utilize insulin.

- Drugs: Antihistamines reduce saliva production; phenytoin (anticonvulsant) causes gum inflammation; immune suppressants (organ transplant drugs) may increase the risk of infection.

- Family history of gum disease

- Hormonal changes during pregnancy and menopause

- Poor diet and nutritional deficiencies (vitamin C, B-vitamins, and calcium)

- Poor oral hygiene (not brushing or flossing regularly)

- Smoking or chewing tobacco

SMOKING AND GUM DISEASE

Next to poor oral hygiene, smoking is the most significant risk factor for gum disease. Tobacco use damages the immune system and creates a favourable environment for bacterial growth. Chewing tobacco and exposure to second-hand smoke can also increase risk of gum disease.

DOCTOR'S ORDERS

Practising good oral hygiene is the best defence against gum disease. If you have early-stage gum disease, your dentist may ask you to come in more frequently. Professional cleaning and scaling can remove tartar and bacteria that can't be accomplished with brushing or flossing. Root planing can be done to smooth the root surface and discourage further accumulation of tartar. Antibiotic mouth rinses may be prescribed to control infection.

For advanced periodontitis, you may be referred to a gum specialist called a periodontist, who can offer various treatments such as flap surgery (to reduce pockets), soft tissue or bone grafts, and tissue-regeneration procedures.

SHERRY'S NATURAL PRESCRIPTION

Dietary Recommendations

Foods to include:

- Cranberries and cranberry juice contain antioxidants that prevent bacteria from adhering to teeth and gums. Choose products that are sugar-free or sweetened with xylitol.

- Fish and flaxseed contain fatty acids, which help reduce gum inflammation and may help reduce bone destruction.

- Fruits and vegetables contain vital nutrients that support immune function and gum health. Citrus, berries, peppers, and cantaloupe are good sources of vitamin C, which is used in the synthesis of collagen.

- Garlic supports immune function and helps fight infection.
- Xylitol is a natural sugar present in gum, candy, and toothpaste that helps prevent cavities and may help prevent gum disease.

Foods to avoid:
- Refined, starchy carbohydrates (white bread/rice/pasta) and sugars (candy, sweets) stick on the teeth and lead to plaque and tartar formation.

Lifestyle Suggestions
- Brush your teeth after meals and at bedtime and floss daily.
- Visit your dentist yearly or more often if recommended to have your teeth professional cleaned.
- Don't smoke, and avoid second-hand smoke.
- Support immune system function by getting adequate sleep and reducing stress levels.
- Try an oral rinse that contains folic acid, thyme, chamomile, or bloodroot as these natural ingredients have shown some benefits for gum disease.

CHOOSING THE RIGHT TOOTHBRUSH

There are many different types of toothbrushes available. Dentists recommend soft bristles as hard bristles can injure the gums. Many toothbrushes are angled so that you can reach every tooth easily. Replace your brush every three to four months or even more often if the bristles are worn down. Electric toothbrushes are very effective and may be helpful especially for those with arthritis or problems with dexterity.

USING PROPER TECHNIQUE

To properly brush your teeth, use short, back-and-forth, then up-and-down strokes on the outer surfaces and vertical strokes on the inner surfaces. Use gentle pressure; the tips of the brush do the cleaning, so it isn't necessary to use force. You should spend about three to five minutes brushing your teeth. To properly floss, use about 18 inches of floss, hold the floss taut and bent around each tooth, and scrape up and down each side of each tooth. Each stroke should go slightly below the gum line. Be gentle as you lift the floss toward the gum line as strong pressure may cause the gums to bleed.

Top Recommended Supplements

Calcium: Essential for bone and teeth. Some research has found that it can improve symptoms of periodontal disease (bleeding gums and loose teeth). Dosage: 500 mg two or three times daily with meals.

Coenzyme Q10: A powerful antioxidant that has been studied for gum health. It helps reduce gum pockets and speeds healing after dental surgery. Dosage: 50–100 mg daily.

Vitamin C: Essential for gum health; protects the gums from cell damage, hastens healing, and strengthens the immune system to fight off the bacterial infection that causes gum disease. Studies have found that those who are deficient in vitamin C are at increased risk of gum disease and supplementing can help to reduce symptoms. Vitamin C with flavonoids may offer additional benefits for reducing inflammation. Dosage: 500–1,000 mg daily.

Complementary Supplements

Fish oils: Reduce inflammation and may reduce bone loss. Dosage: 1–3 g daily.

Vitamin E: Antioxidant properties help protect against free radicals produced by white blood cells attracted to diseased gums. Dosage: 400 IU daily.

FINAL THOUGHTS

To improve gum health and reduce the symptoms of gum disease, consider the following:

1. Brush your teeth after meals and floss daily.
2. Get your teeth professionally cleaned at least once a year.
3. Minimize refined starches and sugars.
4. Don't smoke and avoid second-hand smoke.
5. Consider supplements of coenzyme Q10, calcium, and vitamin C.

HAIR LOSS

Hair loss is a concern that affects us all, although we hope it doesn't. When we see more hairs than usual in the shower or the hairbrush, we suddenly wonder whether we might be losing our hair. It's comforting to know that the human body sheds approximately 100 of its 100,000–150,000 strands of hair every day and new ones grow to take their place. As we age, this renewal process may slow where more hairs are lost than grown.

Real hair loss is most noticeable in men. What is commonly known as male-pattern baldness is an inherited condition called androgenetic alopecia and it may begin as early as age 20. Male hair loss is distinguished by a receding hairline or widow's peak and thinning on the crown. The rate of hair loss may be slow, gradual, or fast. By age 50, about 50 percent of men will experience thinning and hair loss. For 40–50 percent of women, hair may begin to thin after age 50 (typically after menopause). This is called female-pattern baldness. Women tend to see their hair thin throughout the head, but most visibly on the crown. Significant hair loss for women before age 50 is rare and usually triggered by hormonal fluctuations, stress, or a secondary health concern.

Other kinds of hair loss include:

Alopecia areata: This form of hair loss is characterized by patchy baldness or bald spots. It affects both men and women equally, both adults and children, but it is rare, affecting less than 2 percent of the population. Hair loss due to alopecia areata is usually triggered by an immune system disorder. Once addressed, the hair usually grows back.

Anagen effluvium: This condition occurs when hair in the growth phase falls out prematurely. Prescription medications used for the treatment of cancer are the most common cause of this condition. Chemotherapy patients may lose up to 90 percent of their hair as a result of anagen effluvium.

Telogen effluvium: A natural part of the hair growth cycle includes a resting phase called telogen, which involves 10 percent of hair at any given time. Telogen effluvium occurs when up to 30 percent of hairs on the head are in the resting phase at any given time. This condition may be caused by physical or emotional stress, and hair growth will return to normal as stress is eased.

The health of your hair is a reflection of the overall state of your health, so it is important to address hair loss from a multipronged approach that includes both the use of standard medical treatments to slow hair loss, and nutritional and lifestyle changes to address and improve health.

SIGNS & SYMPTOMS

- Bald patches
- Scalp irritation
- Sudden, excessive, or increased hair loss
- Visible thinning of the hair around the top and sides of the head

If hair loss is accompanied by other symptoms such as fatigue, cold hands and feet, dry skin and hair, and menstrual fluctuations, it may be the warning signs of hypothyroidism or an underactive thyroid. See your doctor immediately for further tests.

RISK FACTORS

- Age: Hair loss is more common with age
- Burns, injuries, and skin infections such as ringworm
- Drugs used to treat gout, arthritis, depression, heart problems, high blood pressure, and birth control pills can lead to hair loss.
- Genetics
- Hair treatments: Chemicals used for dying, tinting, bleaching, straightening, or perming can cause hair to become damaged and break off if they are overused or used incorrectly; hairstyles that pull your hair too tightly also can cause some hair loss, which is known as traction alopecia.
- Hormonal changes such as pregnancy and menopause
- Immune disorders (lupus, diabetes, thyroid disease)
- Nutritional deficiencies: Inadequate protein, iron, or essential fatty acids
- Severe gastrointestinal disorders
- Stress: Emotional stress, fever, surgery, flu
- Weight problems and extreme dieting

H

Hair Loss

PUT A LEASH ON DHT

DHT stands for dihydrotestosterone, a hormone formed when the enzyme 5-alpha-reductase breaks down testosterone. DHT is the primary underlying cause of male-pattern baldness. DHT shortens the hair growth cycle, causing the hair follicles to shrink and stop production of hair, leading to hair loss. DHT not only affects men but also women, particularly after menopause when levels of estrogen decrease. Some drugs used to treat baldness work by inhibiting the action of 5-alpha-reductase, thus reducing the formation of DHT. High-fat diets can also boost DHT levels.

DOCTOR'S ORDERS

If you experience sudden or excessive hair loss, or bald patches, you should visit the doctor to rule out nutritional deficiencies, thyroid concerns, and other health problems.

Hair loss due to aging and genetics must be treated as early as possible to stabilize hair loss and stimulate regrowth.

The most highly recommended topical solution is minoxidil (Rogaine). Minoxidil is a vasodilator (a drug that causes the blood vessels in the body to become wider) and was originally introduced as a blood pressure–lowering drug. When it was found to have an added benefit on hair loss and regrowth, it was reformulated as a topical 2 percent solution and is now sold over the counter. Minoxidil is applied to the scalp twice daily. It has been shown to benefit approximately 40 percent of people who use it for hair loss as early as two months after the initial application. Studies show hair weight and hair counts increase with the 2 percent solution, and more so with the 5 percent solution where hair weight increased by 45 percent. Minoxidil must be used on a daily basis for life to ensure hair growth. It may cause irritation and itchiness. Discontinue use if symptoms persist.

Another recommended treatment for hair loss is finasteride (Propecia), an oral prescription medication taken once daily for life. Finasteride is only for men. It has been shown to stop hair loss in 83 percent of cases and to stimulate regrowth in 66 percent of cases. Finasteride works by inhibiting DHT.

SHERRY'S NATURAL PRESCRIPTION

Dietary Recommendations

Even though hair is not a living tissue, it is important to supply nutrients to the hair follicles in the scalp. While there are no foods that directly stimulate increased hair growth, choose foods that supply the body with a rich supply of vitamins, minerals, antioxidants, fibre, and protein.

Foods to include:

- Ensure adequate protein intake as protein is necessary for hair growth. Choose lean sources of protein (fish, poultry, lean cuts of meat, beans, nuts, seeds, and soy). Meat, poultry, and fish also contain iron, which is required for proper hair growth.

- Fish and flaxseed contain essential fatty acids necessary for proper hair growth.

- Nuts and seeds; almonds contain magnesium, which is important for hair growth.

- The outer skin of plants such as potatoes, cucumbers, green and red peppers, and sprouts can strengthen hair because they are rich in the mineral silica.

- Whole grains, vegetables, and fruits are good sources of essential nutrients and fibre.

Foods to avoid:

- Caffeine and alcohol can deplete the body of nutrients and also raise adrenal levels, which can trigger hair loss.

- Foods high in sugar can raise cortisol levels (a stress hormone) and cause the body to produce more androgens, promoting hair loss.

- High intake of salt has been linked to hair loss. Foods high in salt include processed and snack foods, deli meats, and the salt shaker.

- Reduce or eliminate pro-inflammatory foods: saturated fat (fatty meats and dairy) and trans fats (processed foods and fried foods). Saturated fat reduces the amount of sex hormone-binding globulin (SHBG), a substance that normally binds to testosterone. With less SHBG, more testosterone can be converted into DHT, which promotes hair loss.

DRASTIC DIETS STUNT HAIR GROWTH

Severely reducing calorie intake (less than 1,200 calories per day) can trigger sudden hair loss (telogen effluvium). When the body is deprived of sufficient protein, through strict dieting and calorie restriction, it will shut down all production of hair in order to divert all of its energies toward conserving vital body organs. The body will save protein by shifting healthy hairs that are in a normal growth phase (anagen) into a sudden resting phase.

Lifestyle Suggestions

- Regular exercise and healthy sleep habits will increase circulatory and overall health, promoting healthy hair.

- Reduce the frequency of washing and drying your hair. Use a gentle shampoo and conditioner. Avoid using hot water and hair dryers or curling irons whenever possible.

- Avoid exposing hair to chlorinated pool water or any other chemical solutions (perms and dyes).

- Do not overbrush your hair. Limit grooming and always be gentle when brushing or combing hair. Keep braids and ponytails loose.

- Give yourself a weekly deep conditioning treatment and scalp massage to protect the hair shaft and stimulate new hair follicle growth.

- Wear a wide-brim hat when outdoors to protect your scalp and hair from the sun's damaging rays.

- Don't smoke. According to one report, smokers were four times more likely to have grey hair than non-smokers and were more prone to hair loss.

Top Recommended Supplements

B-vitamins: Essential for proper hair growth. A deficiency of the B-vitamins biotin and PABA can cause hair loss. Supplements of biotin may strengthen hair, stimulate new hair growth, slow hair loss, and prevent greying, particularly in those who are deficient in this nutrient. PABA (para-aminobenzoic acid) may protect hair roots and help prevent hair loss. It can also reverse greying in cases where the cause is a deficiency of PABA or other B-vitamins. Dosage: Take a B-complex vitamin daily.

Essential fatty acids: A deficiency can cause hair loss; supplements can help improve the health of scalp and hair. Take a blend of fish, flaxseed, and evening primrose or borage oil. Dosage: 2–3 g daily.

Orthosilicic acid: Enhances collagen formation and makes hair stronger and thicker. One study found that it improved brittleness of hair and nails. Taking silicon supplements will not yield the same results as silicon is poorly absorbed. Orthosilicic acid is the bioavailable (usable) form of silicon and is available in Canada under the name BioSil. Dosage: Six to 10 drops daily in juice (to mask the bad taste). Drink immediately.

RESEARCH HIGHLIGHT: ESSENTIAL OILS STIMULATE HAIR GROWTH

A study by Scottish researchers found that essential oils could benefit bald patches caused by alopecia areata. In this study, half of the participants massaged a combination of essential oils of thyme, rosemary, lavender, and cedarwood onto their scalps each day. The other half of participants massaged inactive oils. After seven months, 44 percent of the patients using the essential oils showed significant improvement in hair growth compared to only 15 percent improvement in the placebo group (*Archives of Dermatology*, 1998: 134; 1349–1352).

Complementary Supplements

Grape seed extract: A potent antioxidant that has been shown in preliminary research to stimulate hair growth. Dosage: 50–100 mg daily.

Minerals: Iron, selenium, and zinc are essential for hair growth; a deficiency can cause hair loss. Dosage: Take as part of a daily multivitamin/mineral complex.

Saw palmetto: Used primarily for the treatment of enlarged prostate. It blocks the production of DHT and thus it may be helpful for treating hair loss due to high DHT levels, although this has not been tested in humans yet. Consult with your health care provider before supplementing with saw palmetto.

FINAL THOUGHTS

To improve the health of your hair and prevent hair loss, consider the following:

1. Eat lots of vegetables, fruits, whole grains, fish, nuts, seeds, and ensure adequate protein intake.
2. Reduce or minimize saturated fat, caffeine, sugar, and salt.
3. Get regular exercise and don't smoke.
4. Avoid using harsh chemicals and heat on your hair. Do a scalp massage with essential oils weekly.
5. Consider supplements of B-vitamins, essential fatty acids, and orthosilicic acid.

HEART DISEASE (CARDIOVASCULAR DISEASE)

Heart disease, also known as cardiovascular disease, refers to diseases of the blood vessels and heart. While cancer is highly feared, heart disease is actually the leading cause of death among Canadians.

There are several forms of heart disease, including coronary artery disease (CAD), hypertension, congestive heart failure, congenital heart disease (a defect that you are born with), arrhythmia (irregular heartbeat), cardiomyopathy (enlargement of the heart), heart block, valve disorders, and pericarditis (infection of membrane surrounding the heart).

This chapter focuses specifically on CAD, also known as atherosclerosis or hardening of the arteries. The coronary arteries supply your heart with blood, oxygen, and nutrients. CAD is thought to start when the inner lining of the arteries become damaged. The blood vessel wall reacts to this injury by depositing cholesterol, calcium, and other substances on the inner lining of the artery. The result is a progressive thickening of the blood vessel wall, which reduces the supply of oxygen-rich blood to the heart, leading to chest pain (angina). If the coronary arteries become completely blocked and the flow of blood is cut off, a heart attack (myocardial infarction) occurs, which results in damage to the heart muscle.

High blood pressure, high levels of cholesterol and triglycerides in the blood, and smoking can all contribute to the development of plaque. Chronic inflammation is a recently recognized factor that contributes to CAD. Inflammation causes damage to the arterial walls and further narrows the passageways.

This process does not happen over night. Damage may begin as early as childhood. Years of smoking, stress, high blood pressure and cholesterol, uncontrolled blood sugar (diabetes), and poor diet take a toll on your heart and contribute to the development of heart disease. The good news is that there are many ways to keep your heart healthy and reduce your risk of heart disease.

CHOLESTEROL: THE GOOD AND THE BAD

Cholesterol is a fatty substance manufactured in the liver and also obtained from consuming saturated and trans fats. There are two forms of cholesterol: LDL and HDL. LDL (low-density lipoprotein) is called bad cholesterol because it can build up in the artery walls of the brain and heart, narrowing the passageways for blood flow. HDL is called good cholesterol because it picks up the LDL deposited in the arteries and transports it to the liver to be broken down and eliminated.

SIGNS & SYMPTOMS

- Chest pain and tightness (often triggered by physical or emotional stress); women may notice pain in the back, arm, neck, or abdomen

- Fatigue with exertion

- Shortness of breath

- Swelling in your feet and ankles

- Age

- Diabetes

- Family history of heart disease

- Gender: Men are at greater risk of coronary artery disease than women. However, the risk for women increases after menopause.

- High blood pressure

- High cholesterol: High LDL (bad cholesterol) and low HDL (good cholesterol)

- Inactivity (sedentary lifestyle)

- Obesity

- Poor diet (high in saturated and trans fat; low in fibre)

- Smoking

- Stress

MULTIPLYING YOUR RISK

Most people with heart disease have more than one risk factor, and the more risk factors you have, the greater your likelihood of heart disease and death. For example, obesity often leads to diabetes and high blood pressure and cholesterol. This cluster of problems is called metabolic syndrome, which greatly increases the risk of heart disease.

In recent years, research has identified other factors that may increase your risk of heart disease. They include:

- C-reactive protein (CRP), a marker of inflammation, which is a factor in the development of atherosclerosis. High CRP levels are correlated with an increased risk of heart attack and stroke.

- Fibrinogen, a protein in your blood that is involved in blood clotting. High levels of fibrinogen may promote excessive clumping of platelets, which can cause a clot, leading to a heart attack or stroke.

- Homocysteine, an amino acid made by the body during normal metabolism. Studies suggest that elevated homocysteine increases the risk of heart disease by causing damage to the lining of the arteries and promoting clots. Homocysteine metabolism is controlled by vitamins B6, B12, and folic acid, and a deficiency of these nutrients can increase levels.

- Lipoprotein (a), a substance that forms when a low-density lipoprotein (LDL) cholesterol particle attaches to a specific protein. The protein that carries lipoprotein (a) may disrupt your body's ability to dissolve blood clots, and high levels of this substance may increase the risk of cardiovascular disease.

DOCTOR'S ORDERS

Lifestyle approaches (diet, exercise, not smoking) are essential for the management of heart disease. If these approaches aren't effective, then your doctor will likely prescribe a medication depending on your needs. There are drugs to lower cholesterol or blood pressure, which are mentioned in those sections of this book. Low-dose daily aspirin (81 mg daily) is often recommended to thin the blood and reduce the risk of clotting. It can also help prevent future attacks. For those with angina, nitroglycerin tablets, spray, or patches may be used to open up the coronary arteries and improve blood flow.

There are also various procedures, such as angioplasty and coronary artery by-pass surgery, which can be done to improve blood flow.

SHERRY'S NATURAL PRESCRIPTION

Dietary Recommendations

Foods to include:

- Drink green tea, which contains antioxidants that offer benefits for the heart.

- Fish and flaxseed contain beneficial omega-3 fatty acids that reduce inflammation and LDL cholesterol, prevent blood clotting, and reduce the risk of heart disease. Try to eat three servings per week of fresh coldwater fish such as salmon, trout, herring, mackerel, and tuna. Reduce consumption of toxins by choosing wild (not farmed) fish.

- Garlic helps reduce cholesterol, thin the blood, and has antioxidant properties.

- Margarines, salad dressings, and spreads that contain phytostanols (plant substances) help lower cholesterol.

- Moderate alcohol consumption (one drink for women daily and two for men) has been shown to have heart-protective effects. Alcohol increases protective HDL cholesterol and also helps to thin the blood. Higher amounts can be hard on the liver and increase blood pressure and the risk of heart disease.

- Nuts (almonds and walnuts) help lower cholesterol levels. Nuts contain fibre and nutrients such as vitamin E, alpha-linolenic acid, magnesium, potassium, and arginine, which are important for heart health. Although nuts are high in calories, some studies have found that increasing nut consumption by several hundred calories per day does not cause weight gain.

- Olive oil is a monounsaturated fat that can help reduce blood clots and lower LDL cholesterol. Add it to your salads and recipes in place of other vegetable oils.

- Soluble fibre—which is found in oats, flaxseed, beans, psyllium, and fruits—helps lower cholesterol levels. Insoluble fibre—which is found in whole grains, vegetables, and fruits—does not lower cholesterol, but studies have shown that it helps protect against heart disease. Aim for a total of 35 g of fibre daily. Fruits and vegetables also contain vital antioxidants and studies have shown that those who consume antioxidant-rich diets have lower rates of heart disease. Appendix B lists low-glycemic foods.

- Soy products (tofu, soybeans, miso, and soy protein powder) can help lower cholesterol and triglycerides. Substituting as little as 20 g per day of soy protein for animal protein can significantly lower cholesterol.

- Yogurt and fermented milk products have been shown to lower cholesterol levels.

Foods to avoid:

- Foods high in cholesterol should be minimized (organ meats, egg yolks, and whole milk products). Aim for no more than 300 mg of dietary cholesterol daily. One egg yolk contains 213 mg cholesterol. Egg whites do not contain any cholesterol and are a good source of protein.

- Foods high in sugar and refined starches (white flour) can raise triglyceride and insulin levels, which increases the risk of heart disease.

- Salt causes water retention and increases the pressure inside your arteries. Reducing salt intake reduces blood pressure in most people. Aim for no more than 2,500 mg daily. Avoid adding salt to foods and minimize eating processed and fast foods such as deli meats, snacks (chips, pretzels), french fries, and burgers.

- Saturated fat, which is present in animal foods (beef, pork, and dairy) and certain oils (palm oil), can raise cholesterol levels and is associated with increased heart disease risk. Limit daily consumption of saturated fat to 10 percent of total calories. Read food labels carefully. Dairy products labelled "low fat" can be misleading. For example, 25 percent of calories in 2 percent milk come from fat. The 2 percent refers to the fraction of volume filled by fat, not the percentage of calories coming from fat.

- Trans fatty acids are found in hydrogenated oils, which are present in most margarines, snack foods (chips), and deep-fried foods (french fries). These fats can raise cholesterol levels and increase the risk of heart disease. Look for non-hydrogenated margarines. Many snack food companies are now making products that are free of trans fatty acids.

Lifestyle Suggestions

- Don't smoke, and avoid second-hand smoke, as this increases many risk factors for heart disease.

- Lose excess weight. Losing even 5–10 percent of excess weight can lower cholesterol and blood pressure.

- Exercise regularly. Moderate-intensity activities, such as brisk walking, biking, or swimming, can reduce cholesterol and blood pressure and help with weight management. Aim for one hour daily.

- Reduce stress levels. Stress causes the liver to increase the production of cholesterol, which is used to make stress hormones. Try meditation, exercise, or yoga to promote calming and relaxation.

- Manage your blood sugar levels. If you have diabetes or are at risk for diabetes, work on improving your blood sugar levels with exercise and a low-glycemic diet.

- See your doctor regularly for checkups and to monitor your blood pressure, cholesterol, and blood sugar. Discuss the results with your doctor.

....

SMOKING AND HEART DISEASE

Smoking is a significant risk factor for heart disease as well as cancer. Smoking lowers the good HDL cholesterol, increases blood pressure, and causes serious damage to blood vessels. It is never too late to quit. Within one year of quitting, your risk of heart disease is half of that of a smoker's. After 15 years, your risk is similar to that of someone who has never smoked.

....

Top Recommended Supplements

Aged garlic extract: Helps lower total and LDL cholesterol and triglycerides, reduces blood clotting, and prevents atherosclerosis. Dosage: 600 mg or more daily.

Coenzyme Q10: An antioxidant that has been widely studied and found to lower blood pressure and cholesterol and strengthen the function of the heart. Dosage: 100 mg twice daily.

Fish oils: Lower triglycerides, raise HDL cholesterol, and reduce inflammation and blood clotting. Fish oil contains the beneficial omega-3 fatty acids, eicosapentaenoic acid (EPA) and docosahexaenoic acid (DHA). Dosage: 3–9 g total of EPA and DHA daily, although higher amounts have been used in some studies. Look for a product that provides at least 400 mg EPA and 200 mg DHA per dosage.

Stanols and sterols: Plant substances that have been shown in many studies to lower LDL cholesterol. They are thought to work by attaching to cholesterol in the digestive tract and carrying it out of the body. They also remove cholesterol from substances made in the liver. A sterol ester, called beta-sitosterol, has been shown to decrease cholesterol absorption by about 50 percent. Dosage: Varies depending on the product and potency.

Complementary Supplements

Antioxidants: Protect against free radical damage and oxidation of LDL cholesterol. Vitamin E also protects against blood clotting, and vitamin C is used to make collagen, a substance that strengthens our blood vessels. It is thought that antioxidants may function best when taken together as they offer synergistic and protective effects in combination. For example, taking a product that contains natural vitamin E, vitamin C, beta-carotene, and selenium may provide better results.

B-complex vitamins: Vitamins B6, B12, and folic acid help to lower homocysteine levels, which is a newly recognized factor for heart disease. Dosage: Take a B-complex vitamin daily.

Calcium and magnesium: Several studies have found that these minerals can promote modest reductions in blood pressure. Both are essential for proper muscle contractions and blood vessel health. Dosage: 1,500 mg calcium and 500 mg magnesium daily. Take in divided dosages with meals.

FINAL THOUGHTS

To improve the management of heart disease, consider the following:

1. Boost intake of soluble and insoluble fibre. Eat more fish, garlic, soy, yogurt, and nuts. Drink green tea.
2. Minimize saturated fat, trans fats, sugar, and salt.
3. Get regular exercise and reduce your stress.
4. Don't smoke.
5. Consider supplements of aged garlic extract, coenzyme Q10, fish oils, and stanols.

HEMORRHOIDS

Hemorrhoids, also known as piles, are a form of varicose veins—swollen, enlarged veins that develop in the anal and rectal area. They are very common; almost everyone will have them at some time in their life and approximately 50 percent of those over age 50 have them.

Hemorrhoids are usually caused by increased pressure on the veins in the pelvic and rectal area, which causes pooling of blood in the veins. The swelling veins stretch the surrounding tissue, leading to the development of hemorrhoids.

While they are uncomfortable and even painful at times, there many natural remedies that can help to shrink them and reduce symptoms, and lifestyle modifications, which can help reduce your risk of developing hemorrhoids.

SIGNS & SYMPTOMS

Hemorrhoids can develop either inside the rectum (internal) or outside (external) and symptoms vary and may include:

- Blue or purple skin in the rectal area
- Feeling of fullness in the rectum (with internal hemorrhoids)
- Itching, skin irritation, and discomfort
- Lumpy tissue protruding from the rectum
- Rectal bleeding (blood in stool or toilet paper)

RISK FACTORS

Any factors that increase pressure in the veins in the rectal area can trigger hemorrhoids, including:

- Chronic diarrhea (irritates rectal tissue)
- Constipation
- Dehydration: Not drinking enough fluids or drinking too many diuretic liquids, such as coffee or cola, can cause hard stools and irritate hemorrhoids.
- Diet (lack of dietary fibre; excess dairy consumption)
- Genetic factors (weak rectal vein walls or valves)
- Heavy lifting or straining
- Obesity
- Pregnancy
- Sitting or standing for a prolonged time

HEMORRHOIDS IN DEVELOPING COUNTRIES

Hemorrhoids are very rare in developing countries where people squat to defecate. Less straining is required to defecate in the squatting position, as the muscles of the abdomen work to expel feces, preventing a strain on the anal area.

DOCTOR'S ORDERS

There are several medical options for treating hemorrhoids. Hemorrhoid creams and suppositories contain ingredients such as hydrocortisone, zinc, mineral oil, shark liver oil, and witch hazel, which help shrink hemorrhoids and soothe the pain. Examples include Preparation H and Anusol.

Procedures to reduce or remove hemorrhoids include the following: Banding is a procedure in which a doctor places tiny rubber bands around the base of the hemorrhoid to cut off its circulation and it eventually falls off. Sclerotherapy involves injecting a solution into the vein to shrink the hemorrhoid. For those with severe hemorrhoids, a surgeon will remove the hemorrhoid. This is usually done as an outpatient procedure and requires a few days for recovery.

SHERRY'S NATURAL PRESCRIPTION

Dietary Recommendations

Foods to include:

- High-fibre foods help prevent constipation and ease bowel movements. Eat more fruits, vegetables, and whole grains. Add dried fruits (figs, prunes, raisins) to your yogurt or cereal along with ground flaxseed. Aim for 25–35 g of fibre daily. Make sure to also increase your fluid intake so that the fibre can do its job.

- Yogurt, kefir, and tempeh contain active cultures (good bacteria) that help improve digestion and elimination, and also help your body to absorb vitamin K better, which helps prevent bleeding.

- Aloe vera juice (pure) can help relieve itching and swelling.

Foods to avoid:

- Fast/processed foods are low in fibre and high in saturated fats and chemicals that have a negative impact on bowel function.

- Caffeine (coffee and cola) is dehydrating.

Lifestyle Suggestions

- Develop good bowel habits. Go when you feel the urge; don't hold it in, as this can cause the stool to become dry and harder to pass. Don't strain to push a stool out.

- Exercise regularly to prevent constipation and improve bowel function.

- Don't lift heavy objects, as this can cause excess strain and increase the pressure on the rectal veins.

- Avoid standing or sitting for a prolonged time. Move around. Use a doughnut cushion or pad on your chair.

- Bathe or shower daily to keep the area clean. Soak in a warm (not hot) sitz bath (a basin that fits over the toilet) with Epsom salts after a bowel movement and at night. Don't use soap, as it can irritate the skin.

- Use soft toilet paper or moist towelettes.

- Apply ice packs or cold compresses to external hemorrhoids to reduce swelling.

- Use creams with witch hazel to reduce swelling. Aloe vera, zinc, and calendula are soothing and promote skin healing.

Top Recommended Supplements

Diosmin: A flavonoid that improves vein health and reduces swelling, pain, itching, and bleeding. Numerous studies, including research on pregnant women, have found benefits for hemorrhoids. Dosage: 600–3,200 mg daily of a product standardized to 95 percent diosmin and 5 percent hesperidin.

Fibre: Supplements can be used to complement the diet. Look for a product that contains both soluble and insoluble fibres. Increase fibre intake gradually and take regularly with plenty of water.

Complementary Supplements

Horse chestnut seed extract: Reduces swelling and pain, and promotes vein health. It may take several weeks to notice benefits. Dosage: 300 mg orally three times per day, or use a cream or gel containing 2 percent aescin three or four times daily.

Probiotics: Supplements containing these "friendly bacteria" help to restore the normal gut flora and have been shown in studies to relieve constipation. Look for Kyo-Dophilus. Take one to three capsules daily.

Witch hazel: Strengthens veins and reduces inflammation. It is available in teas, creams, and solutions (to make compresses). Safe for use during pregnancy and breast-feeding.

SPICY FOODS AND HEMORRHOIDS

It is a myth that spicy foods can worsen hemorrhoid symptoms. A recent study confirmed there is no difference in symptoms following consumption of hot peppers (*Diseases of the Colon and Rectum*, 2006: 49 (7); 1018–23).

FINAL THOUGHTS

To prevent hemorrhoids or reduce symptoms:

1. Boost fibre intake from food and/or supplements; drink more fluids.
2. Avoid prolonged sitting or standing; get regular exercise.
3. Use cold compresses and creams or suppositories with witch hazel.
4. Evidence is strongest for diosmin supplements.
5. Probiotics and horse chestnut seed extract are also helpful.

HEPATITIS (VIRAL)

Hepatitis is an inflammation of the liver caused by one of the six hepatitis viruses, namely, hepatitis A, B, C, D, E, and G. The most common forms are hepatitis A, B, and C. When you are first infected with hepatitis, it is called acute hepatitis. The virus attacks the liver, but there are often few or no initial symptoms. Hepatitis can also become a long-term disease known as chronic hepatitis. All forms of hepatitis cause jaundice, liver tenderness, and severe fatigue. In some cases hepatitis can cause severe symptoms and be fatal.

The hepatitis viruses differ in how they are transmitted (spread). Hepatitis A virus (HAV) is usually transmitted via the fecal-oral route. For example, someone with the virus could use the toilet, not wash his or her hands, and then handle the food you eat, thus passing the virus from their stool to your mouth. HAV can also be spread by drinking contaminated water, eating raw shellfish from water polluted with sewage, or being in close contact with a person who is infected. HAV only causes acute infection, which typically lasts a few months.

Hepatitis B (HBV) virus is transmitted through contact with the blood and body fluids of someone who is infected. Most commonly it is spread by sexual contact, sharing needles (IV drugs abusers), and needle-stick injuries (nurses and hospital workers are susceptible). Women with HBV can pass the infection to their babies during childbirth. HBV can survive on personal items, such as toothbrushes and razors, for a few days and remain infectious. Most people infected as adults recover fully from HBV even if their signs and symptoms are severe. Infants and children are much more likely to develop a chronic infection.

Hepatitis C (HCV) is primarily spread by contact with blood. In the past it was transmitted by blood transfusions, but that is rare today because our blood supply is screened for the virus antibodies. Today it is spread by sharing needles, and less commonly, from contaminated needles used in tattooing and body piercing. In rare cases, HCV may be transmitted sexually or through childbirth. HCV is one of the main causes of chronic liver disease. About 60–70 percent of people who have acute HCV go on to develop chronic hepatitis.

Since there are no effective medical treatments for hepatitis, prevention is key—practising good hygiene and safe sex and taking necessary precautions when travelling to high-risk areas. For those who develop hepatitis, dietary approaches and supplements can help prevent liver damage and improve healing.

BE GOOD TO YOUR LIVER

The liver is the largest internal organ and it performs more than 500 important functions in the body, including processing most of the nutrients absorbed from your intestines; removing drugs, alcohol, and other toxins from your bloodstream; manufacturing bile (the greenish fluid stored in your gallbladder that helps digest fats); and producing cholesterol, blood-clotting factors, and certain other proteins. The liver has an amazing ability to regenerate. It can heal itself by replacing or repairing injured cells. However, the liver is prone to a number of diseases, such as viral hepatitis, which can hamper its function. Take measures to protect yourself against contracting hepatitis by practising safe sex and good hygiene (hand washing) and not sharing needles.

SIGNS & SYMPTOMS

Some people with hepatitis have no signs or symptoms, especially in the acute (early) stages. When symptoms do occur, they may include:

- Clay-coloured stools

- Dark urine

- Fatigue

- Muscle and joint aches and pains

- Nausea and vomiting

- Poor appetite

- Tenderness in the area of your liver (right side beneath your lower ribs)

Note: Hepatitis B can damage your liver—and spread to other people—even if you don't have any signs and symptoms.

Most people infected with HCV develop chronic hepatitis. With chronic hepatitis, there may be no symptoms, or people may experience fatigue, yellowing of the skin and eyes (jaundice), and low-grade fever. Chronic hepatitis increases the risk of cirrhosis and liver cancer.

RISK FACTORS

Hepatitis A:

- Hemophilia or receive clotting-factor concentrates for another medical condition

- In rare cases, hepatitis A may be transmitted through blood transfusions

- Sexually active gay or bisexual man

- Sharing needles

- Travel or work in regions with high rates of hepatitis A

- Work in a research setting where you may be exposed to the virus

Hepatitis B:

- Exposure to infected blood (health care worker)

- Having a sexually transmitted disease such as gonorrhea or chlamydia

- Having unprotected sex with someone who is infected with HBV

- Received a blood transfusion or blood products before 1970, the year the blood supply began to be tested for HBV

- Receiving hemodialysis for end-stage kidney (renal) disease

- Sharing needles

- Travelling to regions with high infection rates of HBV, such as sub-Saharan Africa, Southeast Asia, the Amazon Basin, the Pacific Islands, and the Middle East

Hepatitis C:

- Having an organ transplant before 1992

- Health care worker who has been exposed to infected blood

- Receiving clotting-factor concentrates before 1987 or have the clotting disease hemophilia and received blood before 1992

- Receiving hemodialysis for kidney failure

- Sharing needles

DOCTOR'S ORDERS

Conventional medicine has little in the way of treatment for acute hepatitis.

No specific treatment exists for hepatitis A. The goal is to ensure adequate nutrition and avoid permanent liver damage.

If you are exposed to HBV, call your doctor immediately. Receiving an injection of hepatitis B immune globulin within 24 hours of coming in contact with the virus may help protect you from developing hepatitis B. You should also receive the first in a series of three shots of the hepatitis B vaccine.

For those with chronic hepatitis B or C, the treatment depends on the severity of the signs and symptoms and liver damage. For those who have liver damage, doctors may recommend injections of a drug called interferon alpha, combined with an oral antiviral drug to clear the virus from your bloodstream. Side effects from interferon include severe flu-like symptoms, irritability, depression, poor concentration, memory problems, and insomnia. Antiviral drugs can cause a low red blood cell count (anemia), gout, and birth defects. Both drugs can cause extreme fatigue.

For those with end-stage liver disease, a liver transplant may be necessary. This can be a risky procedure, and difficult to have since there is a shortage of organs available to meet the demands. Newer procedures include the donation of liver segments from a relative. A liver transplants does not cure HCV. Most people who have transplants will experience a recurrence of the virus. Transplant recipients are also at greater risk of developing cirrhosis within five years than are people with HCV who don't receive a transplant.

VACCINES FOR HEPATITIS

Vaccines are available for the prevention of hepatitis A and B. The hepatitis A vaccine (Havrix) may protect you for up to 20 years. It contains inactivated forms of HAV and is safe for children older than two years as well as for most adults, including those with compromised immune systems. The hepatitis B vaccine (Engerix-B) provides more than 90 percent protection for both adults and children. The vaccine generally protects against HBV for at least 15 years. Twinrix is a vaccine that protects people age 18 and older against both HAV and the hepatitis B virus (HBV). Studies have shown Twinrix to be as effective as the separate HAV and HBV vaccines. The vaccines cause minor side effects (pain at injection site, headache, and fatigue), although allergic reactions can occur.

SHERRY'S NATURAL PRESCRIPTION

A healthful diet is important to support liver function and protect against further damage.

Dietary Recommendations

Foods to include:

- Choose organics as much as possible to avoid ingesting pesticides and chemicals, which are hard on the liver.

- Drink vegetable juices—beets and carrots are particularly good.

- Eat small, frequent meals of brown rice, steamed vegetables, whole grains, fish, chicken, and legumes.

- Green tea contains catechins, which aid detoxification.

Foods to avoid:

- Alcohol is hard on the liver and speeds the progression to liver disease.

- Fast foods, processed foods, and snack foods contain chemicals that are taxing to the liver.

- Saturated and trans fats are hard on digestive function and stressful to the liver.

HEPATITIS PREVENTION

To avoid contracting any of the hepatitis viruses:

- Practise safe sex. Use condoms and ask your partner whether he or she has any of the viruses or has been tested.

- Don't share needles or other drug paraphernalia. Contaminated drug paraphernalia is responsible for more than half of all new hepatitis C cases.

- Avoid body piercing and tattooing or if you do undergo piercing or tattooing, be absolutely certain the equipment is sterile.

- Talk to your doctor if you're travelling internationally to areas where hepatitis A or B is endemic, and discuss the benefits and risks of vaccination.

- If you're travelling in regions where hepatitis A outbreaks occur, you can help prevent infection by peeling and washing all your fresh fruits and vegetables yourself and by avoiding raw or undercooked meat and fish. Drink bottled water and avoid ice cubes in beverages. If bottled water isn't available, boil tap water for at least 10 minutes before drinking it. Don't forget to use bottled water for tooth brushing.

Lifestyle Suggestions

To improve your health, if you have hepatitis:

- Avoid medications that may cause liver damage, such as Tylenol. Talk with your pharmacist before taking any over-the-counter (OTC) medications.

- Get regular exercise.

If you have hepatitis, take measures to prevent passing the virus to others:

- Tell your sexual partner if you have hepatitis and that he or she should be tested.

- Practise safe sex (use condoms). Avoid oral-anal contact.

- Wash your hands with soap and water after using the toilet.

- Those with hepatitis A should keep their utensils separate from those used by other members of their household. Wash utensils and dishes in a dishwasher or with plenty of hot, soapy water. Don't prepare food for others while you are actively infected.

- Help prevent others from coming in contact with your blood. Cover any wounds you may have and don't share razors or toothbrushes. Don't donate blood, body organs, or semen, and advise health care workers that you have the virus.

Top Recommended Supplements

Milk thistle: Contains a compound called silymarin, which aids healing and regeneration of the liver. It stimulates the production of antioxidant enzymes that help the liver neutralize toxins. It also seems to increase the production of new liver cells and may even improve the severe scarring of cirrhosis. Dosage: 600–1,000 mg silymarin daily.

SAMe (S-adenosylmethionine): A nutrient that is naturally occurring and involved in numerous body processes, including detoxification. Studies show that it supports liver function and may help in the treatment of chronic hepatitis. Specifically it can help improve cholestasis, a problem that occurs when bile backs up into the liver. Dosage: 800–1,600 mg daily.

Complementary Supplements

Catechin: A type of flavonoid (antioxidant plant compound) that has been shown to benefit those with acute viral hepatitis and chronic hepatitis. Dosage: 500–750 mg three times daily, under doctor supervision.

Cordyceps: Helps reduce fibrosis and improve liver and immune function in those with chronic hepatitis B, including those with cirrhosis. Dosage: The usual amount taken is 3–4.5 g twice daily as capsules or simmered for 10–15 minutes in water to make tea.

Thymus extracts: Made of proteins from the thymus gland; some research shows that these supplements can benefit those with chronic hepatitis B by improving liver function. Dosage: 200–300 mg three times daily, under doctor supervision.

H

Hepatitis (Viral)

FINAL THOUGHTS

To manage hepatitis, consider the following:

1. Eat a healthful diet with lots of vegetables, brown rice, fish, chicken, and legumes. Choose organic foods.
2. Drink vegetable juices and green tea.
3. Avoid alcohol, processed foods, fast foods, and saturated and trans fats.
4. Avoid medications that are hard on the liver, such as Tylenol.
5. Consider supplements of milk thistle and SAMe to promote healing.

HIGH BLOOD PRESSURE (HYPERTENSION)

Blood pressure is a measure of the force that blood exerts on the walls of arteries and veins as it is pumped through the body. High blood pressure, or hypertension, occurs when the pressure on your blood vessels is elevated.

Our blood pressure is regulated by a complex system involving the heart, blood vessels, brain, kidneys, and adrenal glands. It fluctuates from moment to moment, typically increasing in response to physical activity or stress. When blood pressure stays elevated, even when you are at rest, it can damage the arteries and delicate organs like the brain, heart, and kidneys.

In about 90–95 percent of people with high blood pressure, there's no identifiable cause. This is referred to as essential hypertension or primary hypertension, which tends to develop gradually over many years. A combination of factors may be at play, such as diet, lifestyle, stress, and smoking.

The other 5–10 percent of high blood pressure cases are secondary hypertension as they are caused by another underlying condition, such as kidney or adrenal diseases or heart defects. Certain medications can also cause secondary hypertension, as noted below.

High blood pressure is known as a silent killer because you can have it for years without knowing it, and then suddenly have a heart attack or stroke. Uncontrolled blood pressure can also cause organ damage, leading to increased risk of stroke, heart attack, and kidney failure. If you have high blood pressure, it is critical to be under a doctor's supervision. Do not stop taking any prescribed medications. The strategies outlined in this chapter are not meant as a substitute for medical care. Lifestyle approaches, such as proper nutrition, exercise, stress management, and supplements, can be used to complement your medical care.

SIGNS & SYMPTOMS

- Dizziness
- Dull headache
- Flushed cheeks
- Nosebleeds
- Sweating
- Visual disturbances

GET CHECKED

Almost half of people with high blood pressure aren't aware they have it because in the initial stages, there are no obvious signs or symptoms. Uncontrolled high blood pressure can greatly increase your risk of heart disease, stroke, and kidney damage, so it is important to have your blood pressure checked regularly and discuss the results with your doctor.

- Age: It is more common with age; men often develop it between age 35 and 55 and women are more likely to develop it after menopause.

- Chronic conditions such as high cholesterol, diabetes, kidney disease, and sleep apnea are associated with an increased risk of high blood pressure.

- Diet: High intake of sodium and alcohol; low intake of potassium and fibre

- Family history

- Illicit drugs such as cocaine and amphetamines

- Lack of physical activity

- Medications (birth control pills, cold remedies, and decongestants)

- Obesity: Those with a body mass index (BMI) of 30.0 or higher are more likely to develop high blood pressure.

- Race: It is more common in Blacks.

- Smoking

- Stress

RESEARCH HIGHLIGHT

A survey of more than 24,000 workers aged 18–64 found that the more hours people worked, the more likely they were to have high blood pressure. People working more than 51 hours a week had a 29 percent higher incidence of high blood pressure. Researchers tied the higher risk for workers with longer hours to unhealthy eating, less exercise, more stress, and less sleep. In Canada, one in four people work 50 hours or more per week; in 1991 it was one in 10 people working these long hours (*Hypertension,* 2006: 48; 744).

DOCTOR'S ORDERS

The first line of approach to the management of high blood pressure is lifestyle changes, including a healthy diet and regular exercise. If this is not successful, then your doctor will likely prescribe a medication. There are several types of medications that are used depending on the stage of your blood pressure and whether you have other medical conditions. A combination of medications may be necessary. All of these drugs can cause side effects and sometimes your doctor may change the drug and/or dose a few times in order to get your blood pressure properly regulated with the least amount of side effects.

The main classes of medications include the following:

Angiotensin-converting enzyme (ACE) inhibitors: Relax the blood vessels, which reduces blood pressure. Examples include ramipril (Altace) and enalapril (Vasotec). A common side effect is chronic coughing.

Angiotensin II (A-II) receptor blockers (ARBs): Work the same as the drugs above, but do not cause coughing. Examples include losartan (Cozaar) and valsartan (Diovan).

Beta-blockers: Reduce the workload on the heart, slowing your heartbeat, which lowers the pressure. They are often given with a diuretic. Examples include propranolol and acebutalol.

Calcium channel blockers: Relax the muscles of the blood vessels and some slow the heart rate. Examples include diltiazem (Cardizem) and nifedipine (Adalat).

Diuretics: Act on the kidney to help your body eliminate sodium and water, thereby reducing blood volume. Examples include hydrochlorothiazide and furosemide.

SHERRY'S NATURAL PRESCRIPTION

Dietary Recommendations

Foods to include:

- Cold-water fish contains beneficial fatty acids that can help reduce blood pressure and lower the risk of heart disease.

- Garlic and onions contain antioxidants that help lower blood pressure and cholesterol.

- Green tea contains antioxidants that offer benefits for the heart.

- Soy foods can help lower blood pressure. Incorporate soy milk, tofu, soy protein (make shakes), and soy nuts into your diet.

- Stevia is a natural, plant-based sweetener that can actually help lower blood pressure, according to some studies. Use stevia instead of sugar or artificial sweeteners. It is available in liquid or powder form for baking.

- Whole grains, vegetables, fruits, beans, and legumes contain lots of fibre along with potassium, magnesium, calcium, and other nutrients that help lower blood pressure. Apples, oranges, tomatoes, and bananas are a particularly good source of potassium.

Foods to avoid:

- High caffeine intake can increase blood pressure. Limit yourself to 1 or 2 cups of coffee per day. Avoid soft drinks because they contain high amounts of caffeine and provide no nutritional value.

- Limit alcohol to one or two drinks per day; red wine can offer some health benefits due to the antioxidants and is a better choice than beer or spirits.

- Reducing salt intake reduces blood pressure in most people. Salt causes water retention and increases the pressure inside your arteries. Avoid adding salt to foods and minimize eating processed and fast foods such as deli meats, snacks (chips, pretzels), french fries, and burgers. Limit salt intake to 2,500 mg per day.

- Saturated fat (red meat and dairy) and trans fats (deep-fried and snack foods) can increase blood pressure and clog your arteries, increasing the risk of heart disease.

Lifestyle Suggestions

- Don't smoke and avoid second-hand smoke. Smoking greatly increases the risk of heart disease.

- Get regular exercise—aim for one hour of moderate-intensity activity daily. Try brisk walking, biking, swimming, or dancing.

- Maintain a healthy body weight. Being overweight increases blood pressure and stress to the heart.

- Manage your stress levels by finding ways to promote calming and relaxation. Regular exercise, breathing techniques, and meditation are a few ways to reduce the effects of stress.

- Acupuncture and yoga have been shown to lower blood pressure in many studies.

- See your doctor regularly. Get your blood pressure and cholesterol checked and discuss the results with your doctor.

Top Recommended Supplements

Coenzyme Q10: An antioxidant that has been widely studied and found to lower blood pressure and cholesterol and strengthen the function of the heart. Dosage: 100 mg twice daily.

Fish oils: Over 30 studies have shown that the omega-3 fatty acids in fish oil can help lower blood pressure, reduce atherosclerosis, and protect against heart attack. Dosage: 3 g of EPA plus DHA three times daily.

Garlic: Helps lower blood pressure and cholesterol, reduces clotting, and prevents plaque formation in the arteries. Most of the research showing benefits has been done on aged garlic extract (Kyolic). Dosage: 600 mg twice daily.

••

POTASSIUM LOWERS BLOOD PRESSURE

Numerous studies have shown that potassium can lower blood pressure, but the dose used in studies is quite high (2,400 mg daily). The highest dosage sold without a prescription in Canada is 100 mg. Potassium can cause stomach irritation in high doses and should not be combined with potassium-sparing diuretics or taken by those with kidney disease. Talk with your doctor about whether this is a good choice for you. Potassium is found naturally in apples, bananas, oranges, and tomatoes.

••

Complementary Supplements

Calcium and magnesium: Several studies have found that these minerals can promote modest reductions in blood pressure. Both are essential for proper muscle contractions and blood vessel health. Dosage: 1,500 mg calcium and 500 mg magnesium daily. Take in divided dosages with meals.

Vitamin C: Helps to lower blood pressure. Several studies have shown that it offers modest benefits. It also helps the body eliminate heavy metals, such as lead, which can contribute to high blood pressure. Dosage: 500 mg twice daily.

FINAL THOUGHTS

To improve the management of high blood pressure, consider the following:

1. Boost intake of fibre, eat more fish, potassium-rich foods, garlic, soy, and onions and drink green tea instead of coffee.
2. Get regular exercise. Aim for one hour of moderate-intensity activity daily.
3. Reduce your stress. Try acupuncture and yoga.
4. Don't smoke.
5. Consider supplements of coenzyme Q10, fish oil, and garlic.

HIGH CHOLESTEROL

Cholesterol is a fatty substance that is found in every cell of our bodies. It is an important component of cell membranes and is used in the formation of various hormones such as estrogen, testosterone, progesterone and cortisol, and bile acids. The liver manufactures the cholesterol that the body needs. We get additional cholesterol from diet when we eat foods containing saturated fat and cholesterol.

Cholesterol is carried through the blood via proteins called lipoproteins. High-density lipoprotein (HDL) is known as "good" cholesterol because it picks up excess cholesterol in the blood and takes it back to the liver. Low-density lipoprotein (LDL) is called "bad" cholesterol because it can build up in the artery walls of the brain and heart, narrowing the passageways for blood flow, a process known as atherosclerosis, the precursor to heart disease and stroke.

High blood cholesterol, known as hypercholesterolemia, occurs when the liver produces too much cholesterol, the body cannot remove LDL cholesterol from the blood efficiently, or excess amounts of cholesterol or saturated fats are obtained from diet.

There are many natural ways to effectively lower cholesterol; following a healthy diet and getting regular exercise are essential. Lifestyle modifications and supplements discussed below can help. In some cases, medication is necessary.

SIGNS & SYMPTOMS

There are no obvious signs or symptoms of high cholesterol. If left untreated, high cholesterol can form plaques inside the arteries (atherosclerosis). This reduces blood flow to the heart, which may cause chest pain, and increases the risk of heart disease. The plaques can rupture and form a blood clot. If this blood clot blocks the flow of blood to the heart, a heart attack occurs; if it blocks blood flow to the brain, a stroke occurs.

RISK FACTORS

- Diabetes: High blood sugar contributes to high LDL cholesterol and low HDL cholesterol, and also damages the lining of the arteries.

- Family history: Genetic defects can cause the liver to produce too much cholesterol and impair the removal of cholesterol from the blood.

- High blood pressure damages artery walls, which can increase the accumulation of fatty deposits.

- Inactivity.

- Obesity.

- Poor diet: Eating too much saturated fat (meat, dairy) and cholesterol-rich foods

- Smoking damages the blood vessel walls, which makes them prone to cholesterol deposits; smoking also lowers HDL levels.

DOCTOR'S ORDERS

The recommended first-line approach to the management of high cholesterol is life-style changes—a proper diet and regular exercise. Drugs are used when lifestyle changes are not enough or if the person is not willing to make the necessary changes. The most commonly used drugs include:

Bile acid-binding resins: These drugs lower cholesterol by binding to bile acids, substances required for digestion. This causes the liver to use excess cholesterol to make more bile acids, which reduces the level of cholesterol in the blood. Examples include Questran (cholestyramine) and Colestid (colestipol). Side effects include constipation and upset stomach.

Cholesterol-absorption inhibitors: This is a new class of drugs that reduces the absorption of dietary cholesterol. The only drug in this class is ezetimibe (Zetia). Side effects include diarrhea, stomach pain, and dizziness.

Statins: These are the most commonly prescribed class of drugs. They inhibit the action of an enzyme in the liver that is required for cholesterol production. They may also help the body reabsorb cholesterol from accumulated deposits on the artery walls. Examples include Lipitor (atorvastatin), Lescol (fluvastatin), Mevacor (lovastatin), Pravachol (pravastatin), Crestor (rosuvastatin), and Zocor (simvastatin). These drugs require close monitoring as they can cause liver toxicity and muscle wasting.

SHERRY'S NATURAL PRESCRIPTION

Dietary Recommendations

Foods to include:

- Fish contains beneficial omega-3 fatty acids, which help to reduce inflammation and LDL cholesterol levels, and raise HDL cholesterol. Salmon, mackerel, and herring are particularly good sources. To reduce consumption of toxins, choose wild (not farmed) fish.

- Garlic helps reduce cholesterol, thin the blood, and has antioxidant properties.

- Margarines, salad dressings, and spreads that contain phytostanols (plant substances) help lower cholesterol.

- Moderate alcohol consumption (one drink for women and two for men) has been shown to have heart-protective effects. Alcohol increases protective HDL cholesterol and also helps to think the blood. Higher amounts can be hard on the liver and increase blood pressure and the risk of heart disease.

- Nuts (almonds and walnuts) help lower cholesterol levels. Nuts contain fibre and nutrients such as vitamin E, alpha-linolenic acid, magnesium, potassium, and arginine, which are important for heart health. Although nuts are high in calories, some studies have found that increasing nut consumption by several hundred calories per day does not cause weight gain.

- Olive oil, which contains monounsaturated fatty acids, helps lower LDL cholesterol.

- Soluble fibre, which is found in oats, flaxseed, beans, psyllium, and fruits, helps to lower cholesterol levels. Insoluble fibre, which is found in whole grains, vegetables, and fruits, does not lower cholesterol, but studies have shown that it helps protect against heart disease. Aim for a total of 35 g of fibre daily.

- Soy products (tofu, soybeans, miso, and soy protein powder) can help lower cholesterol and triglycerides. Substituting as little as 20 g per day of soy protein for animal protein can significantly lower cholesterol.

- Yogurt and fermented milk products have been shown to lower cholesterol levels.

....

Oat bran is rich in a soluble fibre called beta-glucan, which has been shown to lower cholesterol levels. A typical dose of oat bran is 5–10 g taken with each meal. Beta-glucan is also available in supplement form. The recommended intake is 10–15 g of beta-glucan per day.

....

Foods to avoid:

- Foods high in cholesterol should be minimized (include organ meats, egg yolks, and whole milk products). Aim for no more than 300 mg of dietary cholesterol daily. One egg yolk contains 213 mg of cholesterol. Egg whites do not contain any cholesterol and are a good source of protein.

- Foods high in sugar and refined starches can raise triglyceride levels.

- Saturated fat, which is present in animal foods (beef, pork, and dairy) and certain oils (palm oil), can raise cholesterol levels and is associated with increased heart disease risk. Limit consumption of saturated fat to 10 percent of total calories. Read food labels carefully. Dairy products labelled "low fat" can be misleading. For example, 25 percent of calories in 2 percent milk come from fat. The 2 percent refers to the fraction of volume filled by fat, not the percentage of calories coming from fat.

- Trans fatty acids are found in hydrogenated oils, which are present in most margarines, processed, and deep-fried foods. These fats can raise cholesterol levels and increase the risk of heart disease. Avoid margarines that contain hydrogenated oils. Look for non-hydrogenated margarines. Many snack food companies are now making products that are free of trans fatty acids.

Lifestyle Suggestions

- Lose excess weight. Losing even 5–10 percent of excess weight can lower cholesterol levels, and reduce other risk factors for heart disease.

- Don't smoke. Smoking lowers the good HDL cholesterol and causes serious damage to blood vessels. It is never too late to quit. Within one year of quitting, your risk of heart disease is half of that of a smoker's. After 15 years, your risk is similar to that of someone who has never smoked.

- Exercise regularly. Moderate intensity activities, such as brisk walking, biking, or swimming, can reduce cholesterol, support weight loss, and reduce other risk factors for chronic disease.

- Reduce stress levels. Stress causes the liver to increase the production of cholesterol, which is used to make stress hormones. Try meditation, exercise, or yoga to promote calming and relaxation.

- Get your cholesterol levels checked regularly and discuss the results with your doctor.

Top Recommended Supplements

Niacin (vitamin B3): Numerous studies have shown that niacin can lower LDL, triglyceride, and lipoprotein-A levels and raise HDL. Dosage: 1–4 g daily. Niacin can cause liver inflammation at higher dosages (more than 500 mg daily) and requires physician monitoring.

• •

Niacin at dosages of more than 100 mg daily frequently causes skin flushing, itching, upset stomach, and headache. These symptoms can usually be reduced by gradually increasing the dosage over several weeks or by using slow-release niacin. However, slow-release niacin may increase the risk of liver inflammation. Inositol hexaniacinate may also cause less flushing than regular niacin. Taking aspirin along with niacin can also reduce flushing.

• •

Soluble fibre: Glucomannan, beta-glucan, and psyllium help to lower cholesterol. Dosage varies depending on product and amount of fibre per serving. Add gradually to the diet to avoid gas and bloating. Dosage varies depending on the source. Take with plenty of water.

Stanols and sterols: Plant substances that have been shown in many studies to lower LDL cholesterol, but have negligible effects on HDL and triglycerides. They are thought to work by attaching to cholesterol in the digestive tract and carrying it out of the body. They also remove cholesterol from substances made in the liver. A sterol ester, called beta-sitosterol, has been shown to decrease cholesterol absorption by about 50 percent. The dosage varies depending on the product and potency.

Complementary Supplements

Aged garlic extract: Helps to lower total and LDL cholesterol and triglycerides, reduces blood clotting, and prevents atherosclerosis. Dosage: 600 mg or more daily.

Fish oils: Lower triglycerides, raise HDL cholesterol, and reduce inflammation and blood clotting. Fish oil contains the beneficial omega-3 fatty acids, eicosapentaenoic acid (EPA) and docosahexaenoic acid (DHA). The typical dosage is 3–9 g total of EPA and DHA daily, although higher amounts have been used in some studies. Look for a product that provides at least 400 mg EPA and 200 mg DHA per dosage.

Policosanol: An extract from sugar cane that inhibits cholesterol production in the liver. Many studies have shown that it can significantly lower total and LDL cholesterol and raise HDL cholesterol. Dosage: 10–20 mg daily.

FINAL THOUGHTS

To lower cholesterol, consider the following:

1. Eat more soluble fibre, soy, fish, nuts, and garlic.
2. Minimize intake of saturated fat, trans fats, and processed and refined foods.
3. Maintain a healthy body weight and don't smoke.
4. Get regular exercise and reduce stress levels.
5. Consider supplements of stanols/sterols, fibre, niacin, aged garlic extract, fish oils, and policosanol.

HYPOGLYCEMIA

Hypoglycemia occurs when your blood sugar (glucose) levels drop abnormally low. Blood sugar is the body's main source of energy, and when levels are too low, it can cause fatigue and weakness.

During digestion, your body breaks down carbohydrates (which are present in vegetables, fruits, grains and beans) into sugar molecules, such as glucose, which are absorbed directly into your bloodstream. As blood sugar levels rise, the pancreas secretes the hormone insulin, which ushers glucose into your cells to be used for energy. Blood sugar and insulin levels then return to normal.

Hypoglycemia most often occurs as a complication of diabetes. Diabetics take insulin or other medications to manage blood sugar levels and if they take too much medication, eat too little, or exercise too much, blood sugar levels can drop off, causing hypoglycemia.

Hypoglycemia can also occur if the pancreas overproduces insulin. If too much insulin is released in response to a meal, then blood sugar levels can drop down very low. This is called reactive hypoglycemia. There are other factors that can lead to hypoglycemia and they are noted below.

Hypoglycemia can be managed or prevented with lifestyle measures, primarily nutritional strategies that keep blood sugar levels in a normal range.

SIGNS & SYMPTOMS

- Anxiety

- Confusion and inability to think clearly

- Headache

- Heart palpitations

- Hunger

- Sweating

- Tremor and nervousness

- Visual disturbances, such as double vision and blurred vision

The symptoms may come on slowly or suddenly. As it becomes more severe, dizziness, weakness, confusion, seizures, and loss of consciousness can occur.

IS IT HYPOGLYCEMIA?

The signs and symptoms of hypoglycemia are vague and could be caused by other conditions. To determine whether you have hypoglycemia, your doctor can check your blood sugar levels and perform a glucose-tolerance test.

- Alcohol: Excessive consumption can trigger hypoglycemia.

- Chronic diseases: Liver disease, such as hepatitis, and kidney failure can reduce glucose production; disorders of the adrenal glands (Addison's disease) and the pituitary gland can result in a deficiency of hormones that regulate glucose production; tumours of the pancreas can cause excessive utilization of glucose and overproduction of insulin-like substances.

- Diabetes: Taking too much insulin, not eating enough, or exercising too much

- Gender: Hypoglycemia is more common in women and older adults.

- Medications: Side effects of certain drugs such as quinine, isoniazid, phenylbutazone, propoxyphene, haloperidol, tricyclic antidepressants (amitriptyline), sulfa drugs, SSRIs (fluoxetine and sertraline), thiazide diuretics, ACE inhibitors, and others

- Overproduction of insulin (reactive hypoglycemia) may be caused by a disorder of the pancreas.

- Pregnancy

ALCOHOL AND HYPOGLYCEMIA

Avoid drinking alcohol on an empty stomach as this can trigger hypoglycemia. Heavy drinking can block glucose production and promote the release of insulin, factors that will lower your blood sugar levels and induce hypoglycemia. When having an alcoholic beverage, do so with a meal as food delays the absorption of alcohol.

DOCTOR'S ORDERS

The immediate treatment of hypoglycemia involves measures that raise blood sugar levels. Drinking a glass of juice or taking glucose tablets or candy will raise blood sugar levels within a few minutes. Those with diabetes or who are prone to hypoglycemia should carry some form of sugar with them at all times.

Those with severe symptoms who are unable to take anything by mouth will require immediate medical attention, which involves intravenous glucose or an injection of glucagon. If hypoglycemia is severe and untreated, it can result in serious consequences such as coma, heart problems, and death.

If the hypoglycemia is not caused by diabetes or overproduction of insulin, it is important to work with your doctor to determine the underlying causes and develop a treatment. For example, if it is caused by a medication you are taking, your doctor may recommend changing the medication. If it is due to a tumour or glandular disorder, a surgical procedure may be necessary.

SHERRY'S NATURAL PRESCRIPTION

The recommendations in this section are geared toward diabetics and those with reactive hypoglycemia. Those with organ disease or other serious health problems need to work with their health care provider for specific recommendations.

Dietary Recommendations

Foods to include:

- Eat quality proteins (tofu, eggs, fish, and poultry) and healthy fats (fish, nuts, and seeds) with your carbohydrates as this will slow down the rate of digestion.

- Eat small, frequent meals (every two or three hours).

- High-fibre, low-glycemic carbohydrates such as fruits, vegetables, whole grains, and legumes are digested slowly and therefore promote better blood sugar balance. Refer to Appendix B for more information.

- Sweeteners such as xylitol and stevia are better compared to sugar.

MEASURING CARBOHYDRATES

The glycemic index (GI) is a measure of how quickly carbohydrates are broken down into sugar. Those that break down quickly have a high glycemic index and those that break down slowly have a low glycemic index. Eating low-GI foods helps to promote steady blood sugar levels and prevent hypoglycemia. Appendix B provides a list of the GI of common foods.

Foods to avoid:

- Alcohol can impair blood sugar control and trigger hypoglycemia by interfering with normal glucose utilization and increasing insulin secretion. Avoid drinking on an empty stomach, and limit alcohol to one drink per day.

- Caffeine can trigger hypoglycemia, so it should be minimized. Caffeine is found in coffee, tea, and soft drinks.

- Refined and processed flour products (white bread/bagels/pastries) and foods high in sugar break down quickly into sugar and this can be followed by hypoglycemia.

Lifestyle Suggestions

- Regular exercise helps to improve blood sugar control and improve insulin sensitivity. Try brisk walking, swimming, or cycling for 30 minutes to an hour each day. Have a light snack 30 minutes before exercising to sustain your energy levels and prevent hypoglycemia.

- Reduce stress as this can trigger hypoglycemia. Try meditation, acupuncture, massage, and other relaxation techniques.

- Get adequate sleep to support overall health.

Top Recommended Supplements

B-vitamins: Play a role in metabolizing carbohydrates and converting blood glucose into energy. Look for a B-complex that provides 20–50 mg each of B1, B2, B3, B5, and B6 and 100 mcg of vitamin B12.

Chromium: A cofactor to insulin, chromium is essential for the body's utilization of glucose, and helps prevent hypoglycemia. Look for chromium GTF or chromium picolinate. Dosage: 200 mcg daily.

Fibre: Soluble fibre forms a gel in your stomach and slows the rate of digestion and absorption. Look for products that contain glucomannan, pectin, psyllium, or oats. Mix with water and take two or three times daily.

Complementary Supplements

Fish oils: May help improve insulin sensitivity. Dosage: 1–3 g daily.

Magnesium: May help prevent blood sugar levels from falling low. Dosage: 300–400 mg daily.

Vitamin C: Plays an important role in blood sugar regulation; levels are depleted by chronic stress, which is a factor in hypoglycemia. Dosage: 500 mg three times daily.

FINAL THOUGHTS

To improve blood sugar control and prevent hypoglycemia, consider the following:

1. Eat small, frequent meals of low-glycemic carbohydrates along with quality proteins and fats.
2. Minimize or avoid alcohol and caffeine.
3. Exercise regularly, but not on an empty stomach.
4. Take B-vitamins, chromium, and fibre supplements.
5. Consider fish oils and magnesium.

H

Hypoglycemia

HYPOTHYROIDISM

The thyroid gland is located at the base of your neck, below your Adam's apple. It produces two hormones, triiodothyronine (T3) and thyroxine (T4), which circulate through your bloodstream and control metabolic activity in every cell in the body, from your heartbeat to body temperature to how fast you burn calories. Hypothyroidism or underactive thyroid occurs when the thyroid gland cannot produce enough thyroid hormones to meet the body's demands. This causes all bodily functions to slow down and you feel tired, sluggish, achy, and gain weight.

Decades ago, the most common cause of hypothyroidism was iodine deficiency. Iodine is required for the production of thyroid hormone. When iodine was added to table salt, deficiency became a rare problem. However, today people are encouraged to reduce salt intake for health reasons (hypertension), and most of the salt that we get comes from processed foods that contain non-iodized sodium, so it is possible that low iodine levels are again partly contributing to thyroid disease.

The most common cause of hypothyroidism is Hashimoto's disease, which is an autoimmune disorder in which the body makes antibodies that attack the thyroid gland. This impairs the production of thyroid hormone. People with Hashimoto's develop a lump on their thyroid called a goiter.

Hypothyroidism can also result from treatment of Graves' disease (hyperthyroidism) with radioactive iodine, which destroys the thyroid gland, leaving it unable to produce hormones, and from surgical removal of the thyroid gland due to thyroid cancer. A baby can be born without a thyroid gland (congenital hypothyroidism).

Diseases of the hypothalamus or pituitary gland can also cause hypothyroidism. These glands are involved in the regulation of the thyroid gland and the amount of thyroid hormone that is released. The hypothalamus releases thyrotropin-releasing hormone (TRH), which signals your pituitary gland to make thyroid-stimulating hormone (TSH). The amount of TSH released depends on how much T3 and T4 are in your blood. The thyroid gland regulates its production of hormones based on the amount of TSH it receives.

Hypothyroidism is easily treated today with thyroid hormones, supplements, and various lifestyle approaches.

THYROID DISEASE IN CANADA

According to recent studies, 30 percent of Canadians suffer from a thyroid condition, of those, as many as 50 percent are undiagnosed. Many people do not realize that they have low thyroid because in the early stages the symptoms can be very mild and vague, such as fatigue.

SIGNS & SYMPTOMS

- Anemia and easy bruising
- Cold intolerance (sensitivity to cold)
- Constipation

- Depression, irritability, and anxiety
- Dry, brittle nails
- Dry eyes and droopy eyelids
- Dry, itchy skin; dry hair and hair loss (including eyebrow hair loss)
- Fatigue and sluggishness
- Headaches
- High cholesterol
- Hoarse voice
- Insomnia
- Joint aching
- Low libido
- Memory loss
- Menstrual irregularities
- Muscle swelling or cramps
- Slow heart rate
- Tingling or numbness in hands and feet
- Weight gain

Note: Hypothyroidism is rare in infants and young children. It may cause a large, protruding tongue, choking, yellowing of the skin and whites of the eyes, constipation, poor muscle tone, and excessive sleepiness. If untreated it can lead to physical and mental retardation.

RISK FACTORS

- Age: It is most common after age 40
- Family history
- Gender: It is 10 times more common in women
- History of hyperthyroidism, Graves' disease, or thyroid cancer
- Hormone imbalance (high estrogen and cortisol)
- Iodine deficiency
- Medications (lithium, estrogen)
- Poor diet: Lack of iodine or selenium
- Pregnancy: The body produces antibodies that attack the thyroid gland, increasing the risk of miscarriage, premature delivery, pre-eclampsia, and damage to the fetus.
- Stress

DOCTOR'S ORDERS

Hypothyroidism is often a chronic problem that requires lifelong treatment. Doctors typically prescribe synthetic thyroid hormone (T4), such as Eltroxin or Synthroid. Blood tests are done to check your T3, T4, and TSH levels, and it often takes a few dosage adjustments to find your ideal level. Too much thyroid hormone can cause symptoms of racing heart, increased appetite, insomnia, and shakiness.

Some people do not convert T4 to T3 adequately and do better with a form of T3, which is called Cytomel.

Natural thyroid hormones can be compounded by a pharmacist to provide T3 and T4 or just T3, depending on your needs. Compounded thyroid hormones are available through a compounding pharmacy with a doctor's prescription. The advantage of this form is that the dosage can be tailored to your needs and many people do better with the natural over the synthetic form.

Calcium and iron supplements may reduce the absorption of thyroid hormone, so take these products six hours away from your thyroid medication.

THYROID CHECK

Borderline hypothyroidism, also called compensated hypothyroidism, is very common, and often undiagnosed. Blood tests may show thyroid hormone levels (T3 and T4) that are slightly low or even in the normal range and normal or slightly elevated TSH levels. A person may have no symptoms or vague symptoms, such as fatigue, dry skin, or weight gain. Anyone at risk of hypothyroidism or who has any of the symptoms should consider testing beyond basic bloodwork. Measurement of T3 in a 24-hour urine sample correlate better with patient symptoms than serum TSH levels. These tests can be ordered through a doctor or pharmacy. See Appendix E for more information. You can also check your basal (resting) body temperature. The thyroid regulates metabolism and low body temperature can indicate hypothyroidism. Here is what you do:

- Place a digital thermometer, paper, and pen beside your bed.

- When you wake up in the morning (before you get up or do anything), put the thermometer under your armpit and hold your elbow close to your side.

- Record the temperature and date.

- Repeat this for three mornings.

- A reading between 97.6 and 98.2°F is normal. Readings below 97.6°F may indicate hypothyroidism.

SHERRY'S NATURAL PRESCRIPTION

Dietary Recommendations

Foods to include:

- Essential fatty acids are important for proper thyroid function. Eat more fish and flaxseed.

- Sea vegetables such as kelp, nori, dulse, and wakame contain iodine, which is used by the body to make thyroid hormone. Shellfish and saltwater fish also contain iodine. Iodine through food or supplements is helpful only if you are deficient this nutrient.

Foods to avoid:

- Broccoli, Brussels sprouts, cabbage, cauliflower, collard greens, and kale contain goitrogens, which interfere with thyroid hormone synthesis. Cooking usually inactivates these goitrogens, so this is the rare case where cooked is preferred over raw.

- Tap water contains fluorine and chlorine, which can inhibit the body's ability to absorb iodine.

SOY AND YOUR THYROID

Soy contains isoflavones that in animal studies have been shown to suppress thyroid function. Soy may also have these effects in humans, although more research is needed. Other factors that may worsen the effects of soy on thyroid function are iodine deficiency, consumption of other goitrogens, and other problems synthesizing thyroid hormones. Soy can also reduce absorption of thyroid hormone. Until more is known, if you have hypothyroidism, limit intake of soy foods and avoid supplements containing soy.

Lifestyle Suggestions

- Don't smoke, as smoking can worsen hypothyroidism.

- Avoid fad dieting. Drastically reducing your calorie intake can lower metabolism, which can make weight management more difficult.

- Get regular exercise. Physical activity stimulates the thyroid to secrete more hormone and makes the body more sensitive to any thyroid hormone that is circulating.

- Manage your stress levels. Stress triggers the release of cortisol, which can suppress thyroid function.

Top Recommended Supplements

Compounded thyroid hormones: Provide the body with biologically active, natural hormones. Both T3 and T4 can be made into delayed-release capsules and tailored to your needs. Compounded hormones are available by prescription at compounding pharmacies.

Guggul: Increases production of thyroid hormone (T3). Dosage: 25 mg of guggulsterones (active component) three times daily.

Multivitamin/mineral complex: Many nutrients are required to produce thyroid hormone, such as vitamin C, E, A, and the B-vitamins. Selenium is required for the conversion from T4 to T3. Many people are deficient in selenium, which may hamper thyroid hormone levels, so a complete multivitamin can ensure that all essential nutrients requirements are met.

Complementary Supplements

Ashwaganda: An herbal product that helps boost thyroid function and also reduces stress. Dosage: 500 mg three times daily.

Tyrosine: An amino acid involved in the synthesis of thyroid hormone. Dosage: 500 mg twice daily on an empty stomach.

FINAL THOUGHTS

To manage hypothyroidism, consider the following:

1. Eat more sea vegetables and saltwater fish if you are low in iodine. Fish and flax-seed provide essential fatty acids.
2. Minimize eating raw goitrogens (broccoli, Brussels sprouts, etc.) and soy foods.
3. Don't smoke.
4. Get regular exercise and reduce your stress levels.
5. Consider compounded thyroid hormones and guggul, and take a daily multivitamin/mineral complex.

INFERTILITY

Many couples take fertility for granted, assuming that it will happen once they start trying to conceive. However, the reality is that infertility is becoming a common concern. An estimated 10–15 percent of couples are infertile, which means they are unable to conceive after one year of frequent, unprotected intercourse. While once thought of as primarily a woman's problem, infertility can affect men too.

Infertility may be due to a single cause in either you or your partner, or a combination of factors. To become pregnant, a woman's egg needs to connect with a man's sperm. When a woman's body is functioning as it should, each month the ovaries prepare an egg, which is released during ovulation. This occurs around day 14 of the menstrual cycle and during this time a woman is fertile and can conceive. The egg travels through the fallopian tube and can be fertilized about 24 hours after its release. Conception is more likely to occur when intercourse takes place one to two days prior to ovulation. Sperm are capable of fertilizing the egg for up to 72 hours and must be present in the fallopian tube at the same time as the egg for conception to occur. If fertilized, the egg moves into the uterus where it attaches to the uterine lining and begins a nine-month process of growth.

If something in this whole process doesn't happen properly, it can affect the ability to conceive. Some of the most common causes of infertility in men are:

- Erectile dysfunction or retrograde ejaculation
- Genetic defects, such as blockage of epididymis or ejaculatory ducts
- Impaired production or function of sperm (low sperm count, impaired shape, or slow movement)
- Low testosterone levels
- Sexually transmitted disease (chlamydia and gonorrhea)
- Undescended testicle

In women, infertility can result from:

- Benign uterine fibroids and pelvic adhesions
- Early menopause
- Endometriosis, polycystic ovary syndrome (PCOS)
- Fallopian tube damage or blockage
- Hormonal problems: Elevated prolactin levels, low thyroid function, high estrogen-to-progesterone ratio
- No ovulation or problems with ovulation

I

Infertility

HOW LONG DOES IT TAKE?

Most pregnancies occur during the first six months of intercourse in the fertile phase. According to statistics, after 12 months of unprotected intercourse, approximately 85 percent of couples will become pregnant. Over the next 36 months, about half of the remaining couples will go on to conceive spontaneously.

SIGNS & SYMPTOMS

- Inability to get pregnant

RISK FACTORS

- Age: After about age 32, a woman's fertility gradually declines; older women are also more likely to have health problems that may interfere with fertility; the risk of miscarriage also increases with a woman's age; a gradual decline in fertility is possible in men older than 35.
- Alcohol: Heavy alcohol consumption (binge drinking) is toxic to sperm; alcohol also impairs female fertility.
- Caffeine: Some studies have linked caffeine to infertility, especially high amounts (greater than 3 cups per day); caffeine also increases the risk of miscarriage.
- Cancer or chemotherapy
- Excessive exercise: Exercising more than seven hours a week can affect ovulation.
- Exposure to pesticides and other chemicals.
- Obesity causes hormonal changes that hamper fertility.
- Radiation and chemotherapy impair fertility in men and women.
- Smoking affects both men and women.
- Stress interferes with hormones needed to produce sperm.
- Underweight: Women with eating disorders or very low body fat have hormonal problems and deficiencies of nutrients that can affect fertility.

AGING AND FERTILITY

Beyond age 35, a woman's chances of conceiving are drastically lowered.

According to several studies, by age 35 over one-third of women could not conceive within a year. With age, there are hormonal changes and a reduced quantity and quality of eggs. Women are born with about 400,000 eggs. Each month, during the reproductive years, usually only a single egg matures. The quantity of eggs starts to diminish in childhood and continues into adulthood. Ovulation contributes to the decrease, but the majority of eggs are slowly absorbed by the body. By the fifth or sixth decade of life, most women will have depleted the egg supply they were born with.

DOCTOR'S ORDERS

The treatment of infertility depends on the underlying cause, your age, and personal preferences. For many couples, timing is the issue. In order to determine when you are ovulating, you can check your basal body temperature. Take your temperature when you wake up in the morning and record this every day. There is a slight rise in your body temperature when you ovulate. There are also ovulation kits available that measure hormones in urine to detect ovulation.

There are fertility drugs that can help women with ovulation disorders. The most commonly used drug is clomiphene (Clomid and Serophene), which stimulates the pituitary gland. There are also injectable drugs that can stimulate the ovaries to mature egg follicles. Both oral and injectable drugs can cause multiple births. Surgical procedures can correct blockages in the fallopian tubes.

For women with estrogen dominance (high estrogen-to-progesterone radio), natural progesterone cream can be used to restore hormonal balance. This is available by prescription in compounding pharmacies. Saliva tests can be done to check hormone levels. Refer to Appendix E for more information.

Depending on the cause of male infertility, there are medications, hormones, and surgical options.

For couples who are unable to conceive naturally, there are many other options available such as in-vitro fertilization. It is important to discuss all your options with your doctor.

Proper nutrition and a healthy lifestyle can make a difference in your ability to conceive. These recommendations are not intended to replace the medical advice from your physician.

Dietary Recommendations

Foods to include:

- Choose lean cuts of poultry (free range) and wild fish.

- Eat a healthful diet with whole grains, vegetables, fruits, nuts, and seeds.

- Men should eat pumpkin seeds as they contain zinc, which is important for male reproductive fluids.

Foods to avoid:

- Alcohol is toxic to sperm and can impair fertility in both men and women.

- Avoid farmed fish as it contains PCBs, dioxins, mercury, and other chemicals that can impair fertility.

- Caffeine may impair female fertility and also increase the risk of miscarriage. Minimize or avoid coffee, tea, and soft drinks.

- Fast foods and processed foods are full of chemicals that can cause hormonal imbalances.

Lifestyle Suggestions

- Reduce your stress, which can affect libido and cause hormonal changes that affect ovulation. Try yoga, tai chi, meditation, and massage.

- Acupuncture helps reduce stress and may improve fertility. Some research found it particularly helpful for the treatment of female infertility due to problems with ovarian function.

- Get regular exercise to promote good circulation.

Infertility

- Men should avoid hot tubs.

- Maintain a healthy body weight. Being too thin or too heavy can impair fertility.

- Don't smoke. The more women smoke, the less likely they are to conceive.

- Avoid taking any unnecessary medications.

- Reduce your exposure to phthalates (chemicals used to make plastics soft), which can impair fertility by disrupting hormones. They are found in medical supplies (IV tubing), some flooring material, soft plastic food storage containers, and some cosmetics and perfumes. Contact the manufacturer to find out if their products contain phthalates.

Top Recommended Supplements

For men:

Antioxidants: Neutralize free radicals, which can be damaging to sperm. Some studies have found benefits with vitamins E and C for improving sperm count and activity. Dosage: 400 IU vitamin E and 1,000 mg vitamin C. These are higher amounts than are typically found in multivitamin formulas.

L-carnitine: Numerous studies have shown that it can improve sperm function and enhance male fertility. Dosage: 2 g daily.

Zinc and folate: Essential nutrients for cell division, synthesis of genetic material, and numerous body processes. Two studies of zinc combined with folate have found that the supplements can improve sperm count and the percentage of healthy sperm in men with impaired fertility. Dosage: 15 mg elemental zinc with 5 mg folate. Take along with a multi-vitamin/mineral complex containing copper to prevent a copper deficiency.

RESEARCH HIGHLIGHT

In a double-blind study, 60 men with abnormal sperm function were given either carnitine (as L-carnitine 2 g/day and acetyl-L-carnitine 1 g/day) or placebo for six months. The results showed significant improvement in sperm function in the treated group as compared to the placebo group (*Fertility and Sterility,* 2004): 81; 1578–1584).

For women:

Chasteberry (vitex): Very helpful for infertility due to irregular ovulation. It works by increasing production of luteinizing hormone, which in turn boosts secretion of progesterone during the last 14 days of the menstrual cycle. It also suppresses production of the lactation hormone prolactin, creating a hormonal environment more conducive to ovulation. Dosage: 160–246 mg daily. Discontinue if conception occurs.

Multivitamin/mineral complex: Ensures that your body will get all essential nutrients. The B-vitamins play a key role in reproductive health and also in early fetal development. Folic acid, especially, can prevent certain birth defects. Even a subtle deficiency of nutrients such as iron can impair fertility. Look for a formula designed for women of child-bearing age and take daily.

Vitamin C: Supplements may be helpful for women with infertility due to luteal phase defect. With this hormonal abnormality the uterine lining does not develop and mature properly, likely because of a deficiency of progesterone. One study of women with luteal phase defect found significant benefits with vitamin C supplements for six months. Dosage: 750 mg daily.

Complementary Supplements

Bee propolis: Recommended for women with endometriosis. Preliminary research found that supplementing with 500 mg twice a day for six months significantly increased pregnancy rate in a group of women with infertility and mild endometriosis. The mechanism is not known; more research is needed.

Panax ginseng: Preliminary research found that it improved sperm function. Dosage: 100–200 mg daily.

Essential fatty acids: Fish oils and primrose or borage oil should be taken daily by women to promote the healthy functioning of the uterus and help regulate hormone production. Dosage: 1 g three times daily.

Vitamin B12: Deficiency can lead to reduced sperm counts and lowered sperm mobility. Vitamin B12 supplementation has been tried for improving fertility in men with abnormal sperm production. A few studies have shown benefits. Dosage: 400 mcg sublingually daily.

FINAL THOUGHTS

To improve your chances of conceiving, consider the following:

1. Eat a healthful diet with organic whole grains, vegetables, fruits, nuts, seeds, wild fish, and free-range poultry.
2. Minimize caffeine; avoid alcohol and fast foods, processed foods, and junk foods.
3. Get regular exercise, reduce stress, and don't smoke.
4. Men should take antioxidants, L-carnitine, and a multivitamin/mineral complex containing adequate zinc and folate.
5. Women should take a multivitamin/mineral complex and consider extra vitamin C and chasteberry.

Infertility

INSOMNIA

Insomnia is characterized by persistent difficulty falling asleep, waking up too early, awakening frequently during the night, or waking feeling tired and not refreshed. Approximately 30 percent of adults suffer occasionally from insomnia and 10 percent experience chronic insomnia.

Sleep is vital for physical and mental health, yet it often gets sacrificed when we are busy. While it is thought that sleep is relaxing and passive, actually quite a lot happens in the body during sleep. During the deepest stages of sleep our bodies' major organs and regulatory systems are busy working on repair and regeneration and secreting certain hormones.

Short-term or transient insomnia is common and usually lasts only a few days. This may result from temporary situations, such as jet lag, stress at work, a brief illness, or a change in environment. When the precipitating factor disappears, the condition goes away, usually without medical treatment.

Insomnia is classified as long term or chronic when it lasts more than three weeks. Possible causes include stress; depression; use of alcohol, caffeine, or nicotine; snoring or sleep apnea; and other medical conditions as noted below.

The exact amount of sleep needed varies among individuals, but is between seven and nine hours. Getting less than six hours is associated with health problems, such as memory loss, poor concentration, depression, headache, irritability, increased response to stress, high blood pressure, depressed immune function, low libido, and weight gain.

SIGNS & SYMPTOMS

- Daytime fatigue or irritability
- Difficulty in falling asleep or staying asleep
- Waking too early
- Waking feeling tired and fatigued

RISK FACTORS

- Age (the incidence increases with age)
- Diet (high intake of caffeine, refined and processed foods; overeating)
- Exposure to noise and light
- Gender: Women are more likely to suffer insomnia; this may be due to hormonal changes that occur during the menstrual cycle, pregnancy, and menopause.
- Lack of exercise
- Medical conditions (depression, anxiety, cancer, alcoholism, restless legs, hypothyroidism, sleep apnea, bladder problems)
- Medications (blood pressure, antidepressants, decongestants, long-term use of sleeping pills)

- Pain (back pain, headaches, arthritis, fibromyalgia)

- Poor sleep habits (going to bed at different times)

- Smoking (nicotine is a stimulant)

- Snoring (disrupts deep sleep)

- Stress and muscle tension

- Travelling to a different time zone or working shifts can upset one's internal clock and lead to sleep disturbances.

- Vitamin deficiencies (vitamin B12 and iron)

DOCTOR'S ORDERS

There are several types of medications that are used to promote sleep, called sedatives and tranquilizers. The most commonly used class is the benzodiazepines, including Ativan (lorazepam), Restoril (temazepam), and Valium (diazepam). These drugs are recommended only for short-term use (a few weeks), as they cause a number of side effects, including loss of short-term memory. When used over the long term, they become less effective, can result in dependency, and actually worsen sleep quality. Abruptly stopping use of these drugs can cause withdrawal symptoms therefore they should be weaned off slowly (reduce dosage and take every other night) under doctor supervision.

SHERRY'S NATURAL PRESCRIPTION

There are a number of lifestyle tips and natural remedies that can greatly improve sleep quality. In most cases insomnia is temporary and can be improved with good sleep hygiene habits.

Dietary Recommendations

Foods to include:

- A small snack before bed of food that contains tryptophan (an amino acid) stimulates the release of serotonin, a brain chemical that facilitates sleep. Examples include: turkey, soy nuts, or whole-grain crackers or cereal.

- A glass of milk can also promote relaxation, as it contains calcium, which helps promote relaxation.

Foods to avoid:

- Caffeine (coffee, tea, pop, and chocolate) can affect sleep quality, and should be avoided eight hours before bed.

- Alcohol may help you fall asleep, but it causes nighttime wakening and reduces sleep quality, so minimize or avoid completely.

- Go easy on sugary foods, especially in the evening, as they can cause a sugar rush and affect your ability to fall asleep.

Insomnia

Lifestyle Suggestions

- Set aside at least seven to eight hours for sleep. Leaving only five or six hours may make you feel stressed and affect your ability to fall asleep.

- Establish a regular bedtime and wake time.

- Do relaxing activities before bed—read a book, have a warm bath, or meditate.

- Reserve your bedroom for intimacy and sleep only; don't work in your bedroom.

- Make your bedroom dark, quiet, and comfortable.

- Exercise regularly early in the day.

- Don't smoke, as nicotine is a stimulant and impairs your ability to fall asleep and have a restful sleep.

- Consider acupuncture, massage, yoga, or meditation for relaxation.

Top Recommended Supplements

Melatonin: A hormone that is naturally secreted by the brain in response to darkness and regulates sleep/wake cycles. Supplements reduce the time needed to fall asleep, reduce nighttime wakening, and improve sleep quality. It is particularly helpful for those who work shifts or travel to different time zones (jet lag). Dosage: 1–6 mg one hour before bed. Dosages up to 10 mg have been used in studies.

Suntheanine: An extract of theanine, an amino acid present in green tea. It helps improve sleep quality and reduce stress. Dosage: 50–100 mg 30 minutes before bed.

Valerian: An herb that is widely used for insomnia; it improves many aspects of sleep and is non-addictive. Some formulas combine valerian with hops, passion flower, and other herbs that promote relaxation. Dosage: 600 mg half an hour to one hour before bed, or 2 mL of a tincture.

Complementary Supplements

Calcium and magnesium: Important minerals for muscle and nervous system relaxation. Dosages: 500 mg of calcium and 250 mg of magnesium in the evening.

Chamomile: Teas made with this herb are soothing and calming.

5-Hydroxytryptophan: Increases serotonin and melatonin levels, which promote relaxation and improved sleep. Dosage: 100–200 mg one hour before bed.

Note: Supplements that promote sleep should be used only occasionally, as it is important to address the underlying factors causing insomnia.

FINAL THOUGHTS

For a good night sleep, consider the following:

1. Set aside at least seven hours for sleep and try to go to bed at the same time.
2. Get regular exercise early in the day.
3. Avoid alcohol, caffeine, and smoking.
4. Relax before bed with meditation or stretching.
5. Consider supplements of melatonin, valerian, and Suntheanine.

Insomnia

IRRITABLE BOWEL SYNDROME (IBS)

Irritable bowel syndrome (IBS) is a very common disorder, affecting about one in five Canadians. It is also one of the most common reasons for a doctor's appointment, especially among women. It is characterized by abdominal pain or cramping and changes in bowel function, such as bloating, gas, diarrhea, and constipation, which makes it a sensitive topic to discuss. In the past IBS has been called mucous colitis, spastic colon, and irritable colon, but these terms are misleading because the problem is not limited to the colon.

The walls of the intestines are lined with layers of muscle that contract and relax as they move food from your stomach through your intestinal tract to your rectum. Normally, these muscles contract and relax in a coordinated rhythm. With irritable bowel syndrome, the contractions are stronger and last longer, causing food to be forced through your intestines more quickly. This causes gas, bloating, and diarrhea. In some cases, the opposite occurs and food passage slows, causing dry, hard stools and constipation.

Several factors have been implicated in causing IBS, such as infection, food intolerances, abnormal bowel motility, and nervous system dysfunction. Since women are two or three times as likely as men to have IBS, hormonal changes may also play a role. While the actual cause of IBS is unknown, there is a particular phenomenon in all cases of IBS, and the disorder is increased and intensified by stress.

For most people, IBS is a chronic condition, although there are times when the symptoms will disappear for weeks or months. Although there is no known cure, there are a number of dietary strategies, supplements, and lifestyle measures that can greatly help to manage this condition.

SIGNS & SYMPTOMS

- Abdominal pain or cramping
- Depression and anxiety
- Diarrhea or constipation that may alternate
- Gas and bloating
- Headache and fatigue
- Mucus in the stool
- Nausea

The severity and type of symptoms can vary from one episode to another.

RISK FACTORS

- Age: IBS typically begins around age 20 and rarely appears after age 50.
- Gender: Two to three times as many women as men have the condition.
- Genetics: Many with IBS have a family member with the disorder, suggesting a possible genetic cause.

There are also a variety of factors that can trigger an episode such as emotional stress. Many people find that their symptoms worsen when they eat certain foods, such as milk, caffeine, wheat, alcohol, artificial sweeteners, or food preservatives. Other illnesses, such as an infection, can trigger IBS.

DOCTOR'S ORDERS

The medical treatment of IBS focuses on dietary strategies and drug therapy to reduce symptoms. Drugs that regulate gut motility, namely Dicetel (pinaverium bromide) and Modulon (trimebutine maleate), are often prescribed. They are well tolerated and help to restore normal contractions of the bowel.

Anti-diarrheal medications, such as Imodium (loperamide), and laxatives should be used cautiously and only occasionally when under recommendation by your doctor.

Fibre supplements, when taken along with adequate fluids, can help control constipation and improve bowel function.

Anti-spasmodic drugs, such as Bentylol (dicyclomine) and Buscopan (hyoscine), block the transmission of nerve impulses and reduce muscle activity, thus slowing the movement of food through the intestinal tract.

SHERRY'S NATURAL PRESCRIPTION

Dietary Recommendations

Foods to include:

- Cultured products, such as live yogurt, kefir, and sauerkraut, can help restore normal gut flora, aid digestion, and reduce symptoms of IBS.

- Drink lots of fluids, such as water, herbal tea, and vegetable and fruit juices, throughout the day.

- Eat small, frequent meals (four or five meals daily), chew food thoroughly, and eat slowly. This will help regulate bowel function and improve digestion.

- Fibre can help regulate bowel function and reduce constipation, but it can also cause gas and cramping. Add high-fibre foods to the diet gradually to minimize gas and bloating, and drink plenty of water. Recommended fibre-rich foods include oats, brown rice, milled flaxseed, psyllium, and vegetables.

Foods to avoid:

- Alcohol, caffeinated beverages, and spicy foods stimulate the intestines and can make diarrhea and pain worse.

- Artificial sweeteners, such as sorbitol or mannitol, cause reactions (gas and diarrhea) in some people. Sorbitol and mannitol are found mainly in diabetic and low-carbohydrate foods and snacks.

- Carbonated drinks (pop and soda water) can produce gas and should be avoided.

- Chewing gum causes ingestion of swallowed air, which contributes to intestinal gas.

- Concentrated amounts of fructose (fruit sugar) in dried fruit and fruit juice can ferment in the colon, causing gas and bloating.

- Gas-producing foods, such as beans, lentils, onions, broccoli, cabbage, cauliflower, pickles and peppers, should be minimized.

- High-fat foods, such as whole milk, cream, cheese, ice cream, butter, and fatty meats (prime rib, sausage, deli meats), can trigger IBS in some people.

- Wheat and lactose-containing foods (dairy) are common food allergens that can trigger reactions in those with IBS. If you suspect food allergies, consider an elimination diet. See Appendix D for more information.

IBS AND FOOD ALLERGIES

Several studies have drawn a correlation between food sensitivities and IBS. The most commonly implicated foods include wheat, dairy, sugar, and artificial sweeteners.

Standard blood tests to evaluate allergies are usually not helpful because IBS food sensitivities may not be true allergies but rather an intestinal reaction. Following an elimination diet (see Appendix D) and using a food and symptom diary can help determine which foods should be avoided.

Lifestyle Suggestions

- Stress can trigger and worsen IBS symptoms so it is critical to find ways to reduce stress, such as deep breathing, meditation, and counselling.

- Acupuncture can provide relief from chronic pain, promote relaxation, and improve bowel function.

- Regular exercise will help reduce stress and also stimulate normal contraction of the intestines. Try walking, biking, yoga, and stretching.

- Don't smoke, as nicotine can irritate the stomach lining.

Top Recommended Supplements

Digestive enzymes: Help improve food digestion and reduce bloating and gas. Look for a full-spectrum enzyme that contains proteolytic enzymes, lipase and amylase. Dosage: One or two capsules with each meal.

Flaxseed: Ground flaxseed contains insoluble and insoluble fibres that help reduce constipation and promote bowel regularity. Flaxseed also contains fatty acids that help reduce inflammation. One study found that flaxseed reduced constipation, abdominal pain, and bloating in those with IBS. Dosage: 1–2 tbsp daily. Mix with water or sprinkle on yogurt or cereal.

Peppermint: Contains oils that directly affect the smooth muscle of the digestive tract and reduce spasms. Several studies have found it helpful for reducing pain, bloating, stool frequency, and gas. Take one to three capsules of peppermint oil three times daily, about 15 minutes before meals. Choose a product that is enteric-coated to reduce the risk of heartburn.

Probiotics: Beneficial bacteria are part of normal gut flora and may be depleted in those with IBS. Probiotics aid digestion and several studies have shown reduced symptoms of IBS, such as gas, bloating, and pain. Dosage: one capsule (providing at least 1 billion viable cells), two or three times daily with food. Look for a product that is stable at room temperature with guaranteed potency, such as Kyo-Dophilus.

FLAXSEED FOR IBS

Flaxseed provides a good source of fibre and fatty acids that can improve bowel function and reduce IBS symptoms. In one study, 55 people with chronic constipation caused by IBS received either ground flaxseed or psyllium seed daily for three months. Those taking flaxseed had significantly fewer problems with constipation, abdominal pain, and bloating than those taking psyllium. The flaxseed group had even further improvements in constipation and bloating while continuing their treatment in the three months after the double-blind study ended. The researcher concluded that flaxseed relieved constipation more effectively than psyllium (*Gastroenterology,* 1997: 112; A836).

Complementary Supplements

Evening primrose oil: Contains gamma linolenic acid, a fatty acid that helps reduce inflammation. Preliminary research has shown that it can help reduce pain. Dosage: 1000 mg three times daily.

Melatonin: Plays a role in the regulation of gastrointestinal function and sensation. A few small studies have shown that it can reduce pain and improve sleep in those with IBS. Dosage: 3 mg at bedtime.

Other herbs: Lemon balm, spearmint, ginger root, slippery elm, and turmeric may help reduce some of the symptoms of IBS, although the evidence is preliminary.

FINAL THOUGHTS

To reduce the symptoms of IBS, consider the following:

1. Eat small, frequent meals and eat slowly.
2. Gradually increase fibre intake. Try milled flaxseed.
3. Avoid caffeine, alcohol, carbonated beverages, fatty or spicy foods, and other known food triggers.
4. Reduce stress levels and get regular exercise.
5. Try peppermint oil capsules, probiotics, and digestive enzymes.

Irritable Bowel Syndrome (IBS)

KIDNEY STONES

The kidneys are two bean-shaped organs, about the size of your fist, that are located behind your abdomen on each side of your spine. The main function of the kidneys is to remove excess fluid and wastes from your blood in the form of urine. Kidney stones, known medically as renal lithiasis, occur when minerals and other substances in the urine form crystals inside your kidneys. Over time, these crystals may combine to form a small, hard mass or stone.

Kidney stones have become increasingly common today. It is estimated that 10 percent of North Americans are affected by kidney stones. Poor diet and lack of fluids are the major underlying causes. Crystals can form in the urine when there is a high concentration of substances such as calcium, oxalate, uric acid, and, rarely, cystinem, or phosphate, or a low level of substances that help prevent crystal formation, such as citrate and magnesium. Crystals also may form if your urine becomes too concentrated or is too acidic or too alkaline.

Small kidney stones pass into your bladder without causing any pain or symptoms. However, in some cases, these stones can be large and cause excruciating pain and bleeding in the urine, and even permanent damage. Fortunately, there are a number of medical interventions and natural products that can help eliminate kidney stones, as well as lifestyle measures that can be undertaken to prevent them from occurring.

• •

Roughly 70–80 percent of all kidney stones contain a combination of calcium and oxalate. The actual cause is not always known. Some people have higher levels of calcium in their urine than others, increasing the risk of stone formation. Genetics may play a role. Calcium levels may also be higher in those with cancer, kidney disease, or those taking certain diuretics and thyroid hormones. It was once thought that a diet high in calcium increased your risk for developing kidney stones, but this has been disproven. Oxalates are compounds naturally occurring in some fruits and vegetables, such as rhubarb, spinach, and tomatoes. Eating lots of these foods may increase your risk for stone formation.

• •

SIGNS & SYMPTOMS

- Bloody, cloudy, or foul-smelling urine

- Fever and chills (if there is infection)

- Frequent need to urinate

- Intense pain that may be intermittent and can occur in your lower back or your side (under your ribs); it may radiate to your lower abdomen, groin, and genitals

- Nausea and vomiting

Note: If a large kidney stone is left untreated, it could block the flow of urine, causing pain, bleeding, infection, and the risk of kidney damage. Small kidney stones can partially block the ureters (thin tubes that connect each kidney to the bladder) or the urethra (tube that carries urine out of the body). If left untreated, these stones may also cause recurrent urinary tract infection or kidney damage.

- Climate: Living in hot, dry areas or working in a hot environment increases risk due to increased likelihood of dehydration; kidney stones are also more common during the summer months.
- Dehydration: Not drinking enough fluids, especially water, makes the urine more concentrated.
- Diet: High intake of animal protein and salt and a low intake of calcium and magnesium increases the risk of some types of stones.
- Gender: Men are at greater risk.
- History of kidney stones: If you have had a stone in the past, you're at greater risk; having a family history also increases your risk.
- Imbalance in urinary pH (acid and base balance).
- Lack of activity: Limited activity causes your bones to release more calcium, which can increase the risk of calcium stones.
- Medical conditions: Having kidney disease, gout, chronic urinary tract infections, and hyperparathyroidism
- Medications: Certain diuretics can increase your risk.
- Race: Caucasians are at greater risk.

DOCTOR'S ORDERS

The treatment of kidney stones depends on the type of stone, the underlying cause, and the severity of symptoms. In some cases, a small stone can easily be passed by drinking lots of water (half a gallon to three-quarters of a gallon) and being physically active.

Stones that are too large to pass or causing bleeding, infection, or kidney damage may require treatment by an urologist, a doctor who specializes in the treatment of urinary tract problems. There are various procedures that can break up and remove a kidney stone. Extracorporeal shock wave lithotripsy uses shock waves to break up the stone. Percutaneous nephrolithotomy involves removal of the stone through a small incision in your back using a nephroscope. A stone that is lodged in a ureter can be broken down with ultrasound or laser energy and removed with a small instrument called an ureteroscope.

Depending on the type of stone, there are medications that can be used to change the pH of your urine to prevent and treat the problem.

SHERRY'S NATURAL PRESCRIPTION

Dietary Recommendations

Foods to include:

- Apples, green leafy vegetables, kelp, seeds, legumes, and figs are good sources of magnesium, and a magnesium deficiency can increase the risk of stones.

- Drink lots of water to help flush out your kidneys and prevent dehydration. Add some lemon slices or juice to your water. Lemon contains citric acid, which acidifies the urine and can help assist the passage of calcium oxalate stones.

- Eat lots of vegetables, fruits, and whole grains. Fish, beans, seeds, and poultry provide good sources of protein.

- Oranges, bananas, raisins, avocado, and artichokes contain potassium, which reduces urinary calcium excretion. Boosting intake of potassium has been shown to reduce the risk of stones.

- Pumpkin seeds have been shown in preliminary research to reduce the risk of stone formation.

Foods to avoid:

- Foods high in oxalic acid increase the risk of stone formation, so minimize intake of spinach, rhubarb, beet greens, nuts, chocolate, tea, bran, almonds, peanuts, and strawberries. Other foods contain some oxalic acid, but only these have been found to be a problem.

- Grapefruit juice has been linked to increased risk of kidney stones.

- Studies have shown that a diet high in animal protein increases the risk of stone formation. Animal protein increases the excretion of calcium, causing a buildup of calcium in the urine.

- Reduce sodium intake as a high sodium intake can promote calcium excretion and also lead to dehydration. Limit sodium to 2,000 mg daily. Foods high in sodium include snack foods, deli meats, condiments, and processed foods. Avoid using the salt shaker.

- Sugar has been linked to increased risk of oxalate stones. Limit intake of sweets, candy, and soft drinks. Soft drinks also contain phosphoric acid, which also increases the risk of stones.

Lifestyle Suggestions

- Get regular exercise.

- Acupuncture may help reduce pain and ease the passage of a stone.

- Have a warm bath with mineral salts and add a few drops of lavender or chamomile oil to promote relaxation and ease pain.

Top Recommended Supplements

IP6: Inositol hexaphosphate is a naturally occurring component of plant fibre. Studies have shown that it reduces urinary calcium levels and may reduce the risk of forming a kidney stone. Dosage: 120 mg daily.

Potassium citrate: Helps prevent stone formation by various mechanisms. Citrate binds with calcium in the urine, thereby reducing the amount available to form calcium oxalate stones. It also prevents calcium oxalate crystals from forming into larger stones. Lastly, it makes the urine less acidic, which inhibits the development of both calcium oxalate and uric acid stones. Several studies have demonstrated significant benefits in those at risk of stone formation. Consult your health care provider for individualized dosage recommendations as too much potassium can cause side effects (upset stomach) and interact with medications.

CALCIUM SUPPLEMENTS AND KIDNEY STONES

For years, those with or at risk of calcium oxalate stones were told to avoid calcium-rich foods and supplements. However, recent studies have shown that high-calcium diets actually help prevent stones because dietary calcium binds with oxalates in the gastrointestinal tract so that oxalates can't be absorbed from the intestine and excreted by the kidney to form stones. Calcium supplements seem to have the same protective effect as dietary calcium, but only if they're taken with meals. When taken on an empty stomach, the calcium can't bind with the oxalates in food, thus increasing the risk of stone formation.

Complementary Supplements

Calcium: Helps bind to oxalate and reduce the risk of calcium oxalate stones. Dosage: 500 mg with meals three times daily. Choose calcium citrate as the citrate also has a protective effect.

Magnesium: May help to prevent calcium oxalate stone development. Dosage: 100–200 mg with meals. Choose magnesium oxide or magnesium hydroxide.

Vitamin B6: May help prevent calcium oxalate stones. A deficiency of vitamin B6 increases the amount of oxalate in the urine, and some research has shown that those with a high intake of B6 are at a lower risk of stone formation. Dosage: 50 mg daily as part of a B-complex.

FINAL THOUGHTS

To manage kidney stones and prevent them from occurring, consider the following:

1. Drink plenty of water (half a gallon to three-quarters of a gallon per day) with lemon. This is important for treatment and prevention.
2. Boost intake of potassium- and magnesium-rich foods (oranges, bananas, raisins, apples, and leafy green vegetables).
3. Reduce intake of foods high in oxalic acid, such as rhubarb, spinach, and beet greens.
4. Get regular exercise.
5. For prevention, consider IP6 and potassium citrate supplements.

LICE

For parents of school-aged children, head lice are an inconvenient fact of life. One in 10 Canadian school children get head lice each year.

Head lice are small insects approximately 1–2 mm in length. Head lice bite and consume the blood of their host, causing itching and irritation. An adult louse looks like a small, brown-black, flat-backed beetle. Younger lice, called nymphs, are miniscule and have a spider-like appearance. The eggs or nits are extremely tiny, often shiny or translucent globules found cemented to the hair shaft, usually within 1 in of the scalp. While adult lice and some nymphs may be removed using a fine-toothed or special lice comb, the eggs must be manually removed by pinching them and drawing them off the entire length of the hair strand.

The life cycle of a louse is approximately one month. Only female lice can reproduce. Eggs take up to a week to hatch, and the nymphs a week to become adults, which can then reproduce for the remaining two weeks of their lifespan. Adult females may lay five or more eggs per day. In order to stop the spread of head lice, the adults, nymphs, and nits must all be killed and removed from the hair.

Head lice live only on the scalps of their human hosts (no other area). Off the head, they will die within 48–72 hours unless they find a new host. Head lice have strong legs and claws, which help them cling to the hair during exposure to showers, combs, brushes, and hair dryers. Head lice cannot fly or jump and can pass to others only through direct human contact. They do not infect family pets.

There are many things that can be done to prevent the spread of head lice and to get rid of this problem.

SIGNS & SYMPTOMS

- Persistent scratching of the scalp (especially behind the ears and base of the neck) may indicate lice

- Seeing adult lice or nits (eggs) in the hair, on a brush, or in the tub after a bath or shower

RISK FACTORS

- Head lice are more common in girls likely because girls are more likely to have close contact during play (not because they have longer hair).

- Head-to-head contact (cuddling, hugging, wrestling, etc.)

- Sharing brushes, combs, hats, hooded sweatshirts, head scarves, etc.

DOCTOR'S ORDERS

Most health professionals recommend using an over-the-counter pharmaceutical lice treatment shampoo at the first sign of lice infestation.

Products such as Nix and R & C are commonly used. These shampoos are made with strong chemicals (pesticides) that are designed to kill the lice. None of these products are 100 percent effective in killing the eggs, so a second treatment is often required. Another problem is that lice can be resistant to these pesticides. Use these pesticides only if you or your child have a confirmed case of head lice. Follow the product instructions carefully. Possible side effects of these treatments can include dry scalp, itching, and irritation. They can also trigger asthma and allergies in certain individuals.

NITPICKING

The term "nitpicking," which means "to be critical of inconsequential details," is derived from the process of picking nits out of a person's hair. This is because actual "nitpicking" is a painstaking process of examining each hair strand for a minuscule egg.

SHERRY'S NATURAL PRESCRIPTION

For those concerned about the harsh pesticide chemicals in the pharmaceutical lice treatments, there are various natural products available.

Lifestyle Suggestions

- All school-aged children should be educated about the spread of lice and taught to avoid sharing articles of clothing, combs, and brushes.

- Get into the habit of inspecting school-aged children once a week for lice. Breaking the cycle of lice is significantly easier if it is caught in the early stages when fewer eggs have been laid on the hair follicles.

- Use a natural shampoo and conditioner containing tea tree (if tolerated) or the essential oils of eucalyptus, marjoram, and rosemary to help prevent an outbreak.

- Spray a combination of water and lavender essential oil, which is a natural insect repellant, on the base of the neck and hair each day.

BEATING LICE

Whether you are using a pesticide or natural product to control a lice outbreak, take the following steps:

1. Treat the infected person immediately, according to the product instructions.

2. After treatment, use a lice comb to remove any remaining lice and nymphs. Be patient as this may take up to two hours depending on the length of hair. For children with very fine hair, a lice comb may not be adequate to remove all the eggs. In this case, you can loop a piece of thread through the comb to help pull out the eggs.

3. Examine the scalp of all other members in the household. Treat only those confirmed cases.

4. Strip all bedding in the home and wash in hot water. Dry in a hot dryer for at least 45 minutes.

5. Remove all articles of clothing, including hats, worn in the last week and wash and dry thoroughly.

6. For any items that cannot be washed—such as blankets or pillows or large sleeping bags, quilts, or bulky coats—seal them in garbage bags and place in a cold environment such as garage or basement for at least one week.

7. Inspect the hair daily for at least two weeks to ensure that all nits and lice have been removed; a magnifying glass and bright light may be helpful. Whether you use the pharmaceutical or the natural treatment, the key to success is diligence in removal of all lice and eggs.

Top Recommended Product

LiceBGone: A natural product derived from sugar cane. It contains enzymes that affect the exoskeleton (outer covering) of live lice and also softens the glue that holds the nits to the hair shaft so that they can be easily removed with a nit comb. Studies with schoolchildren have shown a 100 percent success rate. This product is sprayed onto dry hair until saturated. After one hour, the lice and nits are removed with a lice comb and then the hair is rinsed. Most cases require only one application. The product is also effective on scabies. It is available in health food stores and pharmacies, and has been sold worldwide for nine years.

Complementary Treatments

Citronella: A volatile oil extracted from *Cymbopogon nardus* or *Cymbopogon winterianus*. Preliminary research has shown that it can help eliminate lice and prevent recurrence. In this study, a lotion containing 3.7 percent citronella or placebo was sprayed on the hair every morning for six days. After two and four months, those using citronella lotion had fewer cases of head lice.

Resultz: A branded product that contains 50 percent isopropyl myristate (active ingredient) and 50 percent ST-cyclomethicone. It works by dissolving the wax that covers the head lice, dehydrating them and causing them to die. In one preliminary study, 28 out of 29 participants were lice-free after using Resultz. The product is applied to dry hair and left on for 10 minutes, then rinsed away with warm water. The application is repeated seven days later.

Tea tree: Heavily promoted for head lice, but the scientific evidence that it works is lacking. It is said to degrade the bond of the lice to the hair shaft and help dislodge them from the scalp. Regular use may help prevent an outbreak, but there are some concerns with using this on the scalp as it can cause adverse effects (skin rash and irritation). Test a small patch of skin prior to use and consult with your health care provider.

LICE HOME REMEDIES

Various home remedies have been tried over the years to get rid of lice such as applying mayonnaise, petroleum jelly, olive oil, or thick hair gel. Applying these thick products to the hair and scalp and leaving on overnight will theoretically reduce the attachment of lice, but there are no clinical studies supporting the efficacy of these products.

FINAL THOUGHTS

The best way to prevent and to cope with an outbreak of lice is to stay vigilant.

1. Check school-aged children once a week for lice. Use a fine-toothed lice comb.
2. Keep a natural lice treatment product in your medicine cabinet.
3. Use shampoos and conditions containing tea tree oil regularly for prevention.
4. Spray the base of the neck, as well as jackets and knapsacks, with a combination of water and essential oil of lavender.
5. To eliminate a head lice outbreak, consider LiceBGone as a natural remedy.

LOW LIBIDO

Low libido is an absence or deficiency of sexual fantasy and desire for sexual activity. This is also referred to as inhibited sexual desire. It is difficult to define "normal" sexual desire as it varies among individuals, gender, and age. However, surveys have found that approximately 30–40 percent of all adults complain of a low sex drive.

This may be a primary condition (a person never felt much sexual desire) or secondary (a person used to possess sexual desire, but no longer has an interest).

There are many factors that affect one's libido—psychological, physical, medical, and even lifestyle. While this is a sensitive topic for some to discuss, it is an important one because lack of desire for a partner can have troubling consequences for the relationship. As well, studies have found a correlation between sexual desire and overall happiness.

SYMPTOMS

- Loss of interest in or desire for sex

RISK FACTORS

There are many potential causes and risk factors for low libido, including:

- Health conditions: Cushing's syndrome, fatigue, menopause, postpartum depression, diabetes, hysterectomy, and obesity

- Hormonal imbalance: Low thyroid, estrogen, testosterone, or DHEA

- Nutritional deficiency in zinc

- Physical problems: Vaginal dryness, vulvodynia, impotence (ED), and inability to reach climax

- Prescription drugs: Beta-blockers (for blood pressure), birth control pills, antidepressants, tranquilizers, Proscar (for prostate enlargement), Tamoxifen (for breast cancer)

- Psychological issues: Stress, depression, relationship conflict, negative or traumatic sexual experiences

- Use of alcohol or marijuana

Note: Low libido affects more women than men. This could be due to hormonal changes (PMS, child birth, and menopause).

DOCTOR'S ORDERS

Consult with your doctor if you are taking medications or have a condition that could be affecting your libido, as this could be easily remedied by a change in therapy.

There are no specific drugs to treat low libido. However, there are medications that can treat the underlying cause. For example, hormones such as thyroid, estrogen, testosterone, or DHEA can be given to those deficient. For women with low estrogen, testosterone, or progesterone, a compounding pharmacy can prepare a topical cream in an appropriate dosage that is better tolerated than oral pills.

SHERRY'S NATURAL PRESCRIPTION

Dietary Recommendations

Foods to include:

- Eat a healthy, whole foods diet as outlined in Chapter 1.

- Many foods are claimed to enhance libido, but science is lacking in this area. For example, oysters are high in zinc, which raises sperm and testosterone production, yet studies showing that oysters raise libido have not been done.

Foods to avoid:

- Refined carbohydrates, sugar, processed and fast foods, and caffeine can trigger mood swings, irritability, and anxiety.

- Saturated and trans fats (red meat, high-fat dairy, deep-fried and processed foods) can impair blood vessel health.

- Alcohol may reduce inhibitions; however, it can also act as a depressant and negatively affect sexual function.

....

An aphrodisiac is a food, drink, drug, scent, or device that can arouse or increase sexual desire. Named after Aphrodite, the Greek goddess of sexual love and beauty, there is a long list of purported aphrodisiacs, including anchovies, oysters, adrenaline, licorice, chocolate, and Spanish fly. According to the Food and Drug Administration, the reputed sexual effects of aphrodisiacs are based in folklore, not fact. In 1989, the agency declared that there is no scientific proof that any over-the-counter aphrodisiacs work to treat sexual dysfunction.

....

Lifestyle Suggestions

- Exercise: Aerobic activities such as walking and cycling can reduce stress, improve mood, increase energy, and improve circulation (improved blood supply to the pelvic area may help to improve sexual sensation and satisfaction).

- Maintain a healthy body weight.

- Women with vaginal dryness can try a lubricant such as Replens or Astroglide.

- Don't smoke as smoking causes damage to nerves and blood vessels, which can affect sensation.

- Relax—try massage, meditation, yoga, breathing exercises, or a warm bath. Aromatherapy oils known to inspire romance include rose, clary sage, sandalwood, and jasmine.

- Set aside time to be intimate with your partner and work on improving communication.

Top Recommended Supplements

Arginine: An amino acid that is involved in many body processes including hormone secretion and the production of nitrous oxide (substance that relaxes blood vessels). Several studies have found it helpful for improving sexual desire and function in both men and women. It is often combined with other products such as yohimbe, ginkgo biloba and damiana. Dosage: 2–8 grams per day.

Ginkgo biloba: Increases blood flow to the brain and sexual organs (improves sexual sensation); has been shown to alleviate sexual problems caused by antidepressant drugs, such as low libido, arousal, and orgasm. Dosage: 120 mg daily.

Muira puama: Also known as potency wood, clinical studies have found it beneficial for enhancing libido and other aspects of sexual function in both men and women. Dosage: Tincture: 2–4 mL of a 4:1 extract twice daily.

• •

Researchers at the Institute of Sexology in Paris studied the effects of a product containing muira puama and ginkgo biloba in 202 women with low sex drive. Various aspects of their sex life were rated before and after one month of treatment. Significant improvements occurred in the frequency of sexual desires, sexual intercourse, sexual fantasies, satisfaction with sex life, intensity of sexual desires, excitement of fantasies, ability to reach orgasm, and intensity of orgasm. Reported compliance and tolerability were good (*Advances in Therapy*, 2000: 17(5): 255–262).

• •

Complementary Supplements

Zinc: Required for the production of testosterone; levels are depleted by many drugs, including ACE inhibitors, oral contraceptives, and methotrexate. Dosage: 25–50 mg daily.

One double-blind, placebo-controlled study looked at the effects of a combination therapy of **arginine, ginseng, ginkgo, damiana, multivitamins**, and **minerals (ArginMax)** in 77 women with poor sexual function. After four weeks of supplementing, 73.5 percent of those given the supplements reported superior sexual satisfaction scores compared to those given a placebo. Improvements were seen in libido, orgasm, vaginal lubrication, and clitoral sensation (*Journal of Sex and Marital Therapy*, 2001: 27; 541–549). Another double-blind placebo-controlled study using the same product formulation was conducted in 108 women with low sexual desire. After four weeks, both pre- and post-menopausal women who took the ArginMax noted a significant improvement in sexual desire. (*Journal of Sex and Marital Therapy*, 2006: 32(5); 369–378)

Note: Several products, including maca and horny goat weed, are promoted to enhance libido, yet these claims are based on animal studies or traditional use. In order to recommend these products, proper clinical trials need to be done.

Supplements for erectile dysfunction are listed under that condition in this book.

FINAL THOUGHTS

There are many factors that affect one's libido, so it is important to seek help and identify the underlying cause. Here are some general tips to consider:

1. Eat a healthy diet and reduce intake of processed and refined foods and alcohol.
2. Exercise regularly to improve mood and blood flow.
3. Don't smoke.
4. Promote relaxation with massage, meditation, and essential oils.
5. Supplements of arginine, ginkgo biloba and muira puama may help improve several aspects of sexual interest and function.

LUPUS

Lupus is an autoimmune disease, meaning that the immune system produces antibodies that attack the body's own tissues, causing pain and inflammation. It most commonly affects your skin, joints, kidneys, blood cells, heart, and lungs. The underlying cause of lupus is not known, but researchers believe that it results from a combination of factors, including genetics, environment (sunlight), and hormones.

The word "lupus" comes from the Latin word for "wolf" because doctors once thought the classic lupus rash resembled a wolf's face. It appears across the cheeks and bridge of the nose and is actually more of a butterfly-shaped rash. About 50 percent of people with SLE will have this rash.

There are three main types of lupus:

Discoid lupus erythematosus (DLE): A less serious form that causes only skin rash, triggered most often by sun sensitivity.

Drug-induced lupus: Results from the long-term use of certain prescription drugs, such as the antipsychotic chlorpromazine, high blood pressure medications (hydralazine), the tuberculosis drug isoniazid, and the heart medication procainamide. Beta blockers and arthritis and ulcer drugs have also been associated with lupus. Symptoms (joint pain, swelling, fever, and fatigue) usually disappear after the drug is stopped.

Systemic lupus erythematosus (SLE): The most common and most serious form of the disease. This form causes inflammation and pain throughout the body, affecting the joints, muscles, and skin. Infection with a bacteria or virus is a common trigger.

Lupus is a treatable condition. In recent decades, early diagnosis and treatment have greatly improved the life expectancy and quality of life for those with lupus. Proper medical care and lifestyle strategies can help to manage the symptoms and put the disease into remission.

SIGNS & SYMPTOMS

The signs and symptoms vary greatly among individuals. They may appear suddenly or develop slowly, and may be mild or severe. Most people experience intermittent periods of flare-ups and remission. Typical symptoms include:

- Arthritis: Joint pain, particularly in the fingers, hands, wrists, and knees

- Blood vessel inflammation

- Digestive problems: Abdominal pain, weight loss, nausea, and vomiting

- Fatigue and fever

- Hair loss

- Headaches, dizziness, visual problems, and depression

- Heart problems: Inflammation of the sac around the heart (pericarditis), which causes shortness of breath and chest pain

- Kidney damage: Symptoms may include swelling in the legs

- Lung problems: Pleuritis (inflammation of the lining of the lungs)

- Raynaud's phenomenon: Fingers, toes, nose, and ears turn pale and numb when exposed to cold temperatures

- Skin lesions: Small pimples or flat lesions that can become scaly, crusty, or itchy

- Skin rash (affects one in three people with lupus)

- Sun sensitivity (photosensitivity)

- Swollen glands or swelling around the eyes

- Ulcers in the mouth or nose

Without treatment, complications from lupus can be life-threatening. The disease can cause significant damage to the kidneys, heart, central nervous system, and lungs. Lupus also increases the risk of infection because many of the drugs used to treat the disease suppress the immune system.

RISK FACTORS

- Age: Lupus affects people of all ages, but it is most often diagnosed between the ages of 15 and 45.

- Family history

- Gender: Women are approximately nine times as likely to develop the disease as men, with the exception of drug-induced lupus, which affects more men than women; this is likely because men are more likely to develop chronic conditions that require long-term treatment.

- Hormones: In women lupus often comes on during or right after pregnancy, which leads researchers to believe that estrogen may have a role in the disease; many people with lupus have low levels of the hormone DHEA.

- Race: Black Americans are at increased risk of developing lupus; they also tend to develop lupus at a younger age and have more serious complications; Hispanics, Asians, and Native Americans also are at higher risk of developing lupus.

- Recurrent infection with Epstein-Barr virus.

- Sunlight: Exposure can trigger the disease and flare-ups.

ENVIRONMENTAL LINKS

Researchers are continuing to learn about the factors that are thought to play a role, which include stress, certain foods, the artificial sweetener aspartame, silicone breast implants, mercury dental fillings, hair dye, and pesticides and other toxic chemicals. To date, no clear link has been found between these factors and lupus.

DOCTOR'S ORDERS

The treatment of lupus depends on the severity of your symptoms. Drugs can help manage symptoms and prevent complications, but they all carry the risk of side effects and some drugs can actually worsen lupus symptoms, so it is important to discuss the benefits and risks with your doctor. Here are some of the most commonly used drugs for managing lupus:

Anti-malarials, such as hydroxychloroquine (Plaquenil) and chloroquine (Aralen), are commonly used. There is no relationship between lupus and malaria; however, these drugs seem to help with the management of the skin and joint problems and ulcers and may also help reduce flare-ups. Side effects include upset stomach, diarrhea, and visual problems.

Corticosteroids, such as prednisone, help reduce inflammation and suppress the activity of the immune system. They can cause serious side effects, including osteoporosis, weight gain, high blood pressure, diabetes, and increased risk of infection.

Immunosuppressants, such as azathioprine (Imuran) and cyclophosphamide (Cytoxan), suppress the immune system and help to bring lupus into remission. These drugs are used only for severe cases as they cause anemia and increase the risk of infection and cancer.

Non-steroidal anti-inflammatory drugs help to reduce joint and muscle pain and inflammation. Examples include ibuprofen (Motrin), naproxen (Naprosyn), and celecoxib (Celebrex). These drugs can be hard on the stomach and may cause stomach ulcers. Celebrex has also been linked to heart problems.

SHERRY'S NATURAL PRESCRIPTION

Dietary Recommendations

Below are dietary recommendations that can help offset nutrient deficiencies caused by lupus drugs and support overall health.

Foods to include:

- Cranberries and cranberry juice can help prevent urinary tract infections in those at risk.

- Fish contain beneficial fatty acids that help reduce inflammation. Choose wild (not farmed) fish such as salmon, mackerel, herring, and sardines. Flaxseed, wheat germ, olive oil, nuts, and seeds also contain good fatty acids.

- Include rich sources of calcium, especially if you take corticosteroids, which interfere with the absorption of calcium and can lead to osteoporosis. Foods high in calcium include milk and milk products and, to a lesser extent, broccoli, greens (chard, okra, kale, and spinach), sauerkraut, cabbage, rutabaga, and salmon (with bones).

- Tomato products, especially tomato paste, have high levels of lycopene, which may decrease the risk of heart disease and certain kinds of cancer.

- Vegetables, fruits, and whole grains contain essential vitamins and minerals.

- Vitamin C supports immune function and is essential for the health of our skin, heart, and lungs. Foods high in vitamin C include fresh tomatoes, broccoli, citrus fruits, strawberries, cauliflower, cantaloupe, cabbage, and green peppers.

- Vitamin D aids in the absorption of calcium and reduces the risk of osteoporosis. It also supports immune function and may protect against certain cancers. Good food sources include eggs, fish oils, and whole-grain cereals.

Foods to avoid:

- Alcohol hampers immune function; has negative effects on your liver, kidneys, heart, and muscles; and may interact with your medications.

- Caffeine can affect your sleep, so minimize or avoid coffee, soft drinks, and caffeinated teas.

- Saturated fat (meat and dairy) and trans fats (snack and processed foods) can worsen inflammation and also increase the risk of heart disease.

- Soy, alfalfa sprouts, mushrooms, and beans contain compounds that can aggravate lupus symptoms.

- Sugar can hamper immune function and increase the risk of infections. Avoid candy, sweets, soft drinks, and other high-sugar foods.

CORTICOSTEROIDS AND NUTRIENT DEPLETION

Corticosteroid drugs, such as prednisone, can interfere with the absorption of calcium, which can lead to osteoporosis. These drugs can also stop the absorption of nutrients such as vitamins B6, C, and D, zinc, and potassium and interfere with cells' ability to use them. In addition, corticosteroids can cause loss of muscle protein, change the body's ability to handle blood sugar (glucose), and increase fat deposits and sodium retention. In order to counteract the nutrition-zapping effects of corticosteroids, eat a healthful diet and take a daily multivitamin and mineral supplement.

Lifestyle Suggestions

- Get adequate sleep. Lack of sleep can worsen immune function and stress.

- Wear sunscreen with at least SPF 15 on any sun-exposed areas. Make sure the product provides both UVA and UVB protection. Wear sunglasses and a wide-brim hat when outdoors. Limit time outdoors between 11 a.m. and 4 p.m., when the sun's rays are most intense.

- Get regular moderate-intensity exercise, such as walking. Aim for one hour daily. Regular exercise improves heart and lung function, helps reduce stress, and gives you more energy. Weight-bearing activities such as walking also help to improve bone strength and ward off osteoporosis. Start slowly and gradually increase your time and intensity.

- Find ways to manage your stress. Exercise helps, as does meditation, yoga, and deep breathing. Acupuncture can reduce pain and stress.

- Hot paraffin baths, therapeutic mud treatments, baths with Epsom/mineral salts, and sauna can ease pain and inflammation.

- Light massage with botanical oils (camphor, eucalyptus, pine needle, or rosemary) can help reduce pain and promote relaxation.

- Don't smoke. Smoking causes lung and heart damage, and those with lupus are already at risk of these problems.

Top Recommended Supplements

DHEA (dihydroepiandrosterone): A naturally occurring hormone that is used to make all sex hormones (estrogen, progesterone, and testosterone). Levels are often depleted in those with SLE. Several studies have shown that supplementing with DHEA can reduce symptoms and the frequency of flare-ups. In Canada, DHEA is available only by prescription from a doctor and has to be prepared in a compounding pharmacy. Dosage: The typical dosage for SLE is 50–200 mg daily.

Evening primrose, borage, and blackcurrant oils: Contain GLA, a beneficial fatty acid that may help to reduce skin inflammation. Dosage: 1 g three times daily.

Fish oils: Contain omega-3 fatty acids, which have anti-inflammatory effects. Fish oils have been found useful for rheumatoid arthritis, and two studies also found it effective for reducing the symptoms of SLE. In particular it may help reduce joint pain and swelling. Dosage: 6–10 g of EPA plus DHA daily.

Complementary Supplements

Antioxidants: Help to quench free radicals, which are generated by inflammation. Many people with lupus have low levels of antioxidants, such as beta-carotene and vitamin C. These antioxidants are essential for good health, immune function, and disease protection. Antioxidants may play a protective role against lupus complication such as joint, muscle, and organ damage. Vitamin E has been shown in some research to decrease lupus activity. Look for a product that contains vitamins C and E, beta-carotene, and selenium.

Calcium and vitamin D: Essential for bone health. Those with lupus who are taking corticosteroids are at significant risk of osteoporosis. Supplementing with calcium and vitamin D can help protect against bone loss, plus vitamin D levels have been found to be lower in those with lupus and this vitamin is essential for immune function. Some preliminary research suggests that deficiency of vitamin D may play a role in the development of SLE. Dosage: 1,000–1,500 mg calcium plus 800–1,000 IU vitamin D daily. Look for a product that also contains magnesium and zinc, which are also essential for bone health.

Celadrin: A patented blend of fatty acids that reduces inflammation and pain, lubricates joints, and promotes healing. Several clinical studies have shown benefits. Celadrin is available in capsules and cream; there are no known side effects. Dosage: 1,500 mg daily; cream is applied twice daily.

Flaxseed oil: Some preliminary research suggests that flaxseed might help prevent or treat lupus nephritis. Dosage: 1 g three times daily.

Moducare: A combination of beta-sitoserol and beta-sitosterolin, which help to balance/correct immune function. It does not stimulate the immune system. Studies show that Moducare is helpful for reducing pain and inflammation associated with rheumatoid arthritis. While it has not been specifically studied for SLE, it may offer similar benefits. Dosage: One capsule three times daily on a regular basis.

NATURAL PRODUCTS THAT WORSEN SLE

The herb alfalfa contains a substance called L-canavanine, which can worsen SLE or bring it out of remission. People with SLE should avoid alfalfa completely. Echinacea and soy can also aggravate lupus. If you are taking medications to manage your lupus, consult with your doctor and pharmacist before you start taking any new herbal or other supplements to avoid any potential interactions.

FINAL THOUGHTS

To improve the management of lupus, consider the following:

1. Eat a healthful diet of vegetables, fruits, whole grains, fish, nuts, and seeds.
2. Avoid soy, alfalfa, mushrooms, beans, alcohol, saturated and trans fats, sugar, and caffeine.
3. Get adequate sleep and find ways to reduce stress.
4. Wear sunscreen; don't smoke.
5. Consider supplements of fish oils and GLA and talk to your doctor about whether you can benefit from DHEA.

MACULAR DEGENERATION

Macular degeneration is a chronic disease that occurs when the macula of the eye breaks down or is damaged. The macula is part of the retina, which is located on the inside back wall of the eyeball and is responsible for central vision. Deterioration of the macula results in blurring and loss of central vision, which worsens over time, leading to blindness.

This condition most commonly affects older adults so it is referred to as age-related macular degeneration (ARMD). Macular degeneration is the leading cause of visual loss in people over 60 years and the second leading cause of blindness (after cataracts) in those over 65.

There are two forms of macular degeneration:

Dry: This is the most common form and is responsible for 90 percent of cases. It occurs when the macula breaks down and thins over time due to aging, free radical damage, and lack of blood and oxygen to the macula. Cellular debris accumulates under the retina and central vision slowly deteriorates over time.

Wet: Also known as hemorrhagic macular degeneration, this is less common but more serious, as it develops suddenly and progresses fast. It occurs when blood vessels grow under the macula, pushing against it and leaking fluid, which causes scarring of the macula and permanent damage to central vision.

Early detection and intervention can help to reduce visual loss from macular degeneration. It is possible to slow down the progression and prevent macular degeneration with lifestyle measures and supplements.

SIGNS & SYMPTOMS

The symptoms of dry macular degeneration develop slowly over time while symptoms of the wet form develop suddenly and worsen rapidly. They include:

- Increasing need for light to do close work

- Difficulty reading fine print

- Words, straight lines, and signs appear crooked and wavy

- Colours appear less bright

- Blurring and loss of central vision; grey or blank spots in the centre of the visual field

RISK FACTORS

- Age (most common in those over 60)

- Environmental toxin exposure

- Family history

- Gender (women are at greater risk)

- Heart disease (high blood pressure, coronary artery disease, and stroke)

- Light-coloured eyes (green or blue)

- Nutritional deficiencies of vitamins A, C, E, and zinc

- Obesity

- Race (more common among Caucasians)

- Smoking (the most preventable cause of macular degeneration)

- UV light exposure

SMOKING AND MACULAR DEGENERATION

Smoking a pack of cigarettes a day more than doubles a person's risk of developing macular degeneration. Quitting lowers the risk, but they still have a higher risk than non-smokers.

DOCTOR'S ORDERS

There are a few surgical procedures, such as laser therapy, that can be done for wet macular degeneration, with limited success. These procedures prevent further damage to the macula and further visual loss, but they do not restore vision that is lost.

Currently, there are no medical treatments for dry macular degeneration. A number of treatments are being investigated, including photocoagulation. Research has shown that antioxidant supplements can prevent worsening of this condition and further vision loss. This is discussed below.

SHERRY'S NATURAL PRESCRIPTION

Dietary Recommendations

Foods to include:

- Numerous studies have found that those with high intakes of carotenoids have a lower risk of macular degeneration. Carotenoids are antioxidants found in yellow, orange, and dark green fruits and vegetables. They include beta-carotene, lutein, and zeaxanthin. It is thought that these plant pigments protect the macula against UV light damage by dying the macula yellow (acting as natural sunglasses) and by neutralizing free radicals. Carrots are an excellent source of beta-carotene. Kale, collard greens, spinach, and broccoli are the best sources of the lutein and zeaxanthin.

- Vitamins C and E and selenium can protect against macular degeneration. In one study, those with the highest levels of these antioxidants had a 70 percent lower risk of developing macular degeneration. The best food sources of vitamin C are berries (acai, blueberry, and cranberry), tomatoes, peppers, and citrus fruits. Vitamin E is found in nuts, seeds, whole grains, and vegetable oils. Selenium is found in meat, seafood, grains, and vegetables.

- Some research has found that eating fish at least twice a week can reduce the risk of macular degeneration. Fish provide beneficial omega-3 fatty acids that reduce inflammation and also protect against heart disease.

- There is some evidence that a low-glycemic diet can help improve macular degeneration: minimize refined starches (white flour products) and sugar and boost fibre intake. Refer to Appendix B.

Foods to avoid:

- Fast food and processed foods contain hydrogenated fats (trans fats), saturated fats, and chemicals that can generate free radicals and have been associated with an increased risk of macular degeneration.

Lifestyle Suggestions

- Wear sunglasses with UV protection to shield your eyes from the sun's harmful rays. Wide-brim hats are also recommended.

- Don't smoke, and avoid exposure to second-hand smoke, as this is a major risk factor for macular degeneration.

- Use magnifying glasses to read, and have proper light in your home.

- Avoid driving at night and during bad weather conditions.

Top Recommended Supplements

Antioxidants: Research on a specific combination and dosage of antioxidant vitamins and minerals found that they significantly reduced the progression of macular degeneration and the risk of further visual loss. These nutrients are 500 mg of vitamin C, 400 IU of vitamin E, 15 mg of beta-carotene, 80 mg of zinc (as zinc oxide), and 2 mg of copper (as cupric oxide). Look for a product that contains these ingredients and dosages. Note: 80 mg of zinc is a high dose, and can impair copper absorption, which is why it is important to also supplement with copper.

Lutein: Studies have found that supplements can prevent disease progression and improve vision in those with both early and advanced macular degeneration. Dosage: 6–10 mg daily.

Complementary Supplements

Fish oils: Mounting evidence supports the benefits of fish oil for reducing the risk of macular degeneration. Dosage: 1,000–3,000 mg daily.

Ginkgo biloba: Some research has shown that it can improve vision in those with macular degeneration. Dosage: 60 mg three or four times daily.

FINAL THOUGHTS

1. Don't smoke, and avoid second-hand smoke and chemical exposure.
2. Wear sunglasses with UV protection and wide-brim hats outdoors.
3. Eat more eye-healthy foods: carrots, spinach, broccoli, kale, collard greens, berries, peppers, citrus fruits, nuts, seeds, whole grains, and fish.
4. Maintain a healthy body weight.
5. Take antioxidant supplements and lutein.

MEMORY LOSS

Occasionally forgetting a person's name or an appointment is normal, especially when we are busy and multitasking in our daily lives. These temporary lapses in memory are usually not a cause for concern. While many people fear Alzheimer's disease, only a small percentage of people over age 65 develop this disease.

Memory loss can become more frequent and serious with age, but it is not a consequence of aging. In order for our memory to function well, the brain requires healthy nerve cells and adequate supplies of blood, nutrients, and neurotransmitters (chemicals that relay messages between nerve cells). As we age, nerve cells shrink and damage to blood vessels can hamper circulation, which hampers the supply of blood and nutrients to the brain. This reduces the production of neurotransmitters. All of these factors can result in diminished memory. Memory loss can also result from a stroke. In some cases, this type of loss is reversible with therapy.

There are many things that can be done to prevent age-related memory loss, such as physical and mental exercise, supplements, and dietary changes. Even those who are elderly and have experienced memory loss can take steps to improve their memory.

SYMPTOMS

- Difficulty remembering names, places, and events
- Forgetfulness
- Lack of concentration
- Poor mental focus

RISK FACTORS

- Alcohol and illicit drug use can alter chemicals in the brain and impair memory.
- Allergies
- Atherosclerosis, the buildup of plaque in the blood vessels, is a major cause of memory loss.
- Head injury or trauma
- Fatigue: Not getting enough sleep at night can affect your memory the next day.
- High fever
- Hormonal problems such as thyroid deficiency or menopause
- Low blood sugar
- Medications (sleeping pills, antihistamines, antidepressants, pain relievers)
- Poor nutrition: A diet high in fat and refined carbohydrates and low in nutrients; deficiencies of vitamins B1 and B12 can affect memory.
- Stress increases the cortisol level, which impairs memory.

DOCTOR'S ORDERS

It is important to discuss memory loss with your doctor so that tests can be done to rule out Alzheimer's and/or stroke. Even a small stroke can impair memory, and a proper diagnosis and treatment are necessary to prevent further strokes.

There are a few prescription medications that are used to help improve memory:

Hydergine (ergoloid mesylates) is reported to improve oxygen flow to the brain and improve memory and cognitive impairment.

Eldepryl (selegiline) is a drug commonly used for treating Parkinson's disease, but it also offers benefits for memory and brain function. Eldepryl enhances neurotransmitter levels and helps protect neurons.

SMART PILL

A "smart pill" is known medically as a nootropic drug, a substance that enhances cognitive ability, memory, and facilitates learning. The word "nootropic" comes from the Greek words *noos*, which means "mind," and *tropos*, which means "changed" or "turn." One drug that is used for this purpose is hydergine.

SHERRY'S NATURAL PRESCRIPTION

Diet and lifestyle have a major impact on the function of our brain and our memory.

Dietary Recommendations

Foods to include:

- Brewer's yeast, wheat germs, spirulina, and eggs contain B-complex vitamins, which are essential for memory and cognitive function. Wheat germ and whole grains also contain the antioxidant vitamin E, which helps protect against free radical damage.

- Berries, peppers, and citrus fruits contain the antioxidant vitamin C, which helps to protect against free radical damage.

- Cold-water fish (salmon, mackerel, and sardines) contain beneficial omega-3 fatty acids (DHA). Eat wild or organic fish; avoid farmed fish due to toxins.

- Eat a healthy diet that includes plenty of nutrient-rich vegetables and fruits. In particular spinach, broccoli, and leafy greens have been shown to offer cognitive benefits.

Foods to avoid:

- Alcohol destroys brain cells and alters brain chemistry causing memory loss; minimize or avoid completely.

- Diets high in saturated fat can increase the risk of atherosclerosis, which damages blood vessels and reduces blood flow to the brain and heart.

- Refined carbohydrates (white bread/rice/baked goods) and sugary foods can cause blood sugar imbalances that can worsen memory and cognitive function.

- To determine whether food allergies are affecting your memory, refer to Appendix D for information on how to do an elimination diet.

∙∙∙

EAT YOUR VEGGIES

According to a study published in Neurology, eating vegetables may help slow down the rate of cognitive change in adults. Researchers studied 3,718 individuals over age 65. Of the types of vegetables studied, green leafy vegetables had the strongest association with slowing the rate of cognitive decline. Also, reducing foods high in saturated fat and cholesterol and eating fish with beneficial omega-3 fatty acids, such as salmon and tuna, may benefit brain health (*Neurology*, 2006: 67; 1370–1376).

∙∙∙

Lifestyle Suggestions

- Don't smoke, as smoking damages blood vessels and hampers memory.

- Get regular physical exercise to maintain blood flow to the brain.

- Reduce stress with meditation, breathing exercises, and relaxation techniques. Staying calm and relaxed helps improve concentration and memory. Yoga has been found to improve memory and prevent memory loss.

- Keep your brain active. Challenging the brain with such activities as reading, writing, doing puzzles and crosswords, and playing games stimulates brain cells and the connections between the cells, and may help improve memory and prevent cognitive decline.

- Maintain social interactions, which help to reduce stress and improve mental well-being. Studies have found that loneliness increases the risk of late-life dementia.

- Try acupuncture. Some studies have found that stimulating acupuncture points can improve memory.

- Maintain an ideal body weight. Being overweight increases the risk of high blood pressure and cholesterol, factors associated with memory loss.

Top Recommended Supplements

Acetyl-L-carnitine: An amino acid derivative that crosses into the brain and increases the levels of acetycholine, a brain neurotransmitter essential for memory and learning. Studies have found it helpful for improving memory and cognitive function in the elderly. Dosage: 1 g two or three times daily.

Fish oils: Contain omega-3 essential fatty acids, such as DHA (docosahexaenoic acid), which reduce inflammation and promote efficient transmittal of electrical signals between nerve cells. DHA also stabilizes and protects against the natural breakdown of cell membranes, a process that can compromise brain cells and nerves. In addition, DHA seems to improve concentration and may help reverse memory loss. Dosage: 3–9 g daily. Look for a product that provides at least 400 mg EPA and 200 mg DHA per dosage.

Ginkgo biloba: Improves memory and cognitive function by increasing blood flow to the brain. It is particularly helpful for the elderly and those with atherosclerosis or Alzheimer's. Dosage: 120–240 mg daily, standardized to 6 percent terpene lactones and 24 percent flavone glycosides. It may take six weeks to notice benefit.

Phosphatidylserine: An amino acid-like substance that helps support the structure and health of cell membranes. Several studies involving more than 1,000 people have found it effective in improving memory in both college-age people and the elderly. Dosage: 300 mg daily.

Complementary Supplements

Bacopa monnieri: An herb that has been shown to enhance several aspects of mental function. It increases availability of acetylcholine in the brain, which improves memory and cognition. Antioxidant properties help protect brain cells. Dosage: 200–450 mg daily standardized to contain bacosides.

B-vitamins: Play an important role in brain and nerve function. A deficiency of B1, B6, and B12 is more common among the elderly, and can hamper memory and cognitive function. Take a B-complex vitamin daily. Those with poor intestinal health may require monthly injections of vitamin B12.

Melatonin: A hormone that regulates sleep/wake cycles; having adequate sleep is important for cognitive function. Supplements of melatonin have been found to improve sleep quality, mood, and memory. Dosage: 3–6 mg one hour before bed.

Vitamin E: A potent antioxidant that protects the brain from damage due to oxidative stress and inflammation. Studies in older adults have found that those with higher blood levels of vitamin E have better brain function. Supplements at higher dosages have been found to slow cognitive decline. Dosage: 1,000–2,000 IU daily.

FINAL THOUGHTS

To prevent memory loss and improve cognitive function, consider the following:

1. Eat more fish, vegetables, nuts, seeds, and olive oil.
2. Avoid saturated and trans fats.
3. Get regular exercise such as walking.
4. Keep your brain active with games, puzzles, and exercises.
5. Consider supplements of acetyl-L-carnitine, fish oils, ginkgo biloba, and phosphatidylserine.

MENOPAUSE

Menopause is a natural phase in a woman's life that can be thought of as a time of ovarian retirement. At birth women have about one million eggs in their ovaries. At puberty ovulation starts and eggs are released by the ovaries each month for the purpose of conception. As the years go by, the amount of eggs gradually declines until menopause, when the ovaries shut down and stop producing estrogen and progesterone, the two main female sex hormones. Menopause occurs when ovulation ceases and a woman can no longer conceive naturally.

After menopause the adrenal glands, which supply some sex hormones throughout life, become the primary source. Women who have poor adrenal function, which can be caused by chronic stress, poor diet, lack of sleep, or excessive caffeine, are not able to provide adequate hormone amounts, and may have more severe menopausal symptoms. Estrogen can also be produced in the fat cells from androgens. This is why obese women often experience fewer menopausal symptoms.

There are many lifestyle measures and supplements that can promote hormone balance and ease menopausal concerns.

ARE YOU IN MENOPAUSE?

The milestone of menopause is reached when a woman goes one year without a menstrual period. The average age for menopause is about 51 years, but it can occur naturally between ages 40 and 55. The decade or so before menopause is called perimenopause. During this time hormone levels fluctuate and the menstrual cycle becomes erratic, yet you may still be able to conceive.

SIGNS & SYMPTOMS

Menopausal symptoms are caused primarily by an imbalance of the hormones estrogen, progesterone, and/or testosterone. High cortisol levels caused by stress can negatively impact these hormones as well. The severity and duration of symptoms experienced vary due to genetics, ethnicity, cultural factors, and even attitude. They include:

- Fatigue, foggy head, headache, memory loss

- Fluid retention and weight gain

- Hot flashes and night sweats

- Incontinence, bladder infections

- Low libido

- Mood swings, irritability, anxiety, depression

- Vaginal dryness

MENOPAUSE AND WEIGHT GAIN

There are several factors that can contribute to weight gain in menopause. High estrogen levels, as is common in perimenopause or among those with estrogen dominance (low progesterone levels), can impair thyroid function, which may lead to weight gain because the thyroid gland is involved in regulating metabolic rate. Weight gain around the waist could be associated with stress, which elevates cortisol levels and causes fat to accumulate around the midsection. Stress becomes more common as we age.

RISK FACTORS

Menopause usually happens naturally as women age; however, certain medical treatments can bring it on sooner than expected, such as:

- Exposure to radiation or chemotherapy

- Premature ovarian failure: Approximately 1 percent of women experience menopause before age 40; this may be due to genetic factors or autoimmune disease.

- Removal of both ovaries

DOCTOR'S ORDERS

Hormone replacement therapy (HRT) is no longer routinely recommended for women in menopause because several large studies have found that HRT can increase the risk of heart disease, stroke, and breast cancer. The benefits did not outweigh the risks. One study also found that estrogen caused cognitive decline and dementia in older women.

HRT is now used only for women experiencing severe symptoms that cannot be helped by other measures. When it is necessary, it should be used at the lowest dose for the shortest periods of time (less than five years).

Bioidentical hormones are becoming more widely used as a safer alternative to synthetic hormones, while still providing symptom relief. Bioidentical means that the hormones are exactly the same as the ones your body produces. Compounding pharmacists can make customized hormones in various dosages and forms (creams, suppositories, and capsules) to suit your individual needs. Bioidentical hormones are available in compounding pharmacies, by a doctor's prescription.

Women who experience serious emotional symptoms are sometimes prescribed antidepressants and tranquilizers. However, there are many side effects with these drugs, and it is best to try natural methods first.

Bone-building drugs such as bisphosphonates (Didrocal, Fosamax, and Actonel) or selective estrogen receptor modulators (Evista) are often given to women with osteoporosis or those at great risk. It is still important that women taking these drugs get adequate calcium intake and weight-bearing exercise for optimal bone health.

HORMONE CHECK

Many hormones can be unbalanced during menopause (estrogen, progesterone, testosterone, dehydroepiandrosterone, and cortisol) leading to troublesome symptoms. Saliva tests can be done to find out which hormones are causing your symptoms. While blood tests are common, there are some limitations. Most blood tests measure hormones that are bound to protein, not that which is available to the tissues. Saliva tests measure the amount of hormone that has made it into tissue because hormones pass through the salivary gland tissue before getting into saliva. Saliva tests can be ordered by your doctor. See Appendix E for more information.

SHERRY'S NATURAL PRESCRIPTION

The key to managing the symptoms of menopause and enjoying good health during the post-menopausal years is to address factors causing hormone imbalance (especially stress), make dietary and lifestyle adjustments, and use supplements to optimize health.

Dietary Recommendations

Foods to include:

- Vegetables, fruit, whole grains, and legumes provide essential vitamins, minerals, antioxidants, fibre, and compounds that can reduce the risk of cancer and heart disease and improve overall health. In particular, load up on broccoli, Brussels sprouts, cauliflower, and cabbage, as these vegetables contain compounds that help the liver process hormones while reducing the risk of breast cancer.

- Soy foods (tofu, soy milk, soybeans, tempeh, and soy nuts) contain isoflavones (plant-based estrogens), which help minimize menopausal symptoms, offer protection against breast cancer, and improve bone health. Aim for two servings of these foods daily. It may take several weeks to notice benefits.

- Flaxseed is a rich source of fibre, which promotes bowel regularity and reduces the risk of colon and breast cancer and lowers cholesterol. It also contains lignans (another form of phytoestrogen), which may help balance estrogens and reduce menopausal symptoms.

- Fish, nuts, and seeds contain essential fatty acids that are important for heart and skin health.

Foods to avoid:

- Alcohol, caffeine, and spicy foods can worsen hot flashes.

- Saturated fat (red meat) and trans fat (processed, deep-fried, and fast foods) increase the risk of heart disease.

Lifestyle Suggestions

- Address your stress. Stress can make menopausal symptoms more pronounced and affect your adrenal gland function, reducing hormone production. Meditation, yoga, and breathing techniques can help reduce stress. Massage and acupuncture promote relaxation and studies have shown that acupuncture can reduce hot flashes.

- Get regular exercise. Studies have shown that regular exercise reduces the frequency and severity of hot flashes. It also improves mood and sleep, protects against heart disease, and weight-bearing activities strengthen the bones.

- Don't smoke. Smoking can worsen hot flashes and symptoms of anxiety, irritability, and depression.

- Dress in layers so that you can peel off clothing during a hot flash.

- Consider a support group: it may help to share your experience with others.

- Laughter is good medicine. Watch funny movies, go to comedy shows, and spend time with people who make you happy and laugh.

Top Recommended Supplements

Black cohosh: An herb that has been found in many studies to reduce hot flashes, night sweats, insomnia, nervousness, and irritability. Some research has found it beneficial when combined with St. John's wort to relieve symptoms of depression and anxiety. Dosage: 20–40 mg twice daily. Consult with your doctor if you have liver disease.

Calcium and magnesium: Important minerals for bone health; women over 50 years should have 1,200 mg of calcium and 320 mg of magnesium daily, or more if they have osteoporosis. It is difficult to get this amount from diet alone, so supplements are often necessary. Look for a formula that also contains vitamin D and zinc.

Chasteberry: An herb that helps balance hormones and is particularly helpful during perimenopause. Dosage: 160–240 mg daily.

Fish oils: Help to protect against heart disease by lowering blood pressure and cholesterol, reducing atherosclerosis, and protecting against heart attack. Dosage: 1,000–3,000 mg daily.

Complementary Supplements

Ginkgo biloba: An herb that helps improve memory and cognitive function by increasing blood flow to the brain. It is also an antioxidant. Dosage: 40 mg three times daily.

Melatonin: A hormone that regulates our sleep/wake cycles. Supplements help improve sleep quality by reducing the time needed to fall asleep and nighttime wakening. Dosage: 3 to 6 mg one hour before bed. Dosages up to 10 mg have been used in studies.

FINAL THOUGHTS

Menopause is a natural experience in a woman's life that should be welcomed as an important milestone. While there may be certain symptoms, they are usually short-lived and can often be managed effectively with proper lifestyle measures and supplements.

1. Reduce stress: try meditation, yoga, and massage.
2. Get regular exercise and don't smoke.
3. Eat a diet rich in soy foods, fish, whole grains, fruits, and vegetables.
4. Ensure adequate calcium intake or take a mineral supplement for bone health; consider fish oils for heart health.
5. Black cohosh and chasteberry can help relieve symptoms.

METABOLIC SYNDROME

Metabolic syndrome, formerly known as Syndrome X, is a cluster of conditions (abdominal obesity, elevated blood pressure, triglycerides, high cholesterol and/or fasting glucose, and insulin resistance) that occur together, increasing your risk for heart disease, stroke, and diabetes. Having just one of these conditions increases your risk of disease, but having them in combination multiplies the risk significantly. According to research, those who have three features of metabolic syndrome are nearly twice as likely to have a heart attack or stroke and more than three times as likely to develop heart disease as are those with no features.

There is a great deal of research focused on this problem as it is affecting a growing number of our population. According to reports, over half of people over age 60 meet the criteria for metabolic syndrome, and overall about 25 percent of the entire population are classified as having metabolic syndrome.

Researchers believe that insulin resistance is the key underlying cause of this syndrome and responsible for the metabolic changes that occur. Insulin is the hormone secreted by the pancreas that takes glucose from your blood and moves it into the cells to be used for energy. In people with insulin resistance, cells don't respond to insulin and glucose can't enter the cells. The pancreas reacts by releasing more and more insulin to help glucose get into your cells. This results in higher than normal levels of insulin and glucose in the blood. High insulin levels cause triglycerides and cholesterol levels to rise. It also interferes with kidney function, leading to increased blood pressure. High insulin levels also promote fat storage around the belly, leading to abdominal obesity. These combined factors greatly increase one's risk of heart disease, stroke, diabetes, and other conditions.

The key to the management of metabolic syndrome and the prevention of its consequences is to address insulin resistance. This can be done effectively with lifestyle strategies (diet, exercise, and supplements).

SIGNS & SYMPTOMS

- Abdominal obesity (pot-belly)
- Elevated blood pressure
- Elevated fasting glucose
- Elevated triglycerides and low HDL (good) cholesterol
- Insulin resistance

RISK FACTORS

- Age: Metabolic syndrome is more common in those over age 60; it is not caused by aging, but factors that lead to insulin resistance (lack of activity and obesity) are more common among older adults.
- Having high blood pressure, heart disease, or polycystic ovary syndrome
- History of diabetes: Those with a family history of diabetes or women who experienced gestational diabetes are at greater risk.

- Lack of exercise reduces insulin sensitivity.
- Obesity: Having a body mass index (BMI) greater than 25 increases risk.
- Poor diet: Eating a high-glycemic diet (refined starches and sugars)
- Race: Hispanics and Asians are at greater risk.

CHILDREN AND METABOLIC SYNDROME

Metabolic syndrome is a rising problem among youth, due in large part to the obesity epidemic. Over half of children who are obese have the features of metabolic syndrome, putting them at significant risk of heart disease, diabetes, and premature death. Studies have shown, however, that in as little as 12 weeks, regular exercise and healthy eating can facilitate weight loss and improve blood pressure, cholesterol, and blood sugar. (*Pediatrics*, 2006: 118(5); e 1390–8.)

DOCTOR'S ORDERS

The treatment of metabolic syndrome varies depending on which features a person has. Medications can be used to lower blood pressure, cholesterol, triglycerides, and blood sugar and to improve insulin sensitivity. However, lifestyle changes are absolutely critical. As discussed below, a low-glycemic diet and regular activity can greatly improve insulin sensitivity and the other features of this syndrome.

SHERRY'S NATURAL PRESCRIPTION

Dietary Recommendations

Foods to include:

- Add cinnamon to your cereal, oatmeal, or breakfast shakes. Cinnamon contains compounds that work with insulin to reduce blood sugar levels. One study found benefits with just ½ tsp daily.

- Chromium is essential for blood glucose regulation. It is found in brewer's yeast, whole grains (especially wheat germ), onions, and garlic.

- Eat lean animal protein (poultry, fish) and healthy fats (olive oil, nuts, and seeds) with each meal to further slow the rate of digestion.

- For a natural and healthy sugar substitute, try stevia or xylitol.

- Low-glycemic (slow-release), high-fibre carbohydrates such as whole grains (whole-wheat bread, oats, brown rice), vegetables, fruits, and beans help promote better blood sugar control. Refer to Appendix B.

Foods to avoid:

- Alcohol can cause either high or low blood sugar depending on how much you drink and if you are eating while drinking. Limit alcohol intake to no more than two drinks daily.

- Avoid high-fructose corn syrup, which is found in many processed, convenience foods, and drinks including soda and juice cocktails.

- Avoid processed and junk foods as they are high in calories (especially from fat and refined starches) and low in nutritional value.

- High-glycemic (quick-release) carbohydrates such as white bread and baked goods, refined cereals, potatoes, white rice, and sugar (candy, cookies, soda) cause rapid and profound increases in blood sugar and insulin levels.

- Minimize table salt as it can worsen high blood pressure. Try herbal seasonings instead.

- Saturated fat (animal products such as meat and dairy) and trans fats (hydrogenated margarine) and deep-fried foods can worsen blood glucose control.

Lifestyle Suggestions

- Exercise regularly as this can help improve insulin sensitivity and help with weight loss. Aim for 30 minutes to one hour of moderate-intensity activity daily such as brisk walking, cycling, or swimming.

- Incorporate resistance training. Muscle burns more calories than fat and helps your body use blood sugar and insulin more efficiently. Try different strength-training exercises that focus on the core muscle groups: chest, back, shoulders, abdominals, and quadriceps.

- Lose excess weight. Losing even 5–10 percent of excess weight can help improve insulin sensitivity and reduce blood pressure and cholesterol.

- Don't smoke as smoking worsens insulin resistance and also increases the risk of heart disease.

- Manage your stress. Stress triggers the release of hormones that impair insulin sensitivity. Try yoga, meditation, and other relaxation techniques.

Top Recommended Supplements

Since metabolic syndrome is a collection of medical disorders, recommendations vary depending on which factors are present. Below are some general recommendations for supplements that address a few of the features of metabolic syndrome. For specific recommendations on supplements for obesity, diabetes, high blood pressure, and cholesterol, refer to those sections of this book.

Chromium: Improves blood sugar regulation and insulin sensitivity. It may also help lower cholesterol levels. There are several different forms of chromium. Most research has been done with chromium picolinate. Dosage: 400–1,000 mcg daily.

Fish oils: Help improve glucose tolerance, reduce triglycerides and cholesterol levels, and reduce inflammation. Studies have shown that fish oils play an important role in protection against heart disease. Dosage: Look for a product that provides at least 400 mg EPA and 200 mg DHA per dosage, and take three times daily.

Fibre: Helps improve blood glucose control and weight management. Studies involving fibre supplements of psyllium, oat bran, and glucomannan have shown benefits for diabetics. Dosage: Varies with product and formulation. Follow instructions on label and take with plenty of water.

Phase 2: A white kidney bean extract that reduces starch digestion. Studies have shown that it can lower after-meal blood sugar levels, reduce triglycerides, and help promote weight loss. Dosage: 500–1,000 mg before starchy meals.

Complementary Supplements

Alpha lipoic acid: A potent antioxidant that reduces free radical damage. Studies have shown that it can improve blood glucose control and reduce diabetic complications. Dosage: 100–200 mg three times daily.

Vitamin E: Helps improve glucose tolerance and reduce glycosylation (binding of sugar to proteins in blood vessels). It also helps reduce blood clotting, and as an antioxidant, it may help protect against heart disease. Dosage: 400–800 IU daily.

FINAL THOUGHTS

To reduce the risks of metabolic syndrome, consider the following:

1. Eat small, frequent meals with low-glycemic, high-fibre carbohydrates, protein, and healthy fats. Add cinnamon to your diet.
2. Avoid eating fast/processed/refined/deep-fried foods, alcohol, and saturated fat.
3. Reduce your stress with yoga or relaxation techniques.
4. Boost your activity level. Aim for at least 30 minutes of exercise daily.
5. Consider supplements of chromium, fish oil, fibre, and Phase 2.

MIGRAINE HEADACHES

Migraines are intense, severe, pounding headaches that affect about three million Canadians and are more common in women than men. They can be overwhelming and debilitating, affecting one's quality of life.

For some people, migraines are preceded or accompanied by a sensory warning sign, called an aura, such as flashes of light, wavy lines, blind spots, or tingling in your arm or leg. A migraine attack may last for just a few minutes or continue for up to several days. Episodes can vary in frequency from several times in one week to once every few years. Typically, the intensity and frequency of migraines diminishes with age.

It is thought that migraines may be caused by changes in the nervous system (affecting the trigeminal nerve pathway) and by imbalances in neurotransmitters (brain chemicals) such as serotonin, which plays a regulatory role for pain messages going through this pathway. During a migraine, serotonin levels drop. Researchers believe this causes the trigeminal nerve to release substances called neuropeptides, which travel to your brain's outer covering (meninges) and cause blood vessels to become dilated and inflamed. The result is headache pain.

There have been many advances in the treatment of migraines. There are drugs that can abort a headache, and various natural products that can reduce the severity and frequency of headaches. Lifestyle changes, as discussed below, can also be very helpful.

. . . .

Migraines usually begin on one side of the head. (The name "migraine" comes from the Greek word *hemikrania*, meaning "half the skull"). Migraines can also affect the entire head, including the sinus area.

. . . .

SIGNS & SYMPTOMS

- Nausea and/or vomiting

- Sensitivity to light and sound

- Severe pain that can be throbbing or pulsating, usually on one side of the head

- Visual disturbances that precede or accompany the headache

A migraine typically lasts from four to 72 hours, but can go away faster with treatment. Some people experience an aura 15–30 minutes before the headache begins. An aura may cause you to see sparkling flashes of light, changes in vision (wavy lines and blind spots), tingling, and pins and needles sensation in one arm or leg and, less commonly, weakness or difficulty in speaking. Several hours or a day before the headache, some people experience a prodrome—feelings of elation or intense energy, cravings for sweets, thirst, drowsiness, irritability, or depression.

- Age: Migraines are most common between age 20 and 55
- Family history
- Gender: Women are three times more likely to be affected

Migraines can be triggered by the following:

- Bright lights or sun glare
- Change in weather (humidity)
- Foods: Alcohol, aged cheese, eggs, yeast, chocolate, aspartame, caffeine, monosodium glutamate, fermented, pickled or marinated foods
- Hormonal changes: In women, migraines often begin around the onset of menstruation and occur before or during the period; they may get better or worse with pregnancy or menopause; use of birth control pills can worsen migraine headaches.
- Lack of sleep
- Medications: Estrogen, blood pressure drugs, antihistamines, and decongestants
- Smells: Perfumes, flowers, smoke, and strong chemical odours such as gasoline or paint thinner
- Stress: Emotional (worrying) or physical (intense exercise)

DOCTOR'S ORDERS

There are a variety of drugs that can be used to treat and prevent migraines. The choice of treatment depends on the frequency and severity of your headaches and other existing medical problems.

For a mild migraine, a pain reliever such as Tylenol or Motrin may be helpful. For more severe pain, a prescription drug containing codeine may be prescribed. Codeine and other narcotic pain relievers can be addictive and cause constipation and other problems, so they should be used only when absolutely necessary.

The triptans are a class of drugs that has revolutionized migraine treatment. These drugs are rapid acting and effective in relieving the pain, nausea, and sensitivity to light. Examples include sumatriptan (Imitrex), rizatriptan (Maxalt), naratriptan (Amerge), and zolmitriptan (Zomig). Usually a single dose of these drugs will provide relief.

There are drugs that can be taken regularly to prevent migraines (reduce the frequency). They don't work to relieve a migraine that does occur. Examples include beta-blockers (propranolol), calcium channel blockers (verapamil), and antidepressants (amitriptyline and nortriptyline). These drugs can cause serious side effects, so speak to your doctor and pharmacist.

SHERRY'S NATURAL PRESCRIPTION

Dietary Recommendations

Foods to include:

- Drink plenty of water (dehydration can cause a headache).

- Eat small, frequent meals; skipping meals can cause blood sugar levels to drop, which can trigger a migraine.

- Fish (salmon, mackerel, and herring) contain omega-3 fatty acids, which can help prevent migraines.

- Ginger tea may help reduce nausea that accompanies a migraine.

- Whole grains, nuts, seeds, and green leafy vegetables contain good sources of magnesium, which can help prevent migraines.

Foods to avoid:

- Food additives, preservatives, and dyes can trigger migraines (benzoic acid, tartrazine).

- Phenylalanine, which is found in MSG, aspartame, and nitrates (hot dogs and deli meats), is a common trigger.

- Sodium can also be a trigger. Limit foods high in salt (snack foods, deli meats) and avoid using the salt shaker.

- Sugary foods (candy, sweets, and soft drinks) and high-glycemic carbohydrates (white bread/rice and refined grains) can cause rapid blood sugar changes, which may trigger a headache.

- Tyranine—which is found in cheese, chocolate, deli meats, smoked fish, wine, sausage, sour cream, fermented foods, and vinegar—is a common trigger.

Try an elimination diet to determine if food sensitivities are triggering your migraines (see Appendix D).

Lifestyle Suggestions

- Get adequate sleep (seven to nine hours per night).

- Reduce stress with yoga, breathing exercises, meditation, and massage. Biofeedback is also helpful for alleviating migraines. This relaxation technique uses special equipment to teach you how to monitor and control certain physical responses, such as muscle tension.

- Exercise regularly to help prevent migraines. Do moderate-intensity activities (walking, swimming, and cycling) and warm up slowly because sudden, intense activity can trigger a headache.

- Acupuncture can help relieve headache pain.

- During a migraine, go into a dark, quiet room and apply an ice pack wrapped in a towel to the back of your neck and head for 10–15 minutes.

KEEP A DIARY

Keeping a diary of your migraines can help to identify your triggers. Make a note when your headaches start and how long they last. Record what you ate that day and any factors that you feel could have triggered the event, such as stress, reaction to a smell, or light. Also note what you took to relieve your headache. This information will also be helpful to your doctor in determining a treatment strategy.

Top Recommended Supplements

Butterbur: Reduces inflammation and spasms in cerebral blood vessels. Two studies have found that it significantly reduces the frequency of migraine attacks. Dosage: 75–100 mg twice daily with meals. Look for a product standardized to contain at least 15 percent petasins, the main active ingredient.

Feverfew: Several studies have shown that it can reduce the severity and frequency of migraines. It may work by modulating serotonin release and reducing production of inflammatory substances in the brain. Dosage: Take a product that provides 0.25–0.5 mg parthenolide (active component) twice daily. It may take four to six weeks to notice benefits. Avoid if you are allergic to ragweed.

Magnesium: Those with migraines often have low magnesium levels, which can lead to cerebral artery spasm and increase the release of substances that cause pain. Three studies have found that magnesium supplements can significantly reduce migraine attacks. It may be particularly helpful in preventing menstrual migraines. Dosage: 100–200 mg three times daily with meals.

Complementary Supplements

Fish oils: Reduce inflammation and blood vessel spasms and support healthy brain function. Preliminary research shows the supplements can reduce frequency and severity of migraines. Dosage: 1 g three times daily of EPA and DHA.

5-HTP: Increases serotonin levels and has been shown to reduce the frequency and severity of migraines. Dosage: 200–300 mg twice daily.

Vitamin B2 (riboflavin): Shown to reduce the frequency and severity of migraine headaches. Dosage: 400 mg daily; take along with a B-complex vitamin.

FINAL THOUGHTS

To manage migraines and help prevent them, consider the following:

1. Eat small, frequent meals and include more whole grains, nuts, seeds, and fish in your diet. Drink lots of fluids. Try ginger tea to relieve nausea.
2. Get adequate sleep, exercise regularly, and reduce your stress.
3. Keep a diary of your migraines to identify and avoid your triggers.
4. When suffering with a migraine, use cold packs on the head and neck, rest in a dark room, and use medications only if necessary.
5. Try butterbur or feverfew and magnesium for prevention.

MULTIPLE SCLEROSIS (MS)

Multiple sclerosis (MS) is a chronic, often disabling disease that affects your central nervous system (the brain and spinal cord). It is generally believed that MS is an autoimmune disease; the body mistakenly directs antibodies and white blood cells against proteins in the myelin sheath, a fatty substance that insulates nerve fibres in your brain and spinal cord. This results in inflammation and injury to the sheath and ultimately to the nerves that it surrounds. This results in multiple areas of scarring (sclerosis). Over time this damage can slow or block the nerve signals that control muscle coordination, strength, sensation, and vision, causing fatigue, numbness, loss of balance, impaired vision, and disability.

The actual cause for this autoimmune reaction is not known. It is thought that several factors may be involved, such as genetic predisposition, environment, and exposure to a viral infection. Many researchers believe that MS is related to a protein that mimics the myelin protein, which may be introduced into the body by a virus. Other researchers believe that the immune system overreacts toward myelin proteins in people with MS, which leads to an abnormal tendency to develop autoimmune disease. It is known that lifestyle factors, such as stress and poor nutrition, can exacerbate symptoms. Exposure to environmental toxins (pesticides, heavy metals, and chemicals) can bring on symptoms and cause damage to myelin and DNA. Food allergies can worsen symptoms in some people.

MS occurs in four main patterns:

Primary progressive: People with this form experience a gradual decline in function without periods of remission. This form is not as common, and it often strikes after age 40.

Progressive relapsing: This is primary progressive MS with the addition of sudden episodes of new symptoms or worsened existing ones. This form is rare.

Relapsing remitting: About 70 percent of people with MS have this form, which is characterized by periods of sudden flare-ups followed by periods of near-normal health (remission) that can last for months or years.

Secondary progressive: More than half the people with relapsing remitting MS eventually enter a stage of continuous deterioration referred to as secondary progressive MS.

Canada has one of the highest rates of MS in the world. An estimated 55,000–75,000 Canadians have the disease. MS can affect anyone, at any age, although it is most commonly diagnosed between the ages of 15 and 40.

Great progress has been made over the years in our understanding of MS. Today, people with MS can live healthy, productive lives. There are medications, dietary approaches, and supplements that can help reduce symptoms and promote remission.

MS: FACTS OF INTEREST

MS was first identified and described by a French neurologist, Dr. Jean-Martin Charcot, in 1868. According to the Multiple Sclerosis Society of Canada, Canadians have one of the highest rates of MS in the world and MS is the most common neurological disease affecting young adults in Canada. Every day, three more people in Canada are diagnosed with MS.

SIGNS & SYMPTOMS

Signs and symptoms of MS vary widely, depending on the location of affected nerve fibres, and may include:

- Bladder or bowel incontinence
- Blurred vision, visual loss, and eye pain
- Constipation
- Dizziness
- Electric-shock sensations that occur with certain head movements
- Extreme fatigue
- Forgetfulness, lack of concentration
- Loss of balance and coordination
- Muscle stiffness or spasticity
- Numbness or weakness in one or more limbs
- Paralysis
- Slurred speech
- Tingling or pain
- Tremor

RISK FACTORS

- Dietary factors: Deficiency of vitamin D, a diet high in animal fat, food allergies, and digestive problems
- Environmental toxins: Exposure to organic solvents, heavy metals (mercury), pesticides, and X-rays
- Ethnicity: MS is more common in Caucasian people of northern European origin, especially those of Scottish descent; it is extremely rare among Asians, Africans, and Native Americans.
- Exposure to a virus, in particular Human Herpes Virus Type 6, Varicella Zoster, and retroviruses
- Gender: Women are three times as likely as men to get MS.

- Genetics: Represent a small risk; if one of your parents has MS, the risk of you developing it over a lifetime is less than 5 percent; researchers suspect that the tendency to develop MS is inherited, but the disease manifests only when environmental triggers are present

- Geographical location: Rates of MS are about 10 times greater in higher latitudes; it is most common in Europe, Canada, the northern United States, and southeastern Australia; researchers suspect a connection between low levels of sunshine and vitamin D deficiency, which is common in MS.

- Smoking: Smokers are nearly twice as likely to develop multiple sclerosis as people who have never smoked.

COW'S MILK AND MULTIPLE SCLEROSIS

There is evidence that infants fed only cow's milk during infancy may have a higher risk of MS later in life. Studies have also shown that populations that drink cow's milk have a greater prevalence of MS. Whole milk contains a high amount of saturated fat, which has been shown to worsen or trigger MS symptoms. However, researchers believe that the problem with milk extends beyond the fat. One of the proteins in milk mimics a particular protein affiliated with human myelin. This milk protein could elicit an autoimmune response to myelin, triggering an MS episode. This has been demonstrated in animal studies.

DOCTOR'S ORDERS

If you have a relapsing form of the disease, depending on the severity and frequency of your attacks, your doctor may recommend a disease-modifying medication. These drugs are classed as "partially effective" in reducing relapses and worsening of the disease. They cannot be taken if you're pregnant or may become pregnant. Examples include:

Beta interferons: Interferon beta-1b (Betaseron) and interferon beta-1a (Avonex, Rebif) are genetically engineered copies of proteins that occur naturally in your body. They are taken by injection and help fight viral infection and regulate your immune system. These drugs reduce but don't eliminate flare-ups, they don't reverse damage, and they haven't been proven to significantly alter long-term development of permanent disability. Some people develop antibodies to beta interferons, which may make them less effective. Other people can't tolerate the side effects (flu-like symptoms).

Glatiramer (Copaxone): This drug is an alternative to beta interferons for those with relapsing remitting MS. Glatiramer is thought to work by blocking your immune system's attack on myelin. It is injected once daily. Side effects may include flushing, shortness of breath after injection, bacterial infection, lymphadenopathy, edema, weight gain, and nausea.

SHERRY'S NATURAL PRESCRIPTION

As with many chronic diseases, diet and lifestyle changes, dietary supplementation, and moderate physical exercise all contribute to better quality of life with MS.

Dietary Recommendations

Foods to include:

- Drink plenty of water.

- Drinking cranberry juice can help protect against urinary tract infections.

- Eat fresh, whole, unprocessed foods; choose organic as much as possible to avoid ingestion of pesticides and harmful chemicals.

- Eat lots of fruits, vegetables, and whole grains. These foods are rich in nutrients that can help offset deficiencies and are also high in fibre, which helps to prevent constipation.

- Ensure adequate protein intake. Weight loss is a common concern for many people with MS. Protein is essential to support healthy muscles. Choose beans, legumes, nuts, seeds, fish, and lean poultry.

- Fish contains beneficial omega-3 fatty acids, which support proper nerve function and also reduce inflammation. Choose wild (not farmed) cold-water fish such as salmon, cod, herring, and mackerel.

- Yogurt contains beneficial bacteria that aid digestion and improve intestinal flora.

SATURATED FAT AND MS: THE SWANK DIET

There is some evidence that changing the type and amount of fat in the diet might alter the course of MS. A survey of people in 36 countries found that people with MS who ate foods high in polyunsaturated and monounsaturated fatty acids were likely to live longer than those who ate more saturated fats (*American Journal of Epidemiology*, 1995: 142; 733–737).

In another survey, researchers gathered information from nearly 400 people over three years. They found that people who ate more fish were less likely to develop MS, while those who ate pork, hot dogs, and other foods high in animal (saturated) fats were at greater risk. Saturated fats trigger inflammation and alter immune function while polyunsaturated fats (essential fatty acids) reduce inflammation (*International Journal of Epidemiology*, 1998: 5; 845–852).

Based on observations from population studies linking diets lower in saturated fat to lower rates of MS, Dr. R.L. Swank, MD, a professor of neurology at University of Oregon Medical School, developed a special low-fat diet and tested it in 150 MS patients. This program, now called the Swank diet, involved significantly reducing hydrogenated oils, peanut butter, and animal fat (meat and dairy). Cod liver oil (5 g per day) and linoleic acid (an essential fatty acid) from vegetable oil was allowed. After 34 years, the mortality rate among people consuming an average of 17 g of saturated fat per day was only 31 percent, compared with 79 percent among those who consumed a higher average of 25 g of saturated fat per day. People who began to follow the low-fat diet early in the disease did better than those who changed their eating habits after the disease had progressed (*Nutrition*, 1991: 7; 368–376).

Foods to avoid:

- Consider an elimination diet to detect and avoid potential allergens. See Appendix D.

- Saturated fats can worsen the disease progression. Trans fats are also detrimental to health. Minimize meat, dairy, and deep-fried and processed foods.

- Sugar can hamper immune function, increasing the susceptibility to infection. Limit sweets, candy, and soft drinks.

Lifestyle Suggestions

- Manage your stress levels. Stress can trigger a flare-up. Try yoga, tai chi, meditation, and breathing exercises. Massage and acupuncture can help promote relaxation.

- Get adequate rest to allow your body to recuperate and to improve your ability to handle stress.

- Don't smoke, as smoking contributes to the progression of the disease. It is thought that nitrous oxide, a chemical present in cigarette smoke, may hasten degeneration of nerve fibres. Chemicals in cigarette smoke could also damage the cells that create myelin, a protective coating for neurons, or may predispose smokers to autoimmune responses.

- Get regular exercise, which can help improve strength, flexibility, balance, and coordination. It also helps to relieve stress. Swimming is a good activity for those with MS who are sensitive to heat. Regular exercise can reduce the risk of certain complications, such as bladder and bowel dysfunction, osteoporosis, permanent muscle contractions, ulcerations of the skin, or abnormal blood clotting.

- Avoid extreme heat, which can cause muscle weakness and worsen symptoms in some people with MS.

- Avoid exposure to pesticides, heavy metals (mercury, lead), and other chemicals.

- Consider having mercury dental amalgams removed and replaced with mercury-free material. Several reports have linked mercury-containing amalgams to an increased risk of MS and worsening of symptoms in those with the disease.

- Consider hyperbaric oxygen therapy, which involves exposure to oxygen at higher pressures in multiple sessions. Some reports have shown that treatments weekly or every other week over a period of several years can reduce disease progression.

Top Recommended Supplements

Fish oils: Reduce inflammation and support healthy nerve function. Research found benefits from using a dosage of 20 g daily, which is a very high dose. Consult with your health care provider for guidance.

GLA: An essential fatty acid available in primrose, borage, and blackcurrant oil. It helps reduce inflammation, and preliminary studies have shown that it can reduce symptoms and improve peripheral blood flow and hand-grip strength. Dosage: 500 mg three times daily.

Vitamin B12: Essential for supporting myelin formation; deficiency is common in MS and a lack of B12 can cause neurological problems. B12 has been used for decades for MS to alleviate symptoms and boost energy levels. Dosage: 1 mL by injection (from your health care provider) monthly. Sublingual B12 tablets are an alternative. Dosage: 5–40 mg of B12 daily in the form of sublingual methylcobalamin.

Vitamin D: Aside from its benefits for bone health, vitamin D has immune-modulating activity. Most people with MS are deficient in vitamin D, and studies have shown that low levels of vitamin D increase the risk of MS. As well, research suggests that vitamin D may help those who already have MS. Dosage: 1,000 IU daily.

•••

AVOID IMMUNE BOOSTERS WITH MS

Immune-boosting herbs can worsen MS as they enhance auto-antibody production responsible for demyelinating nerve fibres. Avoid taking echinacea, Asian ginseng, licorice, and other immune-boosting herbs.

•••

Complementary Supplements

Antioxidants: People with MS tend to have lower levels of key antioxidants that are necessary to reduce oxidative stress. Free radicals may contribute to the progression of MS. Supplemental antioxidants support cellular antioxidant defences by scavenging free radicals. Look for a formula that contains vitamins C and E, coenzyme Q10, lipoic acid, beta-carotene, and selenium. Dosage: Take daily.

Digestive enzymes: Many people with MS have poor digestion and inadequate digestive enzyme secretion. Supplements can help improve digestion and gut function. Dosage: Take a broad spectrum enzyme before each meal.

Phosphatidylcholine: Necessary for optimal brain and nerve function. It helps protect the myelin sheath and also increases acetylcholine, which is important for muscle function. Dosage: 500 mg twice daily.

Probiotics: Beneficial bacteria that promote healthy GI flora. Some people with MS have reduced levels of beneficial bacteria and Candida overgrowth. Dosage: Take 1–3 capsules daily with meals.

Threonine: A naturally occurring amino acid that might help reduce the muscle spasticity that often occurs with MS. Two studies have demonstrated positive effects. Dosage: 6 g daily.

FINAL THOUGHTS

To improve the management of MS, consider the following:

1. Eat a healthful diet with fruits, vegetables, whole grains, fish, and yogurt.
2. Avoid or minimize saturated fat, trans fats, and sugar.
3. Reduce stress, get adequate sleep, and regular exercise.
4. Don't smoke and avoid extreme heat exposure.
5. Consider supplements of fish oils, GLA, vitamin B12, and vitamin D.

OBESITY

Obesity has become one of the greatest health threats facing Canadians, as it is linked to many serious diseases that result in premature death. Over two-thirds of adults are overweight and nearly one-quarter obese. Children, and adolescents are becoming increasingly overweight and obese, resulting in diseases and a predicted shortened life expectancy.

There are several methods used to determine whether a person is overweight or obese. The most commonly used method is the body mass index (BMI), which compares your height and weight to a standard. To calculate your BMI, take your weight in kilograms and divide that by your height in metres squared (Kg/m2).

A BMI between 18.9 and 24.9 is considered normal, a BMI between 25 and 29.9 is classified as overweight and a BMI greater than 30 indicates obesity. Studies have shown that the greater the BMI, the greater the risk of developing health problems, such as heart disease and diabetes. A drawback of this method is that it does not look at body composition (amount of fat), which is an important determinant of disease risk. To determine body fat percentage, refer to Appendix A.

Men with greater than 25 percent, and women with more than 30 percent, body fat are considered obese and at significant risk of developing health problems. Recommended ranges of body fat are 15–25 percent for women and 10–20 percent for men.

Numerous studies have found that those who maintain a lean body live longer, suffer less disease, and enjoy a better quality of life. If you are overweight or obese, it is important to know that even small losses can improve your health. Studies have shown that losing 10–15 percent of excess weight can reduce blood pressure, blood sugar, cholesterol, and triglycerides.

APPLES VS. PEARS: WHERE'S YOUR FAT?

An "apple"-shaped body (potbelly) is associated with more health risks compared to a "pear"-shaped body (larger hips and thighs). These risks include: type 2 diabetes, high cholesterol and blood pressure, coronary heart disease, stroke, and early death. Men with a waist circumference greater than 40 inches (102 cm) and women greater than 35 inches (89 cm) have a substantially increased risk of developing these diseases. Abdominal obesity is influenced by a number of factors, including genetics and lifestyle choices. Stress and eating a high-glycemic diet (refined carbohydrates) promote belly fat storage. Increased physical activity, not smoking, following a low-glycemic diet, and using unsaturated fat over saturated fat have been shown to reduce abdominal obesity.

SIGNS & SYMPTOMS

- Fatigue and lethargy
- Increased body fat
- Shortness of breath

Note: Those carrying excess weight are at increased risk of developing heart disease, cancer, diabetes, and the complications that come with these diseases. Excess weight also increases one's risk of breathing disorders, gall bladder disease, sexual dysfunction, osteoarthritis, and stroke. The emotional consequences—low self-esteem, depression, and anxiety—can be just as serious.

RISK FACTORS

- Excess calorie intake; poor dietary choices
- Genetics
- Hormonal imbalances (high insulin; low thyroid, testosterone, DHEA, or growth hormone)
- Lack of physical activity
- Lack of sleep (increases appetite and promotes food cravings)
- Low metabolic rate (rate at which calories are burned at rest)
- Medications (antidepressants and hormones)
- Stress (causes hormonal alterations that increase appetite and reduce metabolism)

DOCTOR'S ORDERS

Lifestyle changes should be the first approach to a weight-loss program. In cases where this isn't enough, your doctor may prescribe a drug to help promote weight loss. Sibutramine is an appetite suppressant. Side effects include high blood pressure, irregular heartbeat, seizures, nervousness, anxiety, tremors, and insomnia. Orlistat is a fat blocker that reduces absorption of fat from meals. This product may cause loose stools, fecal incontinence, abdominal cramps, and nausea.

If a hormonal disorder (such as low thyroid) is suspected, you may be referred to an endocrinologist.

For individuals who are extremely obese and at risk of serious health consequences, and where lifestyle changes or drugs have not helped, a surgical procedure may be done to reduce the size of the stomach.

SHERRY'S NATURAL PRESCRIPTION

Dietary Recommendations

Avoid fad diets. There is no good evidence supporting safety and efficacy, and some can be dangerous. For example, the once popular low-carb diets lead to nutrient deficiencies, constipation, depression, and bad breath.

A detoxification program, such as a juice cleanse, can eliminate stored toxins and help the body recover from addictions, such as sugar. This should be done only for a few days and under the supervision of a health professional because drastically reducing calorie intake can lead to nutrient deficiencies, muscle wasting, fatigue, and a reduced metabolism. Refer to Appendix C for more information.

Foods to include:

- Quality proteins, such as lean meat, poultry, fish, beans, soy products, nuts, and seeds are essential for building and maintaining muscle mass, which drives our metabolism. The recommended amount of protein is based on body weight and activity level. For the average person, a daily intake of 0.8 to 1 g per kilogram, or 0.5 g per pound of body weight is adequate. Body-builders and those involved in intense exercise require more protein.

- Nutrient-dense, low-glycemic carbohydrates such as fresh fruits, vegetables, legumes (beans, peas, and lentils) and whole grains (multigrain breads, brown rice/pasta, oats, and flaxseed) are high in fibre, which fills us up and aids digestion and elimination. Fibre also balances blood sugar and insulin levels, which is important in regulating appetite and energy levels. Aim for five to 10 servings of fruits, vegetables, and legumes and two servings of grains daily. Refer to Appendix B for more information on the glycemic index.

- Healthy fats such as those found in cold-water fish, olive oil, nuts, and seeds provide us with essential fatty acids (healthy fats), which are essential for health and disease prevention.

. . . .

HEALTH TIP

Eat five times daily: three small meals and two snacks between meals. This will help keep metabolism and energy levels high. Do not skip meals as this can increase appetite, reduce metabolism, and lead to binge eating.

. . . .

Foods to avoid:

- Processed and fast foods, candy, cookies, and sweets are high in sugar and fat calories and low in nutritional value.

- Limit refined grains (white bread/pasta/rice) as these foods are broken down quickly into sugar, causing fluctuations in blood sugar and insulin levels, which can increase appetite and promote fat storage.

- Avoid saturated and hydrogenated fats, which are high in calories, promote weight gain, and are linked to heart disease and cancer.

- Reduce alcohol intake as these drinks are high in empty calories.

- Cut down on salt as using the salt-shaker and eating salty snack foods and processed foods can cause fluid retention.

Lifestyle Suggestions

- Boost your activity level: Regular physical activity is essential to achieving a healthy body weight. Aim for 30 minutes to one hour of moderate-intensity activity daily. Do a combination of:

  - Cardiovascular activities such as walking, cycling, and swimming, which promote fat loss by burning calories and stored fat.

  - Resistance activities (working out with weights, exercise bands/tubes, or machines) help to build lean muscle mass, which will elevate your metabolic rate so that you burn more calories.

  - Stretching promotes flexibility and relaxation, and reduces injuries. Spend at least five minutes stretching your muscles after a workout.

- Reduce stress, which can trigger appetite and food cravings and increases the production of cortisol, a hormone that promotes fat storage around the abdomen.

- Get adequate sleep as lack of sleep increases production of the hormone ghrelin, which stimulates appetite and can also reduce production of growth hormone, an important regulator of our metabolism.

- Counselling or support groups: If you find that your eating habits are tied to your emotions, you may benefit from counselling or a support group.

Top Recommended Supplements

Conjugated linoleic acid (CLA): A fatty acid that stimulates the breakdown of stored fat, reduces the number of existing fat cells, and prevents fat storage. Dosage: 3–4 g daily; may cause oily skin and loose stool, but no serious side effects.

Hydroxycitric acid (HCA): A compound derived from the fruit Garcinia cambogia, which supports weight loss by reducing appetite, enhancing the breakdown of fat, and inhibiting fat storage. Dosage: 2,800 mg per day; no known side effects.

Phase 2: A white kidney bean extract that promotes weight loss by neutralizing starch from the diet. Foods high in starch include bread, pasta, potatoes, and rice. Phase 2 inhibits the enzyme alpha-amylase, which breaks down starches into sugar. Studies show that it reduces the amount of sugar absorbed from starchy meals, lowers after-meal blood sugar levels, and promotes fat loss. Dosage: 1,000–1,500 mg before starchy meals; no known side effects.

Complementary Supplements

Fibre supplements: Help reduce appetite and cravings, improve blood sugar balance, and promote weight loss. Follow label directions

Green tea: Promotes weight loss by increasing thermogenesis (the rate of calorie burning) due to an interaction between antioxidants (EGCG) and caffeine. There are no serious side effects; however, high amounts of caffeine may cause restlessness, insomnia, and increased heart rate in some individuals. Supplements vary in potency so check labels for dosage.

Suntheanine: An amino acid present in green tea that may help with weight loss by controlling appetite, cravings, and stress-related eating. There are no known side effects or drug interactions. Dosage: 50–200 mg daily.

FINAL THOUGHTS

If you have decided to lose weight, set reasonable goals, make small, gradual changes to your lifestyle, and be patient as it takes time to lose weight, but the rewards are worthwhile.

Here are the key points to keep in mind:

1. Know your risk—check your BMI and body fat percentage.
2. Develop a regular exercise program, including cardiovascular and resistance activities and stretching.
3. Eat small, frequent meals with quality proteins, high-fibre carbohydrates, and good fats.
4. Get adequate sleep and reduce stress.
5. Consider supportive supplements: CLA, Phase 2, and HCA.

OSTEOARTHRITIS

Osteoarthritis (OA), also known as degenerative joint disease, is the most common form of arthritis, affecting 3 million (one in 10) Canadians.

The disease is caused by wear and tear on the joints and deterioration of joint cartilage, which is a gel-like material that covers and protects the ends of bones. As the cartilage breaks down, we lose the cushion that it provides between our bones. As a result, the bones start to rub against each other, causing a grinding or clicking of the joints, bone damage, inflammation, and pain. As the disease progresses, the pain can become severe and affect one's mobility and quality of life.

SIGNS & SYMPTOMS

The disease can affect any joint, but it is most common in weight-bearing joints such as the knees, hips, ankles, fingers, neck, and spine, and it causes:

- Grinding or clicking in the joints

- Growths (spurs)

- Joint stiffness and pain in the morning or after exercise

- Pain

- Red, warm, swollen joints

- Reduced mobility

In some people, the symptoms remain mild or even go away at times. In others the condition progresses as the joint deteriorates and inflammation sets in. Cold weather and humidity can worsen the symptoms.

RISK FACTORS

- Age: It is more common in those over 45, but can occur at any age

- Family history: Inheriting abnormal joint or cartilage structure

- Obesity: Excess weight puts stress on joints, especially hips and knees

- Injury: Joint damage due to an accident, sports, or occupation (i.e., carpet laying)

- Having another forms of arthritis, such as rheumatoid

DOCTOR'S ORDERS

There are various drugs that doctors use to manage the symptoms of OA, including: analgesics, such as Tylenol, help reduce pain but not inflammation. Use of high doses over a long time can cause liver damage. Codeine is a narcotic used for severe pain. Side effects include drowsiness, constipation, and addiction.

Non-steroidal anti-inflammatory drugs (NSAIDs), such as ibuprofen, naproxen, and indomethacin, help reduce pain and inflammation. They do not prevent joint damage, and can actually accelerate cartilage breakdown. There are numerous serious side effects, including stomach ulcers and bleeding, diarrhea, stomach pain, kidney and liver problems, and worsening of heart failure.

Corticosteroids, such as cortisone, are injected into the joint to relieve severe inflammation. Prednisone is taken orally. These drugs are used only for severe cases, and for the short term because they can damage cartilage and remove minerals from the bone, further weakening the joint.

Viscosupplementation involves a clear gel-like substance that is injected into the joint to lubricate the cartilage, which helps to reduce pain and improve mobility.

Arthroscopic procedures to remove loose bone fragments or a joint replacement (with a plastic, ceramic, or metal joint) may be done for severe cases.

SHERRY'S NATURAL PRESCRIPTION

Dietary Recommendations

Foods to include:

- Asparagus, cabbage, garlic, and onions contain sulphur, which is beneficial for the joints.
- Cold-water fish, olive oil, flaxseed, and hemp are rich in essential fatty acids and can help reduce inflammation.
- Green tea: Several studies have found that the antioxidants in green tea (catechins) can reduce chronic joint inflammation and slow cartilage breakdown.
- Pineapple contains the enzyme bromelain, which can help reduce inflammation.

Foods to avoid:

- Nightshade vegetables (potatoes, tomatoes, peppers, eggplant) contain a substance called solanine, which can trigger pain and inflammation; preliminary studies have found benefits in avoiding these foods.
- Processed, fast, and deep-fried foods contain trans-fatty acids, which trigger inflammation.
- Red meat, milk, cheese, and deep-fried foods contain saturated fat, which triggers inflammation.
- Sugar, refined carbohydrates, alcohol, and caffeine

Lifestyle Suggestions

- Acupuncture offers short-term benefits for pain relief.
- Apply ice or heat packs to the affected joints. Heat relaxes aching muscles and reduces joint pain. Cold helps to reduce inflammation and pain.
- Assistive devices, such as canes, walkers, and joint supports, reduce joint strain.
- Avoid activities that put excess strain on the joints (running, jumping, kneeling, or standing for long periods). Take a load off and rest when doing heavy or repeated tasks such as gardening, shovelling snow, or doing housework.
- Exercise helps reduce pain and prevent further joint damage; strengthens muscles and bones, which will help improve mobility and function; and also helps with weight management. Do a combination of strength-training exercises (work with light weights and machines), low-impact cardiovascular activities (swimming, walking), and stretching. Be sure to wear proper, cushioning shoes.

- Light massage with botanical oils (camphor, eucalyptus, pine needle, or rosemary) can help reduce pain and promote relaxation.

Top Recommended Supplements

Celadrin: A blend of fatty acids that reduces inflammation and pain, lubricates joints, and promotes healing. Several clinical studies have shown benefits. Celadrin is available in capsules and cream; there are no side effects. Dosage: 1,500 mg daily; apply cream twice daily.

Chondroitin: A component of human cartilage, bone, and tendon. It enhances the shock-absorbing properties of collagen and blocks enzymes that break down cartilage. Studies have shown that it reduces pain and inflammation, improves joint function, and reduces the need for NSAIDs. It may also slow the progression of OA. Chondroitin is often combined with glucosamine. It may take several months to work. Dosage: 1,200 mg daily; well tolerated.

Glucosamine: A major component of joint cartilage that provides building blocks for growth, repair, and maintenance of cartilage; helps cartilage absorb water; and keeps joints lubricated. Numerous studies have found glucosamine comparable to NSAIDs, yet better tolerated. It may take six to eight weeks to notice benefits. Avoid if allergic to shellfish. Dosage: 1,500 mg daily.

S-adenosylmethionine (SAMe): A nutrient involved in cartilage formation and repair. It reduces pain and inflammation and stimulates cartilage formation. Numerous studies have found it equally effective as NSAIDs with no major side effects. Dosage: 400–1,200 mg daily.

Complementary Supplements

Boswellia: A tree resin used in traditional Indian medicine; some studies show that it reduces pain and inflammation similarly to NSAIDS, but it does not cause stomach irritation. Dosage: 400 mg three times daily.

Bromelain: An enzyme with anti-inflammatory activity that improves joint mobility. It is well tolerated; however, it may thin the blood, so use cautiously along with blood-thinning medications. Dosage: 2,000–6,000 MCU daily.

Capsaicin: A hot pepper extract that reduces pain. It is available in creams; look for a product with 0.025–0.075 percent capsaicin (Zostrix or Menthacin); wash hands after application to avoid getting in the eyes.

Curcumin: An antioxidant that has been shown in studies to have anti-inflammatory effects comparable to cortisone. Dosage: 400 mg three times daily; no side effects.

Essential fatty acids: Both the omega-3s (fish oil) and omega-6s (borage, primrose oil) help to reduce the pain and inflammation and lubricate the joints. Dosage: 2–4 g daily.

FINAL THOUGHTS

To reduce the pain and inflammation associated with OA and protect your joints, consider the following:

1. Eat more fish, flaxseed, olive oil, and pineapple, and drink green tea.
2. Minimize red meat, dairy, sugar, and refined/processed foods; avoid nightshade foods.
3. Do light strength training and cardiovascular and stretching activities regularly to improve joint function and mobility and to reduce pain.
4. Try acupuncture, massage, and heat to reduce pain.
5. Consider supplements of glucosamine/chondroitin or SAMe and Celadrin.

O

Osteoarthritis

OSTEOPOROSIS

Osteoporosis, which means "porous bones," is a disease that thins and weakens the bones to the point where they can easily fracture or break. Approximately 1.4 million Canadians suffer with the disease, with an estimated annual cost of $1.9 billion. Osteoporosis is much more common in women, but men can get it too.

Bone is living tissue that consists of a matrix of protein fibres (collagen), hardened with calcium, phosphorus, magnesium, zinc, copper, and other minerals. An interconnecting structure gives bone its strength: on the outside there is a tough, dense rind of cortical bone, and on the inside there is spongy-looking trabecular bone.

Bone cells called osteoclasts are constantly breaking down old bone at the same time that other cells, called osteoblasts, are building new bone. The activity of these cells is regulated primarily by the hormones estrogen, testosterone, and parathyroid hormone.

Until about age 24, there is a balance in activity of osteoclasts and osteoblasts. After that point, bone loss begins, and as we age more bone is broken down than is replaced. In women, the rate of loss accelerates for several years after menopause, and then slows again.

The trabecular bone normally looks like a honeycomb, but in those with osteoporosis the spaces in that honeycomb grow larger because more bone is destroyed than replaced. This makes the bones weaker and more susceptible to fractures.

There are many factors that contribute to and accelerate bone loss, and much that can be done to prevent this disease. Since bone health affects our mobility and ability to carry out daily activities, it is important to learn how to prevent osteoporosis and maintain strong, healthy bones throughout life.

BONE MINERAL DENSITY

Bone mineral density (BMD) is a term used to describe the solidity of our bones. This can be determined by a DEXA-scan (dual-energy X-ray absorptiometry). The results are reported as a number, which tells us how far off our BMD is from a healthy adult without osteoporosis. A result of –2.5 SD (standard deviation) or greater indicates osteoporosis. A result between –1 SD and –2.5 SD means there is some bone loss, a condition called osteopenia, which often leads to osteoporosis.

SIGNS & SYMPTOMS

Osteoporosis is referred to as the silent thief because bone loss can occur slowly for many years without symptoms until a sudden strain, bump, or fall causes a bone fracture. It most commonly affects bones in the hip, spine, or wrist. Once the bones have become weakened, osteoporosis may cause back pain, collapsed vertebrae, loss of height, and spinal deformities.

- Age (65 or older)
- Body frame (those with small, thin bones are at greater risk)
- Eating disorders (anorexia, bulimia)
- Ethnicity (Caucasian or Asian)
- Family history
- Gender (women are more susceptible than men)
- High alcohol consumption (more than two drinks per day)
- Medical conditions that affect calcium absorption (Celiac and Crohn's disease, hyper-thyroidism)
- Nutritional deficiencies (low calcium and vitamin D intake; high caffeine intake—more than four drinks per day)
- Osteopenia (mild bone loss)
- Prescription medications—steroids (prednisone), diuretics, and anticonvulsants
- Sedentary lifestyle
- Smoking

DOCTOR'S ORDERS

Proper nutrition and exercise are essential for osteoporosis prevention. For those with osteoporosis or osteopenia with strong risk factors for osteoporosis, drug therapy may be recommended to either slow the rate of bone loss or promote bone development. There are a variety of medications that doctors prescribe, such as hormones and bisphosphonates (such as etidronate).

SHERRY'S NATURAL PRESCRIPTION

Dietary Recommendations

Foods to include:

- Calcium-rich foods are essential to build and maintain strong bones. Examples include canned fish with bones (salmon and sardines), dark-green vegetables (kale, kelp, collards, broccoli, and Brussels sprouts), and calcium-fortified orange juice and soy milk. Some studies have shown that people who get their calcium from plant sources have lower rates of osteoporosis. Green vegetables are also a good source of vitamin K.

- While dairy is a heavily promoted source of calcium, these foods may not be ideal for everyone. Many people have difficulty digesting lactose, the sugar in milk, and some are allergic to the protein in milk. Another concern is that dairy cows can be injected with hormones and antibiotics, which pass into their milk. Those who can tolerate milk should choose fat-free, organic milk and cheese to avoid ingestion of these substances.

- Vegetables and fruits are alkaline and health promoting. Recent research suggests that polyphenols (plant pigments) in fruits, vegetables, green tea, and red wine have a positive effect on bone-building cells.

- Lycopene, a carotenoid in tomatoes and tomato products, is an antioxidant that may offer some bone-preserving benefits.

- Magnesium is also necessary for bone formation and may be deficient in those with osteoporosis. Food sources include leafy green vegetables, whole grains, nuts, seeds, meat, milk, soybeans, tofu, legumes, and figs.

- Vitamin D aids in the absorption of calcium. Food sources include fortified milk products and breakfast cereals, fatty fish, and eggs.

- Soy foods such as tofu, soy milk, roasted soy beans, soy powders, and soy bars can also play a role in the prevention of osteoporosis. Soy contains isoflavones, which are plant-based estrogens that protect against bone loss.

- Organic yogurt contains friendly bacteria necessary to convert vitamin K to its active form, which helps in calcium absorption.

Foods to avoid:

- Caffeine (more than three cups coffee per day) or sodium can increase calcium loss through urination, accelerating bone deterioration.

- Soft drinks may contribute to bone loss due to the phosphoric acid and sugar, which changes the acid balance in the blood.

- Fast food and processed foods are acidifying and can promote bone loss.

- Minimize alcohol (less than two drinks per day).

Lifestyle Suggestions

- Weight-bearing activities, which place stress on the bone, help to strengthen bones and improve bone density. Examples include weight lifting, walking, tennis, and dancing. Exercise also increases muscle strength, coordination, and balance, helping to preserve mobility and reduce the risk of injury and fracture.

- Spend 15 minutes outdoors daily. Your body manufactures some vitamin D through sunlight exposure.

- Don't smoke. Smoking increases bone loss, and the risk of osteoporosis.

Top Recommended Supplements

Calcium: Essential for bone health; since it may not be possible to get adequate amounts through diet, supplements may be necessary. Recommended intake for men and women ages 19–50 is 1,000 mg daily and 1,500 mg over age 50. Those with osteopenia or osteoporosis may be advised to take higher amounts. Many products combine calcium with other nutrients for bone health such as vitamin D and magnesium.

CALCIUM SUPPLEMENTING TIPS

To maximize absorption, take no more than 500 mg of elemental calcium at one time and take with meals. Separate calcium-rich foods and supplements by two hours from iron supplements (calcium reduces iron absorption). Avoid drinking tea with meals, as the tannins in tea reduce calcium absorption.

Ipriflavone: An isoflavone derivative that is used worldwide for the treatment and prevention of osteoporosis. Numerous studies have found that it prevents bone loss and reduces bone pain caused by osteoporosis and fractures. It is most effective when taken along with calcium. Dosage: 200 mg three times daily.

Vitamin D: Aids in the absorption of calcium. Dosage: The Osteoporosis Society of Canada recommends that those aged 19–50 take 400 IU of vitamin D per day. Adults over 50 should take 800 IU. Those who are taking medications or have medical conditions that impair vitamin D absorption may require higher amounts.

Complementary Supplements

Fish oils: Recent research suggests that fish oils increase both calcium absorption and improve calcium's delivery to the bones. Dosage: 1 g three times daily.

Green drinks: Rich in polyphenols and nutrients important for bone health. Take daily for health maintenance.

BONE-BUILDING SUPPLEMENTS

Adequate calcium intake from diet and/or supplements is essential, but it is not the only nutrient necessary for building and maintaining strong bones. Vitamins D, K, B6 and B12, boron, copper, manganese, phosphorus, folate, magnesium, silicon, and zinc are also required. As well, new research suggests that fish oils increase both calcium absorption and improve calcium's delivery to the bones. (Source: Sam Graci, Dr. Letitia Rao, and Dr. Carolyn DeMarco, *The Bone-Building Solution*. Toronto: John Wiley & Sons, 2006.)

FINAL THOUGHTS

Osteoporosis is preventable, not inevitable with aging. To strengthen your bones and protect yourself against this disease, consider the following:

1. Eat a diet that is rich in vegetables, fruits, whole grains, beans, and legumes. Drink green tea rather than coffee.
2. Get regular weight-bearing exercise.
3. Spend at least 15 minutes outdoors.
4. Don't smoke, and minimize alcohol and caffeine intake.
5. Supplement your diet with bone-building nutrients.

OVARIAN CYSTS

Ovarian cysts are fluid-filled sacs that develop within or on the surface of an ovary. The ovaries are two, small almond-shaped organs located on each side of a woman's uterus that produce eggs and female hormones.

There are several different types of cysts that can form on the ovaries. Each month, the ovaries grow tiny follicles (sacs) that hold the eggs. When an egg is mature, the follicle breaks open to release the egg, and then dissolves. If the follicle doesn't break open to release the egg, it forms a follicular cyst. This type of cyst usually disappears within one to three months.

A corpus luteum cyst occurs after the egg is released from the follicle. The follicle becomes the corpus luteum. If pregnancy doesn't occur, the corpus luteum normally breaks down and disappears. If this does not happen and fluid builds up in the corpus luteum, it can form a cyst. These cysts can grow to almost 10 cm and may cause bleeding or twist the ovary and cause pain. This type of cyst usually goes away on its own after a few weeks.

Other types of cysts include:

Cystadenomas: Cysts that develop from cells on the outer surface of the ovary. They are often filled with a watery fluid or thick, sticky gel and can become large and painful.

Dermoid cyst: Ovarian cells are able to make hair, teeth, and other tissues. An abnormal growth of these cells can form a cyst. These cysts typically affect younger women.

Endometriomas: A type of cyst that develops in women with endometriosis, a condition where tissue from the lining of the uterus grows outside of the uterus. The tissue may attach to the ovary and form a cyst, which can be painful.

Polycystic ovarian syndrome: Multiple cysts appear on the ovaries due to hormonal imbalance and high insulin levels. This topic is covered separately in this book.

Many women have ovarian cysts at some time during their lives and most ovarian cysts are benign (non-cancerous) and disappear without treatment. However, some cysts can rupture and cause serious symptoms and consequences. For this reason, knowing the signs and symptoms and having regular pelvic exams is important to preserving ovarian health.

SIGNS & SYMPTOMS

Some women have few or no symptoms, while others experience:

- Abdominal fullness or heaviness
- Menstrual irregularities (heavy bleeding or abnormal cycles)
- Nausea, vomiting, or pelvic tenderness
- Pelvic pain that may radiate down the back and thighs

- Pelvic pain during intercourse
- Pressure on the rectum or bladder

DON'T BE ALARMED

Most ovarian cysts are benign (non-cancerous) and go away within a few months. If you develop sudden and severe abdominal or pelvic pain along with fever or vomiting, seek immediate medical attention.

RISK FACTORS

- Age: Women of child-bearing age are at greatest risk.
- Hormonal imbalances (high estrogen levels)
- Race: Caucasian and Hispanic women are at increased risk.

DOCTOR'S ORDERS

The treatment of ovarian cysts depends on the size and type of cyst, symptoms, and the woman's age. Follicular and corpus luteum cysts are usually just monitored by the doctor and go away on their own. Oral contraceptives or progesterone cream are sometimes given to women who get frequent cysts as a way of controlling hormone levels and preventing cyst growth. Surgery is usually considered as a last resort for women with malignant cysts, those who have very large cysts that do not go away, and those with severe symptoms or infertility.

SHERRY'S NATURAL PRESCRIPTION

Dietary Recommendations

Foods to include:

- Beets, carrots, artichokes, and lemons contain nutrients that support liver health, aiding the detoxification of estrogen.
- Fibre may help the body eliminate excess hormones. Boost intake of fruits, vegetables, and whole grains. Aim for 25–35 g daily.
- Flaxseed, soy, beans, and legumes contain phytoestrogens, which may help reduce the impact of other hormones.
- Choose organic foods as much as possible, to avoid ingestion of estrogen-like compounds.
- Drink plenty of water.

Foods to avoid:

- Meat and dairy products may contain saturated fat, hormones, and chemicals that can affect ovarian health and trigger inflammation.
- Minimize caffeine (coffee, tea, chocolate), as it may worsen menstrual irregularities.

Lifestyle Suggestions

- Get regular pelvic examinations. Report any unusual symptoms or changes in your menstrual cycle to your doctor.

- Reduce stress. Try meditation, breathing exercises, and yoga.

- Exercise regularly to reduce stress levels and improve circulation and overall well-being. Aim for 30 minutes to one hour daily.

Top Recommended Supplements

There is limited research on supplements for the prevention and/or treatment of ovarian cysts. The supplements outlined here may play a role in minimizing symptoms and supporting hormone balance and liver health.

Calcium D-glucarate: Helps the liver detoxify and eliminate excess hormones, particularly estrogen. Dosage: 150–300 mg daily.

Chasteberry: Balances estrogen to progesterone ratio and may help normalize ovulation. Dosage: 150–300 mg daily.

Indole-3-carbinol: A compound found naturally in cruciferous vegetables that aids in detoxification of estrogen, protects liver function, and may protect against hormonal cancers. Dosage: 400 mg daily.

Complementary Supplements

Evening primrose oil: Helps reduce pain and inflammation. Dosage: 3,000 mg daily.

Milk thistle: Supports liver function and aids detoxification. Dosage: 50–100 mg daily.

FINAL THOUGHTS

To manage ovarian cysts and protect ovarian health, consider the following:

1. Get regular pelvic exams and report any changes to your doctor.
2. Boost intake of fibre and eat more eggplant, flaxseed, and beans.
3. Minimize saturated fat (mead/dairy).
4. Get regular exercise and reduce stress levels.
5. Consider supplements of indole-3-carbinol, calcium D-glucarate, and chasteberry.

PARASITES

Our bodies are filled with billions of micro-organisms. Some are harmless and even beneficial for health and others can cause illness and disease. A parasite is an organism that lives on or in a host organism and gets its food from or at the expense of its host.

There are two main classes of parasites that can cause intestinal disease in humans:

Helminths: Derived from the Greek word for "worms," these large, multicellular organisms are generally visible to the naked eye. They can be either free-living or parasitic in nature. In their adult form, helminths cannot multiply in humans. The three main groups of helminths that are human parasites are flatworms (tapeworms), thorny-headed worms, and roundworms (hookworms and pinworms).

Protozoa: Microscopic, one-celled organisms that can be free-living or parasitic in nature. They can multiply in humans, which contributes to their survival and also permits serious infections to develop from just a single organism. The most common protozoa that infect humans are *giardia* and *cryptosporidium*.

Parasites get into the intestine from consumption of contaminated food or water. When the organisms are swallowed, they move into the intestine, where they can reproduce and cause disease. You can also contract parasites from intimate contact (oral-anal) with someone who has them.

In some people, intestinal parasites do not cause any symptoms or the symptoms may be mild. In others they can cause horrible gastrointestinal problems, weight loss, irritability, and more. Parasites can be eliminated with medication and/or natural supplements. There are also a variety of lifestyle measures that can reduce your risk of contracting parasites.

SIGNS & SYMPTOMS

- Abdominal cramping and pain
- Bloody stools; mucus in stool
- Coughing
- Diarrhea and foul-smelling stools
- Fatigue·
- Fever
- Gas and bloating
- Irritability and restlessness
- Itching in the rectal area
- Loss of appetite
- Vomiting
- Weight loss

RISK FACTORS

- Age: Children are more commonly infected
- Contact with infected animals
- Drinking contaminated water
- Dysbiosis (imbalanced gut flora)
- Ingestion of undercooked meat or food containing parasites
- International travel
- Poor hygiene
- Sexual or intimate contact with someone who has parasites
- Weakened immune system (e.g., HIV)

DOCTOR'S ORDERS

If you suspect a parasite, see your doctor for proper diagnosis. Fecal testing (examination of your stool) can identify both helminths and protozoa. It is important to do stool tests before taking any anti-diarrheal drugs or antibiotics. Typically three to five stool samples are needed to find the parasite.

The treatment will depend on the particular parasite that you have. Mebendazole (Vermox) is used for roundworm, hookworms, and pinworms. Metronidazole (Flagyl) is used for giardiasis.

SHERRY'S NATURAL PRESCRIPTION

It is critical to see your doctor for proper diagnosis and treatment. Natural products, while helpful, are not as effective and take longer to work compared to prescription drugs.

Dietary Recommendations

Foods to include:

- Boost intake of fibre, which helps improve elimination. Eat more whole grains, vegetables, and beans.
- Drink lots of purified water.
- Eat more raw garlic, pumpkin seeds, pomegranates, beets, and carrots, all of which have anti-parasitic properties.

Foods to avoid:

- Refined carbohydrates and sugars impair immune function.
- Spicy foods, dairy, alcohol, and caffeine can worsen gastrointestinal symptoms.

Lifestyle Suggestions

To reduce the risk of contracting parasites, consider these tips:

- Wash your hands after using the toilet, changing diapers, handling animals, or before eating or preparing food. Use soap and water and don't forget to scrub under your nails.
- Drink purified or bottled water. When camping, boil stream water for at least 10 minutes.

- When swimming in pools, lakes, or streams keep your mouth and eyes closed and try not to swallow water.

- Practise safe sex. Use condoms and avoid oral-anal sex without protection.

TRAVEL TIPS

To reduce your risk of contracting parasites when travelling to developing countries, avoid drinking tap water and eating uncooked foods, foods prepared by street vendors, ice, and fruits that cannot be peeled. Undercooked (rare) fish, meat, and poultry can also cause parasites. Do not drink untreated stream water while camping as it is almost invariably contaminated with giardia, even in North America. Take probiotic supplements while travelling to help maintain normal gastrointestinal flora.

Top Recommended Supplements

Herbal products: Black walnut, wormwood, oil of oregano, and ginger have anti-parasitic properties. Consult with a natural health care provider for advice and dosage guidelines.

Probiotics: Beneficial bacteria such as Lactobacillus and Bifidobacteria can help in the prevention and treatment of parasites by maintaining healthy gut flora and reducing overgrowth of parasites and other pathogens. Dosage: 1–3 capsules daily with meals. Recommended product: Kyo-Dophilus.

Propolis: A resinous substance collected by bees from the leaf buds and bark of trees. It has antimicrobial properties and may help protect against parasitic intestinal infections. Preliminary research found that propolis extract was helpful in eliminating giardiasis in adults and children. Dosage: 30 drops four times daily.

Complementary Supplements

Berberine: A compound found in many plants, such as Oregon grape and goldenseal. Preliminary studies have shown that berberine can be used successfully to treat giardia infections. Dosage: 200 mg three times per day for adult. Not recommended for children.

Digestive enzymes: Aid digestion and make your intestinal tract less hospitable to parasites. Dosage: Take before meals.

FINAL THOUGHTS

To manage a parasitic infection, consider the following:

1. See your doctor for proper diagnosis and discuss the benefits and risks of drug therapy.
2. Boost intake of fibre, drink lots of purified water, and eat more raw garlic, pumpkin seeds, pomegranates, beets, and carrots.
3. Minimize sugar, refined starches, dairy, spicy food, caffeine, and alcohol.
4. Wash your hands after using the toilet and before touching food, and practise safe sex to avoid spreading the parasites.
5. Probiotics can help in the prevention and treatment of parasites. Discuss the role of herbal products with your health care provider.

PARKINSON'S DISEASE

Parkinson's disease is a progressive nervous-system disorder that affects muscle movement. The disease causes degenerative changes in an area of the brain called the substantia nigra. Nerve cells in this area are responsible for producing the neurotransmitter dopamine. As these nerve cells become damaged and die, there is insufficient dopamine to relay messages between nerve and muscle cells, and it becomes progressively more difficult for the body to move smoothly. This causes characteristic tremors and shaking, which interfere with normal activities such as walking, sitting, and standing.

In Canada, there are approximately 100,000 people or one out of every 100 adults with Parkinson's disease. Parkinson's most often affects older adults and as Canada's population continues to age, the incidence of Parkinson's disease is expected to rise.

Researchers are working to understand the underlying causes of Parkinson's. Everyone loses some dopamine-producing neurons with age, but those with Parkinson's lose around 60 percent or more of the neurons in the substantia nigra. Scientists believe that a combination of genetic and environmental factors is involved.

Unlike some neurological diseases, Parkinson's disease is treatable. Over the years there have been great advances in science that have improved quality of life for those with Parkinson's.

SHAKING PALSY

Parkinson's disease was first described in 1817 by a British doctor, James Parkinson, in a publication titled "Essay on the Shaking Palsy." In the 1960s, it was discovered that dopamine deficiency was responsible for the symptoms of Parkinson's. Soon after, the first effective treatment for the disease was introduced, a drug called levodopa.

SIGNS & SYMPTOMS

In the early stages, symptoms may be subtle, such as mild tremor in the fingers, fatigue, or difficulty sleeping. As the disease progresses, it may cause:

- Dementia: Some people with Parkinson's develop impaired mental function, which affects the ability to think, reason, and remember.

- Difficulty swallowing

- Impaired balance and coordination

- Impaired speech: The voice becomes monotone and soft and speech is slower.

- Loss of automatic movements: The face becomes less expressive; some people lose the ability to blink, smile, make hand gestures, and move their arms while walking.

- Rigid, stiff muscles; often occurs in the limbs and neck

- Slowed movement: A slow, shuffling walk with an unsteady gait and stooped posture; leg muscles may freeze up, making it difficult to walk and move

- Tremor: Often starts in the hands and fingers; sometimes hand tremor causes a back-and-forth rubbing of the thumb and forefinger known as "pill-rolling"; tremor may also develop in the legs; tremor is often worse under stress.

RISK FACTORS

- Age: The risk increases with age. Parkinson's is usually diagnosed after age 60, but some people have developed it in their twenties. It is thought that genetic or environmental factors over time lead to neural damage.

- Environmental factors: Exposure to pesticides and herbicides increases risk. Farmers and those handling these chemicals and those who drink well water are at higher risk. Heavy metal toxicity also increases risk.

- Family history: Having one or more close relatives with Parkinson's increases the chances that you'll also develop the disease, although your risk is still less than 5 percent.

- Free radicals: Some research suggests that Parkinson's may be caused by unstable oxygen molecules that cause cell damage.

- Gender: Men are slightly more at risk.

DRUG-INDUCED PARKINSON'S

Several drugs, when used chronically or in excessive dosages, can cause symptoms of Parkinson's disease. Examples include: haloperidol (Haldol) and chlorpromazine (Thorazine), which are used to treat psychiatric disorders, drugs used to treat nausea, such as metoclopramide (Reglan), and the epilepsy drug valproate (Depakene). Once these drugs are stopped, the symptoms disappear.

DOCTOR'S ORDERS

Drug therapy is used to boost dopamine levels, and this can dramatically improve symptoms. However, with chronic use, the benefits often diminish and it may be necessary to adjust the dosage, switch medications, or take multiple medications. Along with medication, physical therapy, exercise, and proper nutrition are recommended.

When lifestyle changes are no longer enough, your doctor will likely recommend certain medications, either alone or in combination. Some of the most common medications used include:

Amantadine: An antiviral that reduces the side effects that are sometimes caused by taking levodopa for a long time. Amantadine is sometimes used alone or, in the early stages of the disease, along with levodopa.

Anticholinergics: An older class of drugs used before the discovery of levodopa. They help control tremor in the early stages of the disease, but are only mildly beneficial and cause side effects such as dry mouth, nausea, confusion, hallucinations, and urine retention. Examples: trihexphenidyl and benztropine (Cogentin).

COMT inhibitors: Prolong the effect of Sinemet by blocking an enzyme (Catechol-O-methyltransferase) that breaks down dopamine. Example: Entacapone (Comtan).

Dopamine agonists: Drugs that mimic the effects of dopamine in the brain. They are often used for young adults or those in early stages, along with Sinemet. Examples include: bromocriptine (Parlodel), pramipexole (Mirapex), and ropinirole (Requip). Side effects include involuntary movements, hallucinations, drowsiness, and the risk of inflammatory reactions in the heart and lungs.

Selegiline (Deprenyl): Helps prevent the breakdown of dopamine. It is often used early in the disease and later combined with Sinemet to enhance its effects.

Sinemet: A combination of levodopa and carbidopa. Levodopa is a natural substance found in plants and animals that is converted into dopamine by nerve cells in the brain. Carbidopa enhances the amount of levodopa that gets into the brain and helps reduce the side effects of therapy. Side effects include involuntary movements, hallucinations, and low blood pressure when standing.

There are a variety of experimental procedures under development such as stem cell transplants and tissue grafts.

SHERRY'S NATURAL PRESCRIPTION

Dietary Recommendations

Foods to include:

- Boost fibre intake to prevent constipation. Eat more fruits, vegetables, whole grains, and beans. Fruits and vegetables also provide antioxidants that help to neutralize damaging free radicals. Eat organic as much as possible to avoid ingesting toxic pesticides.

- Eat small, frequent meals. Chew food slowly to make it easier to swallow.

- Healthy fats such as olive oil and flaxseed oil and wheat germ contain vitamin E, which is a potent antioxidant, and essential fatty acids that help reduce inflammation.

- Yogurt, kefir, and fermented dairy contain beneficial bacteria that can aid digestion, support immune function, and help in the absorption of nutrients.

Foods to avoid:

- Avoid processed and fast foods and artificial sweeteners, which contain chemicals that may have a negative effect on brain function.

- Diets high in saturated fat (meat and dairy) can increase the risk of Parkinson's due to increased formation of free radicals in the brain and oxidative damage to the nerve cells in the substantia nigra. Minimize saturated fat to less than 10 percent of total calories.

- Eating large amounts of fava beans (broad beans) can boost the action of levodopa and can possibly lead to overdose. Speak with a dietitian before adding fava beans to your diet.

- Minimize or avoid alcohol, as it can impair brain function.

PROTEIN AND PARKINSON'S

Several studies have shown that you can enhance the action of levodopa and improve the symptoms of Parkinson's by consuming most of your day's protein requirement at dinner, while keeping the protein content of breakfast and lunch extremely low (less than 10 g). This is because certain dietary proteins can interfere with the stomach's absorption of levodopa and the body's ability to get it to the brain cells. It is important to consult with a dietitian for proper advice on planning your meals.

Lifestyle Suggestions

- Exercise can help improve mobility, range of motion, and muscle tone and strength. Tai chi is particularly helpful. Weight-bearing activities (walking, dancing) can help strengthen the bones, which helps in the prevention of osteoporosis. Wear proper footwear and consult with a physical therapist or personal trainer to get advice on exercises that can improve balance, coordination, and strength.

- Spend 15 minutes outdoors to allow your skin to make vitamin D, which can help protect against osteoporosis and improve Parkinson's symptoms.

- Manage stress with yoga, breathing techniques, and meditation.

- A speech pathologist can help improve problems with speaking and swallowing.

- Get adequate sleep. The medications may make you tired, so it is important to rest as needed.

- Take measures to reduce the risk of falls (remove scatter rugs, keep walking areas clear, and use handrails on stairs and grab bars around tub and toilet).

Top Recommended Supplements

CDP-choline: A substance that occurs naturally in the body. It increases the amount of dopamine in the brain. Studies have shown it can improve symptoms and enhance the efficacy of levodopa. Dosage: 400 mg three times daily. This is a specialty supplement that is available through natural health care practitioners.

Coenzyme Q10: An antioxidant that is involved in energy production in the cells. People with Parkinson's tend to have low Q10 levels and several studies have shown that supplements can slow the progression of the disease. Dosage: 1,200 mg daily. Lower dosages have been used, but with less benefit.

NADH: Nicotinamide adenine dinucleotide hydrogen is an enzyme that helps to improve neurotransmitter function (boost dopamine levels) and has antioxidant properties. Preliminary studies using high doses of NADH for Parkinson's disease have shown reduced symptoms and improved brain function. Dosage: 5 mg twice daily.

RESEARCH HIGHLIGHT

A double-blind trial of 80 people with early Parkinson's disease compared the effects of coenzyme Q10 (at a dose of 300 mg, 600 mg, or 1,200 mg daily) to placebo for 16 weeks. The 1,200 mg dose of coenzyme Q10 significantly slowed the progression of the disease (*Archives of Neurology*, 2002: 59; 1541–1550).

Complementary Supplements

Amino acids: L-tyrosine, methionine, and acetyl-L-carnitine may help in the management of Parkinson's by nourishing the cells that produce dopamine. Preliminary studies with methionine and L-carnitine have shown benefits for reducing symptoms. L-tyrosine should not be taken with L-dopa as it may interfere with the transport of L-dopa to the brain. Consult with your health care provider before supplementing with amino acids.

Ginkgo biloba: An antioxidant that improves blood flow to the brain. Many studies have shown that it can improve memory and cognitive function in the elderly. Dosage: 120–240 mg daily, standardized to 6 percent terpene lactones and 24 percent flavone glycosides. It may take six weeks to notice benefit.

Vitamin B6: May improve Parkinson's symptoms and enhance the effectiveness of Sinemet. Do not take if you are taking levodopa alone as this can increase the conversion of levodopa to dopamine outside the brain. Dosage: 50–100 mg daily.

Vitamins C and E: Antioxidants that protect against free radical damage in the brain, including key dopamine-producing brain cells. In one study, people with early Parkinson's given a dosage of 750 mg vitamin C and 800 IU vitamin E four times daily were able to delay the need for drug therapy by an average of about two and a half years, compared with those not taking the vitamins.

FINAL THOUGHTS

To improve the management of Parkinson's, consider the following:

1. Boost intake of fibre (whole grains, fruits, and vegetables) along with healthy fats and yogurt. Speak with a dietitian about consuming your daily protein in the evening.
2. Minimize or avoid saturated fat, alcohol, processed and fast foods, and artificial sweeteners.
3. Exercise regularly to improve strength, coordination, and balance. Work with a trainer or physical therapist.
4. Get adequate sleep and manage your stress.
5. Consider supplements of CDP choline, coenzyme Q10, and NADH.

POLYCYSTIC OVARIAN SYNDROME

Polycystic ovary syndrome (PCOS) is a disorder characterized by hormonal imbalance, irregular menstrual periods, excess hair growth, and obesity. Women with PCOS typically have numerous cysts on the ovaries, hence the name. PCOS is the most common hormonal disorder among women of reproductive age, affecting an estimated 5–10 percent.

In PCOS, the body produces an excess amount of androgens, and the ratio of luteinizing hormone to follicle-stimulating hormone is abnormally high. Ovulation occurs less frequently, or the ovaries don't release eggs at all. In the absence of ovulation, the menstrual cycle is irregular or absent, and cysts containing the immature eggs form on the ovaries. This causes the ovaries to enlarge.

Research suggests that PCOS may result from excess insulin, which boosts male hormone production (androgens), leading to menstrual cycle disturbances, acne, and coarse hair growth. Genetic factors may also be at play since this occurs more commonly in those with a family history.

Early diagnosis and treatment of PCOS is important to improving quality of life and reducing the risk of long-term complications, such as diabetes and heart disease.

PCOS AND INSULIN RESISTANCE

Insulin resistance is a common feature of both PCOS and metabolic syndrome. Metabolic syndrome is a cluster of symptoms (abdominal obesity, high cholesterol and triglycerides, and insulin resistance) that greatly increases the risk of heart disease and diabetes. Researchers at Virginia Commonwealth University found that the metabolic syndrome is twice as prevalent in women with PCOS compared to those without this hormonal disorder.

SIGNS & SYMPTOMS

- Acne, oily skin, or dandruff
- Enlarged ovaries with cysts
- Increased hair growth on the face, chest, stomach, back, thumbs, or toes (hirsutism) and thinning or male-pattern baldness on the head
- Infertility
- Irregular or absent menstrual periods
- Obesity (particularly around the waist)
- Patches of thickened and dark brown or black skin on the neck, arms, breasts, or thighs
- Pelvic pain
- Skin tags, or tiny excess flaps of skin in the armpits or neck area

Note: PCOS increases the risk of developing type 2 diabetes, high blood pressure, increased triglycerides, decreased high-density lipoprotein (HDL) cholesterol, and cardiovascular disease. Women with PCOS are also at risk of abnormal uterine bleeding and endometrial cancer because the uterus is exposed to higher amounts of estrogen.

RISK FACTORS

- Family history
- High insulin levels
- Obesity
- Race (women of Mediterranean descent are at greater risk)

DOCTOR'S ORDERS

Healthy eating and regular exercise are critical to reduce the risk of diabetes and heart disease. There are several medications that doctors prescribe to address the symptoms of infertility, hirsutism, and acne.

For those not trying to become pregnant, low-dose oral contraceptives are used to regulate the menstrual cycle, decrease androgen production, improve acne, reduce hair growth, and reduce the risk of endometrial cancer. Oral or topical progesterone for 10–14 days each month is sometimes used to regulate the cycle. Spironolactone is a drug used to decrease androgens and reduce hair growth and acne. Other, non-drug methods of hair removal include electrolysis, laser, sugaring, and waxing.

Drugs such as Glucophage (metformin) are used to improve insulin resistance and reduce androgen levels. For women trying to conceive, fertility drugs such as clomiphene and gonadotropin shots are used to stimulate ovulation, which may result in multiple births. About 30 to 70 percent of PCO women on clomiphene will conceive.

SHERRY'S NATURAL PRESCRIPTION

Dietary Recommendations

Foods to include:

- Boost intake of fruits, vegetables, and whole grains. These foods are high in fibre and low in the glycemic index, which helps to improve blood sugar and insulin levels. Refer to Appendix B for more information on the glycemic index.

- Cinnamon can improve insulin sensitivity. Add ½ tsp daily to cereals, breakfast shakes, or other foods.

- Flaxseed, soy, beans, and legumes contain phytoestrogens, which may help reduce the impact of other hormones.

- The essential fatty acids in fish help balance hormones and improve acne.

- Choose organic foods as much as possible.

- Drink plenty of water.

Foods to avoid:

- Sugar (candy, pop, and sweets) and refined starches (white flour products) cause blood sugar imbalances and trigger high insulin.

- Meat and dairy products may contain saturated fat, hormones, and chemicals that can worsen PCOS and trigger inflammation.

- Minimize alcohol and caffeine products, as they may interfere with hormone function.

Lifestyle Suggestions

- Exercise regularly, which will help with weight loss, which in turn can reduce both insulin and androgen levels, and may restore ovulation. Aim for 30 minutes to one hour daily.

- Reduce stress, as stress can worsen insulin response. Try meditation, breathing exercises, and yoga.

- Follow a good skin care regime. Wash your face morning and night using skin care products containing tea tree oil (10–15 percent) to help reduce acne and oily skin. Minimize wearing cosmetics, and use products design for oily skin.

Top Recommended Supplements

Indole-3-carbinol: A compound found naturally in cruciferous vegetables. Although not specifically studied for PCOS, it aids in detoxification of estrogen, protects liver function, and may protect against hormonal cancers. Dosage: 400 mg daily.

Inositol: A nutrient that has been found to improve certain symptoms of PCOS such as ovulation, infertility, cholesterol, and weight gain. Dosage: 100 mg twice daily.

Complementary Supplements

Calcium D-glucarate: Helps the liver detoxify and eliminate excess hormones, particularly estrogen. Dosage: 150–300 mg daily.

Chasteberry: Balances the estrogen to progesterone ratio and may help normalize ovulation. Dosage: 150–300 mg daily.

Chromium: Improves insulin sensitivity, but not specifically studied for PCOS. Dosage: 200 mcg daily.

N-acetylcysteine: A form of the amino acid cysteine. One study found that it significantly increased efficacy of the fertility drug clomiphene. Dosage: 1.2 g daily.

Zinc: May help improve acne and control inflammation. Dosage: 50–75 mg daily.

FINAL THOUGHTS

To manage PCOS and prevent further health risks, consider the following:

1. Boost intake of fibre-rich fruits, vegetables, whole grains, nuts, and seeds.
2. Minimize refined starches and sugars.
3. Get regular exercise.
4. Reduce stress levels.
5. Consider supplements of inositol, indole-3-carbinol and chasteberry.

PREMENSTRUAL SYNDROME (PMS)

Premenstrual syndrome (PMS) is a group of symptoms linked to the menstrual cycle. It is one of the most common conditions affecting women of child-bearing age. Approximately 85 percent of women have one or more symptoms of PMS.

Years ago, the symptoms of PMS were dismissed as being psychological. Today, however, it is recognized there are a number of factors involved in causing the notorious symptoms, including hormonal and biochemical imbalances, diet, and environment.

While the symptoms of PMS can be distressing, there are a number of lifestyle measures and natural products that can greatly improve both the physical and emotional symptoms.

SIGNS & SYMPTOMS

The symptoms of PMS often start a few days to a week before the menstrual cycle and then disappear after menstruation. They vary greatly among women in both severity and the number of symptoms experienced.

Common signs and symptoms include:

- Breast swelling and tenderness
- Changes in appetite and/or food cravings
- Crying spells
- Depression and anxiety
- Fatigue
- Headache
- Insomnia
- Lower abdominal bloating and pain
- Mood swings and irritability
- Weight gain from fluid retention

PREMENSTRUAL DYSPHORIC DISORDER

Premenstrual dysphoric disorder (PMDD) is a severe form of PMS that can be disabling. Symptoms include severe depression, feelings of hopelessness, anger, anxiety, low self-esteem, difficulty concentrating, irritability, and tension. The symptoms of PMDD typically begin a week before a period.

- Biochemical imbalance: Low levels of serotonin, a brain chemical that regulates emotional well-being

- Depression

- Exposure to environmental toxins and estrogens (xenoestrogens)

- Hormonal imbalance (low thyroid or progesterone levels)

- Nutrient deficiencies in B-vitamins, magnesium, or essential fatty acids

- Poor diet: Eating foods high in sugar, saturated fat, or drinking too much alcohol

- Poor liver function

- Seasonal affective disorder

- Stress

Note: Hormonal imbalances are often difficult to determine through blood tests alone. Saliva testing offers certain advantages and is discussed in Appendix E.

DOCTOR'S ORDERS

There are several medications that doctors prescribe for PMS. Non-steroidal anti-inflammatory drugs (NSAIDs) such as Advil or Motrin are used to relieve cramping and pain. Oral contraceptives are sometimes given for those with severe PMS symptoms and heavy bleeding. Antidepressants such as Paxil, Prozac, or Zoloft are given to those with severe depressive symptoms. All of these drugs have serious side effects and should be used only for the short term and under doctor supervision.

SHERRY'S NATURAL PRESCRIPTION

Dietary Recommendations

Eating small, frequent meals will help to stabilize blood sugar levels, which will have a positive impact on mood and energy levels.

Foods to include:

- Several studies have shown that diets low in fat or high in fibre can help reduce PMS symptoms, so eat more vegetables, fruits, whole grains, nuts, seeds, and fish. These foods are also good sources of vitamins, minerals, and essential fatty acids, which may be depleted in those with PMS.

- Cruciferous vegetables (broccoli, cauliflower, and cabbage) contain indole-3-carbinol, which helps to balance estrogen levels.

- Turkey and salmon contain the amino acid tryptophan, which elevates serotonin production.

Foods to avoid:

- Sugar and refined carbohydrates can cause mood swings, irritability, and worsened PMS symptoms.

- Caffeine has been found in studies to worsen PMS symptoms.

- Processed and fast foods often contain chemicals and preservatives that may upset neurotransmitter levels and mood.

- Alcohol is a nervous system depressant and can affect hormone metabolism. It should be minimized or avoided completely.

Lifestyle Suggestions

- Regular exercise can reduce several symptoms of PMS (breast tenderness, fluid retention, depression, and stress). Aim for 30 minutes to one hour of moderate intensity activity daily, such as brisk walking, cycling, or swimming.

- Acupuncture may offer benefits for PMS by stimulating the production of neurotransmitters that regulate mood.

- Massage and reflexology help relieve stress and tension, and promote relaxation.

Top Recommended Supplements

Calcium: Studies have found that calcium can significantly reduce mood swings, pain, bloating, depression, back pain, and food cravings. Dosage: 1,000–1,500 mg daily.

Chasteberry: An herb that is widely used in Europe. It helps balance hormone levels and reduces symptoms of irritability, depression, headaches, and breast tenderness. Dosage: 150–300 mg daily.

Evening primrose oil: A source of gamma linolenic acid (GLA), which may be deficient in women with PMS. Most studies have found benefits for emotional symptoms and breast tenderness. Dosage: 3–4 g daily.

Complementary Supplements

Ginkgo biloba: Preliminary research has found that it can alleviate emotional symptoms and breast pain. Dosage: 80 mg twice daily.

Magnesium: Some research suggests that it may help emotional symptoms and headaches. Combining magnesium with vitamin B6 may improve results. Dosage: 250 mg twice daily.

Vitamin B6: Has been widely used for PMS, although studies have yielded mixed results. It may work best in those with a deficiency of B6 or when used along with magnesium. Dosage: Take 50–100 mg as part of a B-complex product.

FINAL THOUGHTS

There is good evidence that lifestyle adjustments and supplements can help alleviate the symptoms and improve quality of life. Here are the main points to keep in mind:

1. Boost intake of cruciferous vegetables, fish, whole grains, nuts, and seeds.
2. Minimize sugar, caffeine, processed foods, and alcohol.
3. Exercise every day.
4. Take supplements of chasteberry, calcium, and evening primrose oil.
5. Consider supportive supplements of vitamin B6, ginkgo biloba, and magnesium.

PROSTATE ENLARGEMENT (BENIGN PROSTATIC HYPERPLASIA)

Benign prostatic hyperplasia (BPH) is a non-malignant enlargement of the prostate gland, which is located just below a man's bladder, surrounding the urethra (the tube that drains urine from the bladder). This gland produces seminal fluid, which nourishes and transports sperm. About half of men at age 50 have prostate enlargement and up to 90 percent of men in their seventies and eighties are affected.

At birth, the gland is about the size of a pea. In a man, it is the size of a walnut and stays this size until his late forties when it undergoes a growth phase. The cells in the gland begin to reproduce more quickly, which causes the gland to enlarge. As it enlarges, it compresses the urethra and partially blocks the flow of urine. Prostate enlargement is not related to prostate cancer, but it can cause distressing urinary symptoms, such as difficulty in starting or stopping a stream of urine and the need to void frequently.

The cause of prostate enlargement is believed to be hormonal changes associated with aging. As men age, testosterone levels decline and estrogen levels increase. Levels of another hormone called dihydrotestosterone (DHT) increase. These changes are implicated in triggering growth of the prostate, so treatments for BPH are geared toward correcting the hormonal imbalances. There are a number of medications that are effective, but they can cause unpleasant side effects. Vitamin and herbal supplements can also help.

SIGNS & SYMPTOMS

- Blood in the urine
- Difficulty in starting or stopping urination
- Dribbling
- Inability to empty the bladder completely
- Increased frequency of urination
- Increased nighttime urination
- Recurring urinary tract infections
- Weak urine stream

Note: The signs and symptoms of prostate enlargement vary greatly among men. Only about half of men with prostate enlargement experience urinary symptoms that become troubling enough for them to seek medical treatment.

RISK FACTORS

- Age: It is most common in men over age 60
- Diet: High intake of saturated fat and low intake of fibre
- Ethnicity: It is more common in Caucasian men than in Asian men
- Family history

DOCTOR'S ORDERS

The treatment of BPH depends on the severity of the signs and symptoms. If there are little to no symptoms, your doctor may just monitor your situation to see if it changes. Those with bothersome symptoms may be prescribed medications.

Commonly used medications include alpha blockers, such as terazosin (Hytrin) and tamsulosin (Flomax), which relax the muscles at the neck of the bladder, making it easier to urinate. These drugs work quickly within a day or two, but side effects include low blood pressure, lightheadedness, and dizziness. Finasteride (Proscar) is a drug that works by inhibiting an enzyme that converts testosterone to DHT, thus helping to shrink the prostate gland. It takes longer to work (about three months) and can cause impotence and low libido.

Another approach to management of BPH is heat therapy to destroy the excessive prostate tissue. Examples include microwave heat, radio waves, electric currents, or laser. Heat therapy works better than the drugs, with fewer side effects, but it does require a brief hospital stay and a few days' recovery.

Surgery to remove the excess prostate tissue is reserved for those with severe symptoms and complications, such as frequent infections, bleeding, and kidney damage. Risks of surgery include impotence, retrograde ejaculation, and incontinence.

CAUTION

Over-the-counter decongestants, such as pseudoephedrine (Sudafed) and cold remedies that contain decongestants, can worsen BPH symptoms because they cause the band of muscles that control urine flow from your urethra (urethral sphincter) to tighten, making urination more difficult. Antihistamines can also worsen symptoms by causing urinary retention. Ask your pharmacist for help when looking for a cold or allergy product.

SHERRY'S NATURAL PRESCRIPTION

Dietary Recommendations

Foods to include:

- Drink plenty of water to keep fluid through your urinary tract.

- Fish and flaxseed contain beneficial fatty acids that reduce inflammation.

- Foods rich in soy, such as tofu, contain substances (isoflavones) that may also protect the prostate and ward off cancer.

- Pumpkin seeds contain zinc, an essential nutrient for the prostate.

- Tomatoes contain lycopene, a nutrient that has protective effects on the prostate. Cooked tomato products, such as tomato sauce and ketchup, actually contain more lycopene than fresh tomatoes.

Foods to avoid:

- Alcohol increases urine production and irritates your bladder.

- Caffeine will increase urine production, cause bladder irritation, and aggravate your symptoms.

- Saturated fat (red meat and dairy) can worsen symptoms.

- Sugar hampers immune function and may increase the risk of bladder infections. Limit candy, soft drinks, and sweets.

Limit drinking after 7 p.m. to reduce your need to go to the bathroom during the night.

Lifestyle Suggestions

- Get regular checkups with your doctor. A symptom questionnaire, digital rectal exam, and PSA test are helpful in detecting an enlarged prostate.

- Exercise regularly. Studies show that men who are active have fewer symptoms of BPH.

- Empty your bladder regularly.

PSA TEST

Have your doctor do a PSA test. PSA stands for prostate-specific antigen, which is naturally produced in your prostate gland to help liquefy semen and a small amount circulates in your blood. Having higher than normal levels in your blood could indicate BPH, prostate cancer, or prostatitis (infection or inflammation of the prostate).

Top Recommended Supplements

Beta-sitosterol: A cholesterol-like compound found in many plants. It reduces inflammation and several studies have shown that it can reduce BPH symptoms. Dosage: 60–130 mg daily. It may take four weeks to notice benefits.

Saw palmetto: The most widely researched natural product for BPH. In many countries it is actually prescribed by doctors. Over 10 studies have shown that it can significantly improve urinary flow rate and most other measures of prostate disease. Studies have compared saw palmetto to the drugs Proscar and Flomax and found it equally effective, only better tolerated. Dosage: 160 mg twice a day of an extract standardized to contain 85–95 percent fatty acids and sterols.

Complementary Supplements

Nettle: Contains compounds that may modulate hormones and change the properties of the prostate cells. Some research has shown benefits with supplements made of nettle root. Dosage: 120 mg twice daily.

Pygeum: Thought to reduce inflammation in the prostate, and also to inhibit prostate growth factors. Studies show that it can reduce symptoms such as nighttime urination, urinary frequency, and residual urine volume. Dosage: 50 mg twice daily.

FINAL THOUGHTS

To manage the symptoms of BPH, consider the following:

1. Eat more tomato products, pumpkin seeds, soy, fish, and flaxseed.
2. Avoid or minimize saturated fat, alcohol, caffeine, and sugar.
3. Get regular exercise.
4. Empty your bladder regularly.
5. Consider supplements of beta-sitosterol and/or saw palmetto.

P

Prostate Enlargement (Benign Prostatic Hyperplasia)

PSORIASIS

Psoriasis is a common and recurring condition that affects the life cycle of skin cells. Normally, it takes about a month for our skin cells to move from the lowest skin layer (where they're produced) to the outermost layer (where they die and flake off). In people with psoriasis, the entire life cycle takes only days. With rapid cell growth, the skin cells build up, forming thick, silvery scales and itchy, dry, red patches that are sometimes painful. This is considered a chronic condition as there are persistent periods of remission and then flare-ups.

It is thought that psoriasis is caused by a disorder of the immune system. Specifically, researchers believe that overactive T cells (a type of white blood cell) attack healthy skin cells, causing an increased production of skin cells and other immune responses that lead to an ongoing cycle of rapid skin turnover. Dead skin and white blood cells can't slough off quickly enough and build up in thick, scaly patches on the skin's surface. Researchers are not sure what causes the immune system to malfunction, but it is believed to be a combination of genetic and environmental factors.

Psoriasis can be an uncomfortable and also embarrassing condition to deal with. Fortunately, there are a number of medical treatments and natural approaches that can help improve the symptoms and quality of life for those suffering with this condition.

SIGNS & SYMPTOMS

- Bleeding, itching, burning, and soreness of the skin
- Dry, red patches of skin covered with silvery scales
- Pus-filled blisters
- Small scaly spots
- Swollen and stiff joints
- Thickened, pitted, or ridged nails

Note: The signs and symptoms vary in severity from person to person. Psoriasis most commonly affects areas of the body that are exposed to friction, irritation, or injury, such as the knees, elbows, feet, lower back, and scalp. Psoriasis can affect fingernails and toenails, causing pitting, abnormal nail growth, and discolouration. Severe cases may cause the nail to crumble. It can also affect the armpits and groin (called inverse psoriasis) or the joints (called psoriatic arthritis).

RISK FACTORS

- Family history: About one in three people with psoriasis has a close relative who also has the condition.
- Immune system disorders, such as HIV or diabetes
- Obesity increases risk of inverse psoriasis (psoriasis in armpits, groin, skin folds, and under breasts).
- Stress hampers immune function and increases risk of psoriasis.
- Smoking increases the risk of psoriasis and also makes the disease more severe.

PSORIASIS TRIGGERS

There are certain factors that can trigger or worsen psoriasis, such as a skin injury (cut, bug bite, or severe sunburn) infection, extreme cold weather, smoking, heavy alcohol consumption, and use of certain medications such as lithium, beta-blockers, or anti-malaria drugs.

DOCTOR'S ORDERS

The goal of treatment is to interrupt the cycle that causes an increased production of skin cells, thereby reducing inflammation and plaque formation, and to remove scales.

Topical products are helpful for mild to moderate psoriasis. They work on reducing inflammation and itching. Examples include: corticosteroids, coal tar, salicylic acid, vitamin A and D derivatives, and anthralin. Moisturizers can help reduce itching, scaling, and dryness.

Light therapy (phototherapy) involves use of natural or artificial light. Light causes the activated T cells in the skin to die, thus slowing down skin cell turnover. Drawbacks of light therapy include skin irritation, sunburn, and increased risk of skin cancer.

Oral medication, such as retinoids (vitamin A derivatives), work by reducing the production of skin cells. Methotrexate helps psoriasis by decreasing the production of skin cells, suppressing inflammation, and reducing the release of histamine. There are also immune suppressants (asathioprine and cyclosporine), which are used for more severe cases. All of these drugs carry the risk of serious side effects so it is important to discuss the benefits versus risks with your doctor.

SHERRY'S NATURAL PRESCRIPTION

Dietary Recommendations

Foods to include:

- Essential fatty acids help to reduce inflammation. Eat more cold-water fish (salmon, herring, mackerel, and trout). Choose wild (not farmed) fish to avoid ingestion of toxic chemicals. Flaxseed and flaxseed oil are also good sources of EFAs.

- Fibre-rich foods (whole grains, vegetables, and fruits) aid detoxification.

- Orange, yellow, and green vegetables contain vitamin A, which may be deficient in those with psoriasis.

- Pumpkin seeds provide zinc, which is often deficient in those with psoriasis.

Foods to avoid:

- Alcohol can cause flare-ups and also decrease the effectiveness of treatments.

- Gluten, a protein present in wheat, rye and barley, and triticale, can be a trigger for some people.

- Saturated fat (red meat and dairy products) may worsen inflammation.

To determine if food sensitivities are triggering your psoriasis, try an elimination diet (see Appendix D).

Lifestyle Suggestions

- Work on identifying and avoiding your triggers. Stress, smoking, and food sensitivities are common triggers.

- Bathe daily in warm water to remove scales and calm inflamed skin. Add mineral or sea salts, bath oil (lavender), or oatmeal to the water and soak for at least 15 minutes. Avoid hot water and harsh soaps, which can make your symptoms worse.

- Apply a moisturizer after bathing and reapply as needed. Use a heavy cream or an ointment as they will keep the skin hydrated longer than lotions.

- Do not scratch, pick, or rub at the lesions; this will only make it worse.

- Spend some time in the sun. We produce a powerful form of vitamin D when our skin is exposed to sunlight and this vitamin D can improve skin lesions. However, too much sun (getting sunburn) can worsen the problem. Try 10–15 minutes in direct sunlight. When spending a longer time outdoors, apply a sunscreen to areas not affected with psoriasis to protect against sunburn.

Top Recommended Supplements

Fish oils: Contain beneficial fatty acids that help reduce inflammation. Some studies have found benefits with high doses of fish oils in improving skin lesions. Dosage: Choose a product with a high EPA concentration. One study found benefits with 3.6 g of EPA daily. Some research has also found benefits with applying fish oils (10 percent concentration) directly to the psoriatic lesions twice daily.

Oregon grape: Contains compounds that slow the rate of abnormal cell growth and reduce inflammation. Several studies have shown benefits for reducing symptoms, but it does not appear to be as effective as prescription creams. Dosage: Apply a cream containing 10 percent Oregon grape extract three times daily to the affected areas.

Complementary Supplements

Aloe vera: Helps to reduce inflammation and has antibacterial and antifungal properties. Some research has shown that it can reduce psoriasis symptoms. Dosage: Apply a cream that contains 0.5 percent aloe three to four times daily.

Capsaicin: An extract from cayenne pepper. Creams made from capsaicin are used to treat a number of pain-related conditions. Some research found that capsaicin cream may be helpful for psoriasis. Wash hands after application; avoid contact with eyes.

Celadrin: A blend of fatty acids that reduces inflammation, redness, and pain. Preliminary research suggests benefits for psoriasis. Dosage: Apply cream twice daily.

FINAL THOUGHTS

To improve the management of psoriasis, consider the following:

1. Eat more cold-water fish, pumpkin seeds, colourful vegetables, and whole grains.
2. Avoid alcohol and minimize saturated fat.
3. Reduce stress and don't smoke.
4. Spend 10–15 minutes daily outdoors in the sun.
5. Consider fish oil supplements and Oregon grape cream to reduce inflammation.

RESTLESS LEG SYNDROME

Restless leg syndrome or RLS is a neurological or nervous system disorder causing discomfort and abnormal sensations throughout the legs and sometimes into the pelvis and arms. For some, the sensations may feel as though insects are creeping on or in their legs. People with RLS feel a strong urge to move, stretch, flex, or shake their limbs to ease the discomfort. This restlessness may prevent them from sitting comfortably for extended periods of time. Symptoms of RLS often worsen in the evening, causing serious disruptions to sleep.

RLS may occur spontaneously (referred to as idiopathic) or may be triggered by an existing health condition, such as peripheral neuropathy, damage to the nerves in your hands and feet that is often due to chronic diseases such as diabetes and alcoholism. In many cases, there is no known cause for restless legs syndrome. It is thought that it may be due to an imbalance of the brain chemical dopamine, which sends messages to control muscle movement. Genetic factors may also be involved. Researchers have identified sites on the chromosomes where genes for RLS may be present.

RLS FACTS

Restless leg syndrome is very common—between 2 percent and 15 percent of people around the world suffer with this condition. Over 80 percent of people with RLS also experience uncontrollable movements of the arms or legs during sleep, a phenomenon called periodic limb movements in sleep (PLMS), which usually occur every minute or so throughout the night. These alarming movements wreak havoc on sleep habits.

SIGNS & SYMPTOMS

- Abnormal sensations deep in the legs or arms
- Itching, twitching, burning, throbbing, tugging, tingling, pins and needles, and pain
- Movement may help relieve symptoms temporarily

Note: The symptoms of RLS are worse in the evenings when a person is inactive, such as sitting or lying down or sleeping.

RISK FACTORS

- Age: More common in older adults
- Chronic disease such as diabetes, kidney disease, and Parkinson's disease
- Heredity: About 60 percent of people with RLS report a family member with the same condition.
- Lifestyle choices such as smoking or lack of exercise
- Medications (drugs used for nausea, depression, mood disorders, and seizures)
- Nervous system disorders

- Nutritional deficiencies, particularly low levels of iron, calcium, or magnesium

- Obesity

- Poor diet, such as excess caffeine, alcohol, or sugar

- Pregnancy (particularly the third trimester) and hormonal changes

- Smoking

- Stress

DOCTOR'S ORDERS

Many people do not go to the doctor for RLS until their symptoms have become intolerable, often due to insomnia. Consult with your doctor if you have experienced the symptoms of RLS for more than a week.

RLS is often the sign of an existing health problem, so the standard treatment is to first identify and then treat the underlying cause. This may involve blood tests or a general examination regarding overall health, diet, lifestyle, and prescription drug use. If an underlying cause, such as nutritional deficiencies, is identified and treated, the symptoms of RLS may decrease or disappear altogether.

To counter mild symptoms, a doctor may recommend lifestyle approaches as noted below, and, for severe cases, medication.

There are four types of prescription medications that are used:

Anticonvulsants, such as gabapentin (Neurontin) help ease the abnormal sensations.

Dopaminergic drugs boost dopamine levels, which help central nervous system function. Examples include pramipexole (Mirapex) and ropinirole (Requip).

Muscle relaxants and sedatives help promote relaxation and sleep, but they also cause drowsiness the next day and are addictive. Examples are clonazepam (Rivotril), lorazepam (Ativan), and temazepam (Restoril).

Opioids are narcotic pain killers, such as codeine and oxycodone (Percocet).

All of these medications have potential side effects and drug interactions. Make sure to discuss the benefits and risks with your doctor.

SHERRY'S NATURAL PRESCRIPTION

There are a variety of natural strategies that can be effective in managing the symptoms of RLS.

Dietary Recommendations

Foods to include:

- Eat small, frequent meals to keep blood sugar levels stabilized as hypoglycemia (low blood sugar) can trigger RLS.

- Whole grains, fruits, vegetables, nuts, and seeds contain essential vitamins and minerals that are needed to support the nerves and muscles.

Foods to avoid:

- Alcohol and caffeine can aggravate RLS symptoms. Minimize caffeine-containing products (including chocolate, coffee, tea, and soft drinks) for a few weeks to see if this helps.

- Refined starches (white bread) and sugar (soda pop and candy) can cause blood sugar fluctuations, which can worsen RLS.

Lifestyle Suggestions

- Get regular exercise. Aim for 30 minutes to one hour daily. This will help to reduce stress and improve sleep at night. Do not overdo it because vigorous exercise can exacerbate the symptoms of RLS.

- Do not sit for extended periods of time. Take regular stretching breaks when seated at a desk or in a car.

- Lose excess weight, which may cause or worsen RLS.

- Reduce your stress load. Try acupuncture, meditation, massage, and yoga.

- Don't smoke, as smoking can trigger or worsen symptoms.

- Get adequate sleep. Fatigue can worsen symptoms. Aim for seven to nine hours of sleep per night and establish good sleep hygiene habits (make your bedroom quiet and comfortable, do relaxing activities in the evening, and go to bed and get up at the same time).

- To manage symptoms, try warm or cold packs, or alternating therapies to reduce the sensations.

Top Recommended Supplements

Iron: A deficiency (even mild) can cause RLS. Studies have shown that when iron deficiency is the cause of RLS, supplementing can reduce the severity of the symptoms. Do not take iron supplements unless you have low iron levels (ask your doctor to check this) because too much iron can cause side effects. Dosage: Consult with your health care provider for dosage guidelines.

Magnesium: Helps to promote muscle relaxation and also improves sleep in those with RLS, according to preliminary research. Dosage: 300 mg at bedtime. Take along with 500 mg calcium to avoid loose stools. Calcium is also important for proper muscle and nerve function.

Multivitamin/mineral complex: Ensures that your body is getting all essential nutrients. Low levels of B-vitamins (especially B1, B6, B12, and folic acid) can impair muscle function and nerve health. B12 deficiency can cause peripheral neuropathy, which can trigger RLS. Dosage: Take daily.

Complementary Supplements

Melatonin: A hormone that is naturally secreted by the brain in response to darkness and regulates sleep/wake cycles. Supplements reduce the time needed to fall asleep, reduce nighttime wakening, and improve sleep quality. Melatonin has not been studied particularly for its effects on RLS, but may be helpful for managing insomnia. Dosage: 1–6 mg one hour before bed.

Valerian: An herb that is widely used for insomnia; it improves many aspects of sleep and is non-addictive. It also helps reduce stress and anxiety. Some formulas combine valerian with hops, passionflower, and other herbs that promote relaxation. Dosage: 600 mg half an hour to one hour before bed, or 2 mL of a tincture.

FINAL THOUGHTS

To relieve the discomfort of RLS, consider the following:

1. Eat small, frequent meals with lots of whole grains, vegetables, and fruit. Reduce or eliminate caffeine, sugar, and alcohol.
2. Don't smoke.
3. Get regular exercise and avoid sitting for extended periods of time without stretching.
4. Consider taking iron (if deficient), magnesium, and a multivitamin.
5. Consider taking melatonin or valerian to improve sleep.

ROSACEA

Rosacea is a type of inflammatory skin condition that causes flushing, red splotches, lesions or bumps, and broken blood vessels across the cheeks, chin, forehead, and nose. Rosacea is often mistakenly referred to as "adult acne" or "acne rosacea" because it afflicts adults. While rosacea may resemble acne in that the outbreaks can come and go, triggered by a variety of lifestyle factors, unlike acne, rosacea outbreaks do not cause blackheads or whiteheads, and may often be accompanied by burning, stinging, or chapped, dry skin. Rosacea is also associated with several eye conditions, including swollen, burning, itchy eyes called ocular rosacea. Some estimates suggest that up to two million Canadians suffer from various degrees of rosacea. Since this condition has a traumatic impact on sufferers, it is critical to find ways to control the symptoms and reduce outbreaks.

DON'T IGNORE ROSACEA

If left untreated, advanced cases of rosacea may cause a condition called rhinophyma in which the skin thickens unnaturally. While rare, rhinophyma may cause large warty growths to appear around the nose, and the skin to take on a wax-like appearance.

SIGNS & SYMPTOMS

- Burning, stinging, dry skin
- Facial flushing, with persistent redness (though cheeks are not warm to the touch)
- Itchy, sore eyes
- Red, inflamed pimples or bumps (erythema)
- Swollen nose (mostly in men)
- Visible red veins on the face and blood vessel lines

RISK FACTORS

- Age: Adults between the ages of 20 and 60
- Gender: Women are more commonly affected
- Hormonal changes (pregnancy and menopause)
- Having fair skin
- Heredity

Factors that may trigger or worsen rosacea include: use of birth control pills or drugs that affect blood vessels (vasodilators); caffeine; alcohol; hot or spicy foods or drinks; exposure to sun, wind, or cold temperatures; emotional stress; vigorous exercise; hot baths or saunas.

DOCTOR'S ORDERS

There is no cure for rosacea, but medications are often prescribed to help control symptoms and prevent the skin condition from progressing. For mild rosacea, doctors often recommend topical antibiotic creams. For more severe cases, antibiotic pills may be prescribed in combination with antibiotic creams.

Azelaic acid cream is a new product available in Canada for the treatment of rosacea. This acid is found naturally in wheat, rye, and barley and has antimicrobial effects. Studies have found that it can reduce rosacea symptoms. One study that compared it to metronidazole (a commonly used antibiotic) found that azelaic acid provided better results for improving skin redness and pimples.

For advanced cases of rosacea, cosmetic surgery such as laser surgery or dermabrasion may be recommended. Dermabrasion is a cosmetic procedure that "sands" or "finishes" the top layer of the skin, giving it a smoother appearance.

Do not use over-the-counter products formulated for treating common (teenage) acne as the main ingredients (salicylic acid and benzyol peroxide) can worsen rosacea.

SHERRY'S NATURAL PRESCRIPTION

Dietary Recommendations

Foods to include:

- Drink at least eight glasses of filtered water daily.

- Eat a fibre-rich diet (whole grains, vegetables, and fruits) to support the body's natural elimination and detoxification process. These foods also contain vital nutrients (vitamin C, B-vitamins, and zinc) for skin health.

- Essential fatty acids help reduce inflammation. Eat three or more servings per week of cold-water fish, along with flaxseed and other nuts and seeds.

- Green tea is a potent antioxidant and detoxifier. Drink green tea instead of coffee or black teas. A green food supplement may support improved digestion and detoxification.

- If you are taking antibiotics, eat yogurt and kefir to replenish the friendly bacteria.

Foods to avoid:

- Avoid hot, spicy foods and beverages, as they can worsen symptoms.

- Minimize salt and alcohol, which can dilate blood vessels and worsen symptoms.

- Reduce stimulants in your diet such as chocolate and coffee.

- Saturated fats (red meat and dairy) can worsen inflammation.

Keep a food journal to determine potential triggers.

Lifestyle Suggestions

- Reduce stress; try stress-reduction techniques such as massage.

- Avoid washing with hot water, or using scrub brushes or face cloths.

- Use a gentle cleanser and moisturizer daily. Look for products that contain soothing ingredients such as aloe vera, burdock, calendula, chamomile, rosehips, and vitamin E. Look for the words "safe for sensitive skin" or "hypoallergenic."

- Avoid extended sunlight exposure as the sun is a common trigger. Use sunscreen with at least SPF 15 when going outdoors and wear a wide-brim hat.

- Consider stress-reduction therapies such as massage, yoga, and meditation. Exercise is also a great way to reduce stress and boost confidence.

- Avoid smoking and second-hand smoke as nicotine damages blood vessels.

Top Recommended Supplements

Golden chamomile cream: Also known as *Chrysanthellum indicum*, it helps to reduce redness and inflammation. Look for a product that contains a 1 percent concentration, and apply twice daily.

Green tea: Has antioxidant and anti-inflammatory properties. Some research has shown that green tea cream can reduce redness and pustules. Look for a product that contains 2 percent polyphenone and apply twice daily.

••

RESEARCH HIGHLIGHT

A large study involving 246 people with rosacea examined the safety and effectiveness of a cream containing 1 percent *Chrysanthellum indicum* extract (applied twice a day) or placebo. After 12 weeks, the *Chrysanthellum indicum* cream significantly improved rosacea symptoms, including facial redness, compared to placebo. Adverse reactions were mild and did not differ compared with the placebo group (*Journal of the European Academy of Dermatology*, 2005: 19; 564–568).

••

Complementary Treatments

Digestive enzymes: It is thought that some people with rosacea have digestive problems and low stomach acid. Some research has found benefits with digestive enzymes supplements. Dosage: One or two capsules with each meal.

Essential fatty acids: Help to reduce inflammation. One preliminary study of a topical product called Celadrin (mixture of bovine fatty acids) found that it reduced inflammation and redness. Oral supplements of fish oils, borage, or evening primrose may also be helpful. Dosage: Follow label directions.

Multivitamin/mineral complex: Those with rosacea may be deficient in certain nutrients such as the B-vitamins and zinc. Consider taking a daily multivitamin/mineral formula. Ask your pharmacist for a recommendation based on your age and lifestyle. Follow label directions.

FINAL THOUGHTS

To manage rosacea, consider the following:

1. Identify triggers of your outbreaks and reduce exposure to those triggers.
2. Eat lots of fibre-rich foods such as fruits, vegetables, legumes, nuts and seeds, whole grains, fish, and flaxseed.
3. Reduce stress and minimize sun exposure (wear sunscreen).
4. Use a gentle facial cleanser that contains soothing ingredients such as aloe vera, calendula, and rosehips.
5. Use a topical cream containing golden chamomile or green tea regularly.

SEASONAL AFFECTIVE DISORDER (SAD)

Seasonal affective disorder (SAD) is a form of depression that follows the seasons. It typically occurs during the winter months and goes away during the spring and summer, although a small number of people experience depression during the summer.

Approximately 4 percent of Canadians suffer from SAD. The exact cause is unknown. However, it may result from light deprivation that upsets the body's internal clock, or from seasonal variations in serotonin (levels are lower in the winter and a deficiency of serotonin can cause depression) or melatonin (levels are higher during darker months, which causes sleepiness).

Fortunately, there are a number of lifestyle measures and supplements that can improve emotional well-being and reduce SAD symptoms.

SIGNS & SYMPTOMS

- Cravings for carbohydrates (sweets and starchy foods)
- Depression
- Difficulty concentrating
- Fatigue and increased sleep
- Feelings of hopelessness and sadness
- Increased appetite and weight gain
- Irritability and anxiety
- Loss of interest in sex
- Social withdrawal
- Thoughts of suicide

RISK FACTORS

- Family history
- Gender (women are at greater risk)
- Light deprivation (living in northern areas where there is less sunlight)
- Season: It most often occurs during December, January, and February
- Stress

DOCTOR'S ORDERS

Medical treatment of SAD involves light therapy and/or medication. Light therapy should be tried first, as it is highly effective—80 percent of people experience improvement. A specially made light box providing full-spectrum light is used for 30–60 minutes. Benefits may be noticed in as little as a few days to a week. Light therapy should be used daily during the fall and winter until symptoms subside and enough daylight is available.

If light therapy doesn't help, doctors may recommend medication. The selective serotonin reuptake inhibitors (SSRIs) drugs raise serotonin levels and help alleviate symptoms. However, they cause numerous side effects and drug interactions. Examples include Paxil, Prozac, Zoloft, and Effexor.

SHERRY'S NATURAL PRESCRIPTION

Dietary Recommendations

Foods to include:

- Vegetables, fruits, whole grains, nuts, and seeds provide vitamins, minerals, and essential fatty acids, which may be depleted in those with depression.

- Turkey, chicken, tuna, salmon, legumes, nuts, and seeds contain the amino acid tryptophan, which elevates serotonin production.

- Fish is also a good source of essential fatty acids.

- Eat small, frequent meals to maintain energy levels and mood.

Foods to avoid:

- Sugar and refined carbohydrates may temporarily elevate your mood, but the effect is short term and these foods cause blood sugar imbalances, mood swings, and irritability.

- Caffeine is a stimulant that offers a temporary rush of energy followed by fatigue and irritability, plus it depletes nutrients from your body. Have no more than one cup per day.

- Processed and fast foods often contain chemicals and preservatives that may upset brain chemistry.

- Alcohol is a depressant and should be minimized or avoided completely.

Lifestyle Suggestions

- Regular exercise; engage in fall/winter activities outside to maximize available sunshine. With proper winter clothing, walking, skating, and skiing can be a great way to get exercise and sunshine, plus exercise is a natural mood elevator, improves sleep, and helps combat stress.

- Increase the amount of light in your environment—sit near a window, open blinds, and trim any trees that block your exposure to the sun.

- Try light therapy. Specially made light boxes or light visors are available that provide broad-spectrum light. These are used for 30 minutes to several hours each day. Benefits may be noticed in as little as a few days. However, it may take a week or longer to get the full effect. Light therapy should be used regularly during the fall and winter until symptoms subside and enough daylight is available.

- Acupuncture has been found to be beneficial for depression. It may work by stimulating the production of neurotransmitters.

- Massage and reflexology relieve stress and tension, and promote relaxation.

Top Recommended Supplements

5-Hydroxytryptophan (5-HTP): A substance used by the body to create serotonin. Research shows benefits for depression. It may cause nausea, which can be minimized by taking an enteric-coated product. Dosage: 100–200 mg three times daily.

Fish oils: Rich in omega-3 fatty acids, which are essential for the nervous system and neurotransmitter function. Levels may be depleted in those with depression. Studies show benefits for depression, especially for those not getting an adequate response to antidepressant drugs. Dosage: 3–9 g daily.

S-adenosylmethionine (SAMe): Supports the production of neurotransmitters (serotonin, dopamine, and norepinephrine); is shown to be beneficial for depression. SAMe is well tolerated, has benefits for joint and liver health, and a quick onset of action (two weeks). Dosage: 400–1,600 mg daily on an empty stomach; start with a low dose and gradually increase if needed.

....

AVOID EXCESS SEROTONIN

Be cautious about combining products that elevate serotonin, such as SSRI or MAO-I drugs, St. John's wort, SAMe, and 5-HTP, together. This should be done only under the supervision of a health care professional, as excess serotonin can cause serotonin syndrome. Symptoms include confusion, anxiety, racing heart, nausea, and muscle spasms.

....

Complementary Supplements

B-Complex: B-vitamins (such as B12 and folic acid) may be deficient with SAD. Folic acid works with SAMe to boost neurotransmitter levels. Several studies have found benefits. Dosage: Take 400–1,000 mcg of folic acid along with 50–100 mg of other B-vitamins daily to support brain function.

Vitamin D: Vitamin D is produced by the body in response to sun exposure and levels may be depleted in those with SAD. Preliminary studies have found benefits with supplements. Dosage: 400–800 IU daily.

Note: St. John's wort is helpful for mild to moderate depression. However, it should not be used with light therapy for SAD due to the risk of light sensitivity, skin rash, and eye damage.

FINAL THOUGHTS

To improve mood and reduce the symptoms of SAD, consider the following:

1. Minimize sugar, refined/processed foods, caffeine, and alcohol.
2. Eat more tryptophan-containing foods.
3. Exercise regularly to reduce stress and improve mood and sleep.
4. Maximize your exposure to natural light and try light therapy.
5. Supplements of SAMe or 5-HTP, fish oils, B-vitamins, and vitamin D can reduce symptoms and improve mood.

SHINGLES (HERPES ZOSTER)

Shingles, known medically as herpes zoster, is a viral infection that causes a painful rash and blisters. Shingles is caused by the varicella-zoster virus, the same virus that causes chickenpox. About 95 percent of North American children will contract chickenpox before age 18. After you get chickenpox, the virus lies dormant in your nerves and years later it may reactivate as shingles. About one in 10 healthy adults who have had chickenpox eventually develop shingles. With shingles the virus travels along a nerve pathway to your skin, causing rash and blistering and pain. It typically affects the torso, but it can also affect an area around the eyes, face, or cheeks.

While it can be painful, in most cases shingles clears up in a few weeks. However, about one in five people develop a complication from damaged nerve fibres called postherpetic neuralgia, which causes skin pain and sensitivity that can last for several months.

The best way to help prevent a shingles outbreak is to manage stress levels and follow a healthy lifestyle. Once the virus is reactivated, there are some medical treatments and supplements that can help speed recovery and ease symptoms.

THE HERPES FAMILY

Varicella-zoster is part of a group of viruses called herpes viruses, which includes the viruses that cause cold sores, genital herpes, and chickenpox/shingles. While the symptoms among these viruses vary widely, they all can lie dormant in your nervous system for years after an initial infection and then be reactivated and cause infection.

SIGNS & SYMPTOMS

- Clear, fluid-filled blisters

- Fever, chills, and headache

- Pain, burning, tingling, itching, numbness, or extreme sensitivity in a certain area of the body

- Red rash

- Upset stomach

Note: Shingles can lead to other complications, such as postherpetic neuralgia (nerve pain), inflammation of the brain (encephalitis), and other neurological problems. If shingles occurs on your face, it can cause hearing problems, temporary or permanent blindness, and loss of facial movement (paralysis), which is rare. The blisters can also get infected if they are picked or not properly treated.

CHICKENPOX VS. SHINGLES

While chicken pox and shingles are caused by the same virus, chickenpox often strikes in childhood and shingles in adulthood. They both can cause itching, but chickenpox causes intense itching and the blisters can affect the entire body whereas shingles typically affects only one area. Shingles is also more painful.

RISK FACTORS

- Age: Most commonly occurs after age 50
- Previous infection with chickenpox
- Weakened immune system caused by stress or illness (HIV, diabetes)

SHINGLES IS CONTAGIOUS

A person with shingles can pass the varicella-zoster virus to anyone who hasn't had chickenpox before. This usually occurs through direct contact with the blisters or open sores of the shingles rash. Once infected, the person will develop chickenpox (not shingles). Until the blisters scab over, those with shingles should avoid contact with:

- Anyone who has a weak immune system (HIV, diabetes)
- Anyone who has never had chickenpox
- Newborn babies
- Pregnant women (chickenpox infection can be dangerous for a developing baby)

DOCTOR'S ORDERS

In most cases shingles usually heals within three to five weeks. If the infection is caught early (within the first 48–72 hours), there are medications that can speed healing and reduce the risk of complications. These drugs include acyclovir (Zovirax), valacyclovir (Valtrex), and famciclovir (Famvir).

Painkillers can be used to manage severe pain, such as Tylenol or ibuprofen (Motrin). Topical ointment containing capsaicin (Zostrix, Zostrix-HP) can also help to reduce nerve pain.

SHERRY'S NATURAL PRESCRIPTION

Dietary Recommendations

Foods to include:

- B-vitamins support nervous system function. Good food sources include whole grains, legumes, seeds, poultry, fish, and fortified soy and rice beverages.
- Citrus fruits, berries, broccoli, Brussels sprouts, red peppers, and tomatoes contain vitamin C, which supports the immune system. Orange, yellow, and red vegetables contain beta-carotene, which also supports immune function and skin recovery.

Foods to avoid:

- Sugar can hamper immune function. Minimize candy, sweets, and soft drinks.

Lifestyle Suggestions

- Acupuncture may help reduce the pain of shingles and postherpetic neuralgia.

- Do not pick or squeeze the blisters as this can lead to infection. Keep the affected area clean. Apply cool, wet compresses to relieve pain.

- Get plenty of rest. The viral infection can make you more tired and you will need more sleep to recover.

- Moderate exercise such as walking can help relieve stress and pain and support healthy immune function.

- Reduce stress levels. Stress can trigger an outbreak and hamper recovery. Try yoga, breathing techniques, and tai chi.

- Soak in a tub of lukewarm water with bath salts or oatmeal to help relieve itching. Apply calamine lotion afterward or a product containing calendula, chamomile, or lavender.

SHINGLES AND STRESS

Several studies have linked high levels of stress to outbreaks of shingles.

Stress, which is our internal reaction to external events, can hamper immune function, making you more susceptible to infections. It can also delay recovery. Finding effective ways to cope with stress is essential.

Top Recommended Supplements

Capsaicin cream: Capsaicin is extracted from cayenne pepper. Studies have shown benefits for reducing pain associated with postherpetic neuralgia. Dosage: 0.075 percent cream applied three to four times daily. Wash hands after application and avoid getting in the eyes, as it can burn.

Proteolytic enzymes: Include papain (from papaya), bromelain (from pineapple), and trypsin and chymotrypsin (extracted from the pancreas of various animals). They aid digestion and are thought to benefit shingles by decreasing the body's inflammatory response and regulating immune response to the virus. Dosage: Varies with the product; follow label instructions or consult your natural health care provider.

RESEARCH HIGHLIGHT

A study of 190 people with shingles compared the effects of proteolytic enzymes to the standard antiviral drug acyclovir. Participants were treated for 14 days and their pain was assessed at various intervals. Both groups had similar pain relief, but the enzyme-treated group experienced fewer side effects. Similar results were seen in another study of 90 people with shingles (*Fortschritte der Medizin*, 1995: 113; 43–48 and *Phytomedicine*, 1995: 2; 7–15).

Complementary Supplements

B-complex: Helps to support the nervous system, which is under attack with the herpes zoster virus. Dosage: Take 50–100 mg of B-vitamins daily.

Vitamin C: Supports immune function and aids skin recovery. Dosage: 500 mg twice daily.

Vitamin E: May be helpful for reducing pain associated with postherpetic neuralgia. Dosage: 1,200–1,600 IU daily. Vitamin E oil (30 IU per gram) can be applied to the skin to aid recovery of blisters. Several months of taking vitamin E continuously may be needed in order to see an improvement.

FINAL THOUGHTS

To manage the pain of shingles and speed recovery, consider the following:

1. Eat a healthful diet with lots of colourful vegetables and fruits, whole grains, legumes, seeds, poultry, fish, and fortified soy and rice beverages.
2. Minimize intake of sugar.
3. Reduce stress and get regular exercise and lots of rest.
4. To soothe itching, soak in an oatmeal bath and apply cream containing calendula, chamomile, or lavender.
5. Consider proteolytic enzymes to promote healing and capsaicin cream for treatment of postherpetic neuralgia.

SINUSITIS

Sinusitis is an inflammation of the sinuses, the air-filled hollow cavities around your nose and nasal passages. Sinusitis develops when the mucous membranes of your upper respiratory tract (nose, pharynx, sinuses, and throat) become inflamed. The swelling obstructs the sinus openings and prevents mucus from draining normally. This creates a moist environment that can breed infection. It also makes it difficult for you to breathe and causes pain around the nose, eyes, and forehead.

Sinusitis can be either acute (short term) or chronic. Acute sinusitis often develops as a result of the common cold virus. Most colds resolve within a week or two, but nearly 2 percent develop into acute sinusitis. A virus can damage the tissues in the sinuses and then bacteria can invade, creating an infection. Acute sinusitis can also result from a fungal infection, especially in those with diabetes or compromised immune function.

Sinusitis is considered chronic when it lasts longer than 12 weeks. This is usually a sign of a suppressed immune system, which leads to recurrent respiratory infections and chronic inflammation of the sinuses. Smoking, allergies, and exposure to irritants can also cause chronic sinusitis.

There are many things that can be done from a dietary and lifestyle perspective to prevent and manage sinusitis. Nutritional supplements can also play a role in helping to speed healing and reduce inflammation.

SIGNS & SYMPTOMS

- Bad breath
- Cough
- Difficulty breathing through your nose
- Fatigue
- Fever
- Nasal congestion and greenish-yellow discharge
- Nausea
- Pain under the eyes, around the nose, cheeks, jaw, or forehead
- Redness of the skin over the sinus caused by increased blood flow to the capillaries
- Reduced sense of smell or taste

Note: If untreated, sinusitis may develop into a chronic condition, such as asthma. If it is severe and untreated, it can also lead to meningitis.

SINUS HEADACHE OR MIGRAINE?

According to a study by the Headache Care Center, 97 percent of people who thought they were sinus headache sufferers actually had symptoms of migraine as defined by the criteria of the International Headache Society. Both migraines and sinus headache, which can cause pain in the area round the sinuses and eyes to tear, can be triggered by weather. They differ in the origin of the problem. Sinus pain (headache) is due to inflammation and/or infection of the sinuses. Migraines cause inflammation of nerves and blood vessels in the head. When the trigeminal nerve is affected, it sends signals to the sinus region, causing sinus pain. See your doctor for proper diagnosis as the treatment of these headaches is different.

RISK FACTORS

- Allergies trigger inflammation that may block your sinuses
- Dental infection (abscessed tooth)
- Deviated septum (the wall between the nostrils)
- Having a respiratory infection such as a cold or flu
- Having cystic fibrosis, gastroesophageal reflux disease, or a weakened immune system (e.g., HIV)
- Nasal polyps
- Smoking or exposure to air pollution

DOCTOR'S ORDERS

Most cases of sinusitis subside within a week or two and rarely require antibiotics. If your doctor suspects you have a bacterial infection, then an antibiotic may be necessary. If allergies are suspected, you may be referred to an allergist to identify your triggers and develop a treatment strategy.

Over-the-counter nasal decongestants, such as pseudoephedrine (Sudafed) and oxymetazoline (Dristan), can help relieve congestion and nasal stuffiness. Both oral and nasal decongestants can cause racing heart, increased blood pressure, insomnia, and they can interact with certain medications. They should not be used longer than three days because of the risk of rebound congestion. Saline nasal sprays are a safer alternative. They lubricate the nasal passages and reduce stuffiness without the side effects of the decongestants. If necessary, pain relievers such as Tylenol or Motrin can be taken.

SHERRY'S NATURAL PRESCRIPTION

Dietary Recommendations

Foods to include:

- Drink plenty of fluids (water, juice, and herbal tea) to dilute mucus secretions and promote drainage. Look for herbal teas that contain marshmallow, licorice, and slippery elm.
- Elderberry juice has antiviral activity.

- Fish and flaxseed contain essential fatty acids that help to reduce inflammation.

- Fruits and vegetables (especially berries, citrus, garlic, onions, and ginger) provide important nutrients and compounds that support immune function.

- Horseradish helps break up mucus. Have ½ tsp to 1 tsp of the freshly grated root three times per day.

Foods to avoid:

- Alcohol can worsen swelling in the sinuses.

- Dairy products may worsen mucus secretions.

- Minimize salt as it can be dehydrating.

- Sugar can hamper immune function.

Many people with chronic sinusitis have food allergies. If you suspect food allergies, try an elimination diet (see Appendix D) to determine which foods are triggering your symptoms.

Lifestyle Suggestions

- Don't smoke, and avoid second-hand smoke as tobacco is very irritating to the nasal passages and causes inflammation.

- Minimize exposure to pollution and known allergens and irritants, such as perfumes, chemicals, and preservatives.

- Use an air purifier in your home and a humidifier if the air is dry.

- Do a therapeutic steam inhalation by leaning over a bowl of hot water with a few drops of eucalyptus oil.

- Apply warm compresses around your nose, cheeks, and eyes to ease pain.

- Acupuncture and craniosacral therapy are helpful in clearing the sinuses and relieving nasal congestion and pressure.

Top Recommended Supplements

Bromelain: An enzyme derived from pineapple, which has anti-inflammatory properties and has been shown in studies to reduce symptoms of sinusitis. Dosage: 250–500 mg three times daily between meals.

Echinacea: Helps support immune function, and studies show that it can reduce the severity and frequency of cold symptoms. It may also help prevent a cold from developing into sinusitis. Look for Echinacea purpurea. Dosage: 300–600 mg capsules twice daily or 2–4 mL tincture four to six times daily at the first sign of a cold for seven to 10 days. Some products combine echinacea with astragalus, which also has antiviral and antibacterial properties.

Vitamin C: Supports immune function and helps prevent oxidative damage to the lungs. Studies have shown that it can reduce the severity and duration of the common cold, which may reduce the likelihood of complications, such as sinusitis. Dosage: 500 mg daily.

Complementary Supplements

Aged garlic extract: Contains antioxidant compounds that help support immune function. When taken regularly, it may help prevent colds and bacterial infections. Dosage: 600 mg daily.

American ginseng: Helps to prevent and relieve colds and flu and may help to prevent these respiratory infections from leading to sinusitis. Look for COLD-fX, a patented extract of polysaccharides derived from North American ginseng that has been clinically studied. Dosage: See package for directions.

Fish oils: Contain essential fatty acids that help reduce inflammation. One study in children found that daily fish oil supplements reduced the risk of recurrent respiratory tract infections. Dosage: Children should take 15 mg EPA plus DHA per pound body weight per day; adults should take 1–3 g EPA plus DHA daily.

N-acetylcysteine (NAC): An amino acid derivative that helps break up mucus and clear the sinuses. Dosage: 300–600 mg daily.

FINAL THOUGHTS

To improve healing of sinusitis and prevent it from occurring, consider the following:

1. Eat more fruits, vegetables, fish, onions, garlic, ginger, and horseradish.
2. Drink lots of fluids, especially water and herbal teas.
3. Avoid smoking and being around smoke and other irritants.
4. Do a steam inhalation with eucalyptus oil.
5. Consider supplements of bromelain and vitamin C. Echinacea may help to shorten the duration of a cold.

STRESS

Stress has become an all too familiar complaint today, hence the commonly heard phrase "stressed out." While we think of stress as an outside force, it is actually how we react internally to external stimuli, whether it is family pressures, deadlines at work, or being stuck in traffic.

This innate mechanism was designed to help us cope with short bursts of stress, such as that caused by the attack of a predator. Our bodies have not adapted to handle the chronic stress so common today, which leads to damage and destruction throughout the body.

According to Dr. Hans Selye, one of the founders of the Canadian Institute of Stress, the physical experience of continuous stress has three stages: alarm, resistance, and exhaustion. In the alarm stage, our bodies engage in their biologically programmed fight-or-flight mode. The stress hormones catecholamines (adrenaline and noradrenaline) and glucocorticoids (cortisol) are released. Secreted by the adrenal glands, these hormones prepare the body to fight. When this occurs, the body enters a catabolic state; that is, it begins to break down fuels (fats, stored sugar) to provide energy. Our senses are heightened and heart rate, blood pressure, blood volume, and pulmonary (lung) tone increase to enhance the function of the heart and lungs. At the resistance stage, the body works to heal itself by adapting resistance mechanisms to counter the negative effects of stress. If the stress continues, we may eventually fall into the exhaustion stage. Mental and physical fatigue sets in, and stress-related disorders may surface.

Numerous studies have linked stress to increased risk of heart disease, cancer, diabetes, high cholesterol and blood pressure, anxiety, depression, memory loss, insomnia, muscle tension, obesity, fatigue, low libido, erectile dysfunction, and menstrual cycle disturbances.

It is absolutely critical to find positive ways to handle stress. There are a variety of lifestyle, nutritional, and supplemental approaches discussed in this chapter.

SUPER STRESSED

Did you know that nearly 50 percent of adults suffer adverse health effects from stress? In fact, stress-related ailments account for between 75 percent and 90 percent of all visits to the doctor, and stress is linked to the six leading causes of death—heart disease, cancer, lung ailments, accidents, cirrhosis of the liver, and suicide.

SIGNS & SYMPTOMS

- Changes in appetite and weight
- Decreased concentration, memory problems
- Depression, mood swings
- Digestive problems (upset stomach, ulcers, colitis, constipation, and diarrhea)
- Exacerbation of asthma or arthritis

S

Stress

- Fatigue

- Headaches

- High blood pressure

- Immune deficiency and increased risk of infection

- Infertility

- Insomnia

- Loss of libido

- Muscle tension

- Nervousness, anxiety, irritability

- Skin disorders (rash, hives)

RISK FACTORS

Almost any aspect of life, from the weather to work, traffic, and family relationships, can cause stress depending on how you respond to these events. Even small things such as spilling your morning coffee or being low on gas might trigger stress. Here are some of the most common triggers for stress:

- Being the victim of a crime or being in an accident

- Family demands and disagreements

- Financial concerns and taxes

- Holidays and special events

- Home-related concerns such as renovations, buying or selling, and moving

- Illness or death of a loved one

- Unexpected events or events we cannot control

- Work, new work, or loss of work

DOCTOR'S ORDERS

Doctors frequently see patients only after the negative effects of prolonged stress have started. As a result, they are often left to treat the visible complaint, such as insomnia, blood pressure, ulcers, or depression. In most cases, these secondary health concerns are treated with prescription medications, but healthy eating, sleep, and stress management should be the central focus.

The main class of drugs used to treat anxiety and stress include the benzodiazepines, namely, alprazolam (Xanax), clonazepam (Rivotril), diazepam (Valium), and lorazepam (Ativan). These drugs work quickly (30–60 minutes) to ease anxiety and promote relaxation, but they are addictive and have numerous side effects, including drowsiness, loss of coordination, dizziness, and impaired memory.

People suffering from chronic stress may also want to seek the help of a mental health professional to identify and resolve issues in their life, or to provide support for coping.

SHERRY'S NATURAL PRESCRIPTION

Dietary Recommendations

Foods to include:

- Drink lots of purified water and calming herbal teas containing chamomile, lemon balm, and passionflower.

- Eat a diet rich in low-glycemic carbohydrates such as whole grains, legumes, and fruits and vegetables. These foods provide essential nutrients that are needed to help the body deal with stress.

- Fish and flaxseed contain essential fatty acids that are necessary for proper brain and nervous system function.

Foods to avoid:

- Caffeine and alcohol can trigger and worsen stress. Wean off caffeine slowly to avoid withdrawal symptoms, which can worsen anxiety. Avoid soft drinks, which are high in caffeine, sugar, and alcohol. Limit alcohol to one to two drinks per day.

- Fast foods and processed foods (snack foods) are high in saturated fat and sugar and low in nutritional value. These foods can trigger anxiety and mood swings.

- Sugary foods cause fluctuations in blood sugar, which may cause mood swings and worsen stress. Cut down on candy, baked goods, condiments, and snack foods.

Lifestyle Suggestions

- Develop a positive attitude toward life's many challenges and work on managing anger and hostility. Practise controlling or redirecting your frustrations into something positive.

- Train your mind to react differently to current triggers.

- Learn to be more flexible and let go of things you cannot control.

- Develop strategies to deal with stressful situations or avoid the things that cause the most stress. (For example, listen to music, news, or an audio book while driving; bring a book to the doctor's office and read while you are waiting.)

- Proper time-management and organizational skills help prevent stressful situations from occurring.

- Embrace friends and family. Studies show that close friendships contribute to less stress and a longer life.

- Get regular exercise. Exercise releases nervous energy and induces a calming effect. You can do vigorous exercise such as running or calming exercises such as yoga.

- Get adequate sleep at night. Sleep allows the body to recuperate and regenerate. When we are tired, we are more susceptible to stress.

- Deep breathing calms the body and slows heart rate. Consider meditation or acupuncture to promote calming.

- Massage helps loosen muscle tension caused by stress and improves circulation.

- Don't smoke. Many smokers light up when they are stressed, but smoking actually worsens stress and causes nervous system damage.

Top Recommended Supplements

B-vitamins: Essential for nervous system and adrenal function; a deficiency can cause anxiety and worsen the response to stress. Dosage: Look for a product that provides 50–100 mg of the B-vitamins and take daily.

Calcium and Magnesium: Promote calming and relaxation, and support muscle and nerve function. Levels of these minerals are depleted by stress and anxiety. Dosage: 500 mg calcium and 200 mg magnesium, three times daily with meals.

Lactium: A milk protein that contains bioactive peptide with anti-stress properties. Several studies have shown that Lactium can help reduce the physical and mental effects and symptoms of stress. Dosage: 150 mg twice daily as needed.

Suntheanine: A patented extract of theanine, an amino acid in green tea. It promotes calming and relaxation without drowsiness or addiction. Dosage: 50–200 mg daily.

Complementary Supplements

Panax ginseng: An adaptogenic herb that helps reduce the response to stress. It also supports physical and mental performance, immune function, and adrenal gland function, all of which can be hampered by stress. Dosage: 100–200 mg daily.

Relora: A combination of magnolia and phellodendron, which reduces stress without causing drowsiness. It is non-addictive. Dosage: 250 mg three times daily.

Rhodiola: Helps reduce fatigue and improve mental alertness when under stress. Dosage: 170–185 mg daily, providing 4.5 mg of salidroside.

Valerian: An herb with relaxing and calming properties. It causes drowsiness, so it can be helpful for those with insomnia due to stress. Dosage: 300–500 mg of an extract an hour before bed.

Vitamin C: Helps the adrenal glands in dealing with the stress response. It also helps in the production of important neurotransmitters that are required for mood and proper sleep, and it provides support for cardiovascular and immune function. Dosage: 500 mg twice daily.

FINAL THOUGHTS

To better manage stress and reduce its adverse health effects, consider the following:

1. Eat a healthy diet that is rich in vegetables, fruits, legumes, nuts, and seeds, and choose lean protein and healthy fats.
2. Reduce or eliminate processed fast foods, caffeine, refined starches, sugar, alcohol, and tobacco.
3. Identify your stress triggers and work on strategies to cope more effectively. Try yoga, tai chi, meditation, massage, and acupuncture to promote relaxation.
4. Get regular exercise and adequate sleep.
5. Consider taking B-vitamins, calcium, magnesium, Lactium, and Suntheanine.

STROKE

A stroke, which is also called a brain attack, is sudden loss of brain function that develops when an artery supplying oxygen-rich blood to the brain becomes blocked or ruptures. Without adequate blood flow, brain cells begin to die within minutes. Areas of the brain commonly affected by stroke are those that control movement, speech, vision, and sensation. Stroke is a medical emergency that requires immediate treatment to minimize damage to the brain and disability.

There are two types of stroke: ischemic and hemorrhagic. About 80 percent of all strokes are ischemic strokes. They occur when blood clots or other particles block arteries to your brain and cause severely reduced blood flow (ischemia). This deprives your brain cells of oxygen and nutrients, and cells may begin to die within minutes. Hemorrhagic stroke occurs when a blood vessel in your brain leaks or ruptures. This can result from a number of conditions that affect your blood vessels, such as uncontrolled high blood pressure (hypertension) and weak spots in your blood vessel walls (aneurysms).

Stroke is a major cause of death in Canada, but your chance of surviving a stroke today is much greater than it was a few decades ago. About half of all people who have a stroke recover to some degree, although about one-third of first strokes are fatal, so early detection and prevention are critical. The various factors known to increase your risk of stroke are outlined below. Many of them are lifestyle related and within your control.

SIGNS & SYMPTOMS

- Confusion or memory loss

- Problems with spatial orientation or perception

- Sudden difficulty speaking, seeing clearly, or understanding speech

- Sudden dizziness and loss of balance and coordination

- Sudden massive headache, which may be accompanied by a stiff neck, facial pain, and pain around the eyes

- Sudden numbness, weakness, or paralysis of your face, arm, or leg, which often occurs on one side of your body

Unfortunately, some people have no warning signs of a stroke and it happens suddenly. Some people may have a mini-stroke called a transient ischemic attack (TIA) before a major stroke. A TIA is a temporary interruption of blood flow to a part of your brain. It causes the same signs and symptoms as a stroke, but it lasts for a short time (few minutes to hours) and then disappears. A TIA represents a serious risk that a full-blown stroke may follow.

RISK FACTORS

- Age: More common in older adults

- Diabetes is a major risk factor for stroke because it increases the risk of high blood pressure and atherosclerosis; diabetes also interferes with your body's ability to break down blood clots, increasing your risk of ischemic stroke.

- Estrogen therapy: Taking birth control pills or estrogen therapy for menopause increases your risk; the risk is higher for smokers and those over 35 years.

- Family history: Having a parent or sibling who had a stroke or TIA

- Gender: Strokes affect men and women about equally, but women are more likely to die of stroke than are men.

- Heart disease: Having congestive heart failure, a previous heart attack, an infection of a heart valve (endocarditis), an abnormal heart rhythm (atrial fibrillation), aortic or mitral valve disease, valve replacement, or a hole in the upper chambers of the heart will increase risk.

- High blood pressure weakens and damages blood vessels in and around your brain, leaving them vulnerable to atherosclerosis and hemorrhage.

- High homocysteine level: This amino acid occurs naturally in your blood, but when it is elevated, it increases the risk of heart and blood vessel damage.

- High LDL cholesterol and triglycerides increase your risk of atherosclerosis; in contrast, high levels of HDL (good) cholesterol reduce your risk of atherosclerosis by removing cholesterol from your body through your liver.

- Obesity increases the risk of high blood pressure, heart disease, atherosclerosis, and diabetes, all of which increase your risk of a stroke.

- Personal history: Having one TIA or stroke increases the risk of another one.

- Race: Blacks are at greater risk of stroke partly due to a higher prevalence of high blood pressure and diabetes.

- Smoking contributes to plaques in your arteries and makes your heart work harder by increasing your heart rate and blood pressure; it also reduces oxygen delivery to your tissues, including the brain.

- Stress increases blood pressure, cholesterol, and risk of atherosclerosis, all major risk factors for stroke.

THE FIVE WARNING SIGNS

Stroke is a medical emergency. It is so important to recognize the warning signs and call 9-1-1. These signs are:

1. Weakness: Sudden loss of strength or sudden numbness in the face, arm, or leg, even if temporary.

2. Trouble speaking: Sudden difficulty speaking or understanding or sudden confusion, even if temporary.

3. Vision problems: Sudden trouble with vision, even if temporary.

4. Headache: Sudden severe and unusual headache.

5. Dizziness: Sudden loss of balance, especially with any of the above signs.

(Source: Heart and Stroke Foundation of Canada)

DOCTOR'S ORDERS

Recognizing the early signs and getting immediate medical attention can greatly improve survival and recovery. Treatment depends on the type of stroke. For an ischemic stroke (caused by a blood clot), a doctor can administer a clot-busting drug called TPA (tissue plasminogen activator). This drug can improve your chances of a full recovery, but it is effective only if given within three hours of initial symptoms. This drug does not work for hemorrhagic stroke, and can actually worsen the problem.

If you are at risk of ischemic stroke, your doctor may give you anti-coagulant drugs, such as warfarin (Coumadin) or anti-platelet drugs such as aspirin, clopidogrel (Plavix), or ticlopidine (Ticlid). There are procedures that can open up an artery narrowed by plaque. A carotid endarterectomy involves an incision in your neck to expose your carotid artery and remove the plaques. Angioplasty is another option. This involves insertion of a balloon-tipped catheter into the obstructed artery to open it up.

Surgical procedures can be done for the treatment and prevention of hemorrhagic stroke. Aneurysm clipping involves placing a tiny clamp at the base of the aneurysm to keep it from bursting. This can also prevent rebleeding of an aneurysm that has recently hemorrhaged. There are other procedures that can seal off or remove the aneurysm.

SHERRY'S NATURAL PRESCRIPTION

Stroke is a medical emergency that requires medical treatment. The strategies outlined here can aid recovery and help prevent stroke. Do not stop taking any medication unless advised by your doctor.

Dietary Recommendations

Foods to include:

- Boost fibre intake by eating lots of whole grains, vegetables, fruits, beans, nuts, and seeds, which will help lower cholesterol levels, improve blood sugar control (essential to prevent diabetes), and help with weight management. Colourful fruits and vegetables contain antioxidants that help reduce the risk of atherosclerosis and heart disease. Apples, oranges, tomatoes, and bananas are a particularly good source of potassium, which can help lower blood pressure.

- Cold-water fish contain beneficial omega-3 fatty acids that help reduce cholesterol, inhibit blood clot formation, and reduce the risk of heart disease. Try to eat three servings per week of fresh cold-water fish such as salmon, trout, herring, mackerel, and tuna. To reduce consumption of toxins, choose wild (not farmed) fish.

- Drink green tea, which contains antioxidants and has modest effects in lowering blood pressure and cholesterol.

- Garlic helps reduce cholesterol, thin the blood (prevent clots), and has antioxidant properties.

- Margarines, salad dressings, and spreads that contain phytostanols (plant substances), which help lower cholesterol.

- Nuts (almonds and walnuts) help lower cholesterol levels. Nuts contain fibre and nutrients such as vitamin E, alpha-linolenic acid, magnesium, potassium, and arginine, which are important for heart health. Although nuts are high in calories, some studies have found that increasing nut consumption by several hundred calories per day does not cause weight gain.

- Olive oil is a monounsaturated fat that can help reduce blood clots and lower LDL cholesterol. Add it to your salads and recipes in place of other vegetable oils.

- Soy products (tofu, soybeans, miso, and soy protein powder) can help lower cholesterol and triglycerides. Substituting as little as 20 g per day of soy protein for animal protein can significantly lower cholesterol.

- Yogurt and fermented milk products can help lower cholesterol.

Foods to avoid:

- Foods high in cholesterol should be minimized (organ meats, egg yolks, and whole milk products). Aim for no more than 300 mg of dietary cholesterol daily. One egg yolk contains 213 mg of cholesterol. Egg whites do not contain any cholesterol and are a good source of protein.

- High alcohol intake can increase your blood pressure and contribute to the development of heart disease and stroke. Limit alcohol to one or two standard drinks a day.

- High-glycemic foods (white bread and refined starches) raise blood sugar levels and increase the risk of diabetes. See Appendix B for more information.

- Salt causes water retention and increases the pressure inside your arteries. Reducing salt intake reduces blood pressure in most people. Aim for no more than 2,500 mg daily. Avoid adding salt to foods and minimize eating processed and fast foods such as deli meats, snacks (chips, pretzels), french fries, and burgers.

- Saturated fat, which is present in animal foods (beef, pork, and dairy) and certain oils (palm oil), can raise cholesterol levels. Limit consumption of saturated fat to 10 percent of total calories. Read food labels carefully.

- Trans fatty acids, found in hydrogenated oils, which are present in most margarines, snack foods (chips), and deep-fried foods (french fries), can raise cholesterol levels and increase the risk of heart disease and stroke.

POTASSIUM LOWERS STROKE RISK

Studies have found an association between diets low in potassium and increased risk of stroke. Conversely high potassium intakes have been associated with a lower risk of stroke. Some of the protective effects of potassium lie in its ability to lower blood pressure. Foods high in potassium include bananas, potatoes, oranges, raisins, artichokes, avocados, spinach, nuts, seeds, lima beans, cod, chicken, and salmon.

Lifestyle Suggestions

- Don't smoke, and avoid second-hand smoke. Smoking contributes to atherosclerosis, increases the risk of blood clots, reduces the oxygen in your blood, increases your blood pressure, and makes your heart work harder. In fact, smoking nearly doubles the risk of ischemic stroke.

- Lose excess weight. Losing even 5–10 percent of excess weight can lower cholesterol and blood pressure.

- Exercise regularly. Moderate-intensity activities, such as brisk walking, biking, or swimming, can reduce cholesterol and blood pressure and help with weight management. Aim for one hour daily. Not being active nearly doubles your risk of heart disease and stroke.

- Reduce stress levels. Stress increases the risk of heart disease and stroke. Try meditation, exercise, or yoga to promote calming and relaxation.

- Manage your blood sugar levels. If you have diabetes or are at risk for diabetes, work on improving your blood sugar levels with exercise and a low-glycemic diet.

- See your doctor regularly for checkups and to monitor your blood pressure, cholesterol, and blood sugar. Discuss the results with your doctor.

Top Recommended Supplements

Citicoline: A form of the B-vitamin choline that has neuroprotective properties, citicoline prevents brain damage due to lack of oxygen, helps restore key membrane components called phospholipids, and counteracts the effects of membrane-injuring molecules known as free radicals. Seven studies have shown that treatment with choline within 14 days of onset of ischemic or hemorrhagic stroke can significantly reduce death and disability. Dosage: 500–2,000 mg daily. This is a specialty supplement that is available through natural health care practitioners.

Fish oils: Lower triglycerides, raise HDL cholesterol, and reduce inflammation and blood clotting. Studies have shown that fish oils reduce the risk of stroke. Dosage: The typical dosage is 3–9 g total of EPA and DHA daily, although higher amounts have been used in some studies. Look for a product that provides at least 400 mg EPA and 200 mg DHA per dosage.

Policosanol: Several studies have shown that it can significantly reduce blood clotting (comparable to aspirin). It also lowers cholesterol. Dosage: 20 mg daily. Do not combine with other blood thinners such as aspirin unless advised by your health care provider.

Complementary Supplements

Aged garlic extract: Helps lower total and LDL cholesterol and triglycerides, reduces blood clotting, and prevents atherosclerosis. Dosage: 600 mg or more daily.

B-vitamins: Lower levels of homocysteine, an amino acid linked to increased risk of stroke in many studies. Folic acid, vitamin B6, and vitamin B12 can lower homocysteine levels, but studies have not yet demonstrated whether this will result in a decreased risk of stroke. Consider a B-complex or take a multivitamin that provides 50–100 mg of the B-vitamins.

Ginkgo biloba: Inhibits blood clotting and improves blood flow to the brain. It may be helpful for both the prevention and treatment of stroke (improving recovery). Dosage: 120–240 mg daily, standardized to 6 percent terpene lactones and 24 percent flavone glycosides.

FINAL THOUGHTS

To prevent stroke and aid recovery, consider the following:

1. Know the warning signs and seek immediate medical attention if you suspect a stroke.
2. Eat lots of fruits, vegetables, whole grains, beans, nuts, fish, soy, garlic, and yogurt, and drink green tea.
3. Minimize saturated fat, trans fats, sugar, and salt.
4. Get regular exercise, reduce stress, and don't smoke.
5. Consider fish oils and policosanol for prevention, and citicoline to improve recovery.

THRUSH (CANDIDIASIS)

Thrush is an overgrowth of the fungus, *Candida albicans*. It typically affects the mouth (called oral thrush) or the vagina (called *Candida vulvovaginitis*, or more commonly a yeast infection). This chapter deals specifically with oral thrush; yeast infections are covered in the chapter on vaginitis.

We all have a variety of micro-organisms in our bodies; some are essential for health and others can become a problem when they grow out of control. This is the case with *Candida albicans*. Levels of this fungus are usually kept under control by our normal bacteria (flora). However, when our normal bacteria are depleted, Candida can proliferate, causing thrush, vaginitis, and other problems. Oral thrush can spread throughout the mouth and throat if left unchecked. It may also be passed from infant to the mother's breasts during breast-feeding.

There are a number of dietary and lifestyle suggestions and supplements that can help prevent thrush and improve healing if you are infected.

SIGNS & SYMPTOMS

- Bad breath

- Coated tongue

- Dry mouth

- Inflamed, painful red or white patches in or around the mouth

The lesions can spread into the esophagus, causing difficulty or pain in swallowing and a sensation of food sticking in the throat. In severve cases the infection can spread throughout the body, which is called *systemic candidiasis*. This may cause fatigue, pain, fever, mood swings, chronic infections, allergies, skin conditions, and digestive problems.

Infants with oral thrush may have difficulty feeding or be irritable or inconsolable. When the mother is infected she may have bright red, shiny, sore or painful nipples.

RISK FACTORS

- Age: The very young and the very old are most susceptible.

- Chronic illness such as cancer

- Dry mouth could be caused by a salivary gland disorder, chemotherapy, radiation, or by use of diuretics, antihistamines, or tranquillizers.

- Immune disorders such as diabetes or HIV/AIDS

- Smoking

- Use of antibiotics, corticosteroids, or birth control pills

- Weakened or underdeveloped immune system function

- Wearing dentures

DOCTOR'S ORDERS

Oral thrush in infants is treated with antifungal liquid medication applied directly to the patches. If diaper rash has also occurred, then an antifungal ointment may be used. In healthy babies, oral thrush may clear up on its own and may be left untreated but carefully watched.

Thrush transferred to the mother's breasts is often treated with an antifungal ointment. Breast-feeding should stop during an infection and milk should be pumped and discarded.

Adults with oral thrush are usually treated with either a topical or oral antifungal medication (such as nystatin), depending on the extent of the infection.

Systemic candidiasis is more difficult to diagnose, but it may also be life threatening, particularly for people with weakened immune health or illness. Up to 75 percent of people with systemic candidiasis die from complications. As such, if you suspect you may have a Candida infection, see your doctor immediately.

SHERRY'S NATURAL PRESCRIPTION

Dietary Recommendations

Foods to include:

- Brewer's yeast and flaxseeds

- Eat lots of vegetables and yeast-free whole grains (pita bread); asparagus, Jerusalem artichokes, and soybeans contain substances (FOS) that promote the growth of beneficial bacteria.

- Garlic and onions help reduce fungal growth.

- Vegetable juices/green drinks

- Yogurt with live cultures and other fermented dairy (kefir) provide beneficial bacteria that help to reduce Candida overgrowth.

Foods to avoid:

- Alcohol hampers immune function; beer and wine contain yeasts that can be a problem.

- Dairy products and aged cheese can increase the risk of Candida in some people.

- Fruit and fruit juices are high in sugar and should be minimized; drink vegetable juices, water, and green tea instead.

- Limit foods that contain sugars (candy, sweets, soft drinks) or yeasts (breads) as these foods can encourage growth of Candida.

- Nuts and nut butters may contains moulds.

Note: Food allergies may trigger Candida infections. Try an elimination diet (see Appendix D) to determine if you have food allergies.

Lifestyle Suggestions

- Avoid the use of mouthwash or oral sprays; the alcohol can destroy healthy bacteria in your mouth and cause dry mouth; instead use a saltwater or baking soda solution in warm water and do not swallow.

- Be on the lookout for signs of oral thrush before breast-feeding.
- Clean bottle nipples and pacifiers regularly using hot, soapy water.
- Clean breasts with warm cloth and apply conditioning lotion or oil to nipples after breast-feeding.
- Don't smoke.
- Practise good oral hygiene; clean your mouth and dentures; soak dentures in a denture cleaner nightly and rinse well.

Top Recommended Supplements

Aged garlic extract: Supports immune function and has antifungal properties. Studies have shown that it can reduce *Candida albicans*. Dosage: One capsule twice daily. This clinically studied form of garlic is odourless. It is also available in liquid.

Gentian violet: An old remedy for eliminating thrush that is becoming popular again today. It has antifungal properties and works quickly to relieve thrush. Pharmacists can prepare a 1 percent solution of gentian violet. To use, dip a cotton swab in the solution and apply to the affected areas of the mouth and tongue. Use for up to one week. This product can be used on infants, adults, and mother's breasts. This product will stain fingers and clothing.

Probiotics: Lactobacillus acidophilus and Bifidobacterium are beneficial bacteria that help prevent overgrowth of Candida. It is especially important to take a probiotic after a course of antibiotics. Look for Kyo-Dophilus, a probiotic that is stable at room temperature and of guaranteed potency. Dosage: Take two or three capsules orally daily with meals. It is also available in chewable tablets and powder for children.

Complementary Treatment

Caprylic acid: A fatty acid derived from coconut oil that has antifungal properties. Dosage: 1,000 mg three times daily. Avoid if you have ulcerative colitis.

FINAL THOUGHTS

To reduce oral thrush, consider the following:

1. Eat fermented dairy products (yogurt), vegetables, garlic, onions, yeast-free breads, and foods containing FOS.
2. Avoid sugar, yeast, and alcohol.
3. Don't smoke and avoid alcohol-containing mouthwashes.
4. Inspect your infant's mouth (and your breasts) regularly and see your doctor if there are signs of thrush.
5. Aged garlic extract, gentian violet, and probiotics can help prevent and treat Candida infections.

TINNITUS

Tinnitus is the sensation of ringing, buzzing, roaring, or hissing in the ears. According to the Tinnitus Association of Canada, this condition affects more than 360,000 Canadians. Tinnitus is often associated with hearing loss or noise exposure, although even people with normal hearing develop this problem.

Tinnitus is not a disease, but rather a symptom resulting from a medical condition, injury, or side effect of medication. Inside the inner ear there are thousands of auditory cells that maintain an electrical charge. There are tiny hairs on these cells that move with the pressure of sound waves. The movement triggers the cells to discharge electricity through the auditory nerve and the brain interprets these signals as sound. If these hairs become bent or broken, they move randomly and the auditory cells send random electrical impulses to the brain as noise. Damage to the auditory cells or hair in the inner ear most often results from exposure to loud noise, a blow to the head, or a whiplash injury. Other risk factors for tinnitus are described below.

Although tinnitus can be distressing, it is rarely a sign of a serious health problem. Identifying and treating the underlying cause is essential. For those with irreversible tinnitus, there are a variety of holistic therapies and lifestyle measures that help reduce the symptoms and improve quality of life.

SIGNS & SYMPTOMS

- Hearing loss

- Ringing, buzzing, roaring, or hissing sounds in the ear when no external sounds are present

The symptoms of tinnitus vary in intensity from mild to severe. The sounds may be heard intermittently or continuously. It may be heard in one ear or both, and it can vary in pitch.

KEEP YOUR EARS CLEAN

A buildup of earwax can reduce your ability to hear outside noises and amplify internal noises. If you produce a lot of earwax, speak to your doctor about having excess wax removed. Do not try to remove it yourself unless advised by your doctor. Using cotton swabs improperly can damage the ear and push the wax deeper into your ear.

RISK FACTORS

- Blood vessel disease (atherosclerosis): Buildup of cholesterol in the blood vessels of the inner ear causes loss of elasticity, making blood flow more forceful and easily heard.

- Buildup of wax in the ear canal can cause tinnitus.

- Ear or sinus infection: Usually the tinnitus is temporary once the infection is healed.

- Exposure to loud noises can cause irreversible damage to hair cells in the inner ear.

- Head or neck trauma.

- Insulin resistance: High insulin and blood sugar levels (which precede type 2 diabetes) have been linked to tinnitus in some studies.

- Jaw misalignment: This can often be corrected with treatment.

- Medications: Some drugs are toxic to the ear, such as aminoglycoside antibiotics, the malaria drug quinine, and the cancer drugs cisplatin; others cause tinnitus as a side effect, such as aspirin and anti-inflammatory drugs (NSAIDs), diuretics (furosemide), and some blood pressure and cholesterol-lowering drugs. This effect can be temporary or permanent.

- Tumours can put pressure on auditory nerves, causing tinnitus.

DOCTOR'S ORDERS

The treatment of tinnitus depends on the cause. To determine the cause, your doctor may refer you to an otolaryngologist, otherwise known as an ear, nose, and throat specialist. Another specialist, an audiologist, can measure your hearing and fit you with a hearing aid if needed.

The drug gabapentin (Neurontin) has been used with some success in relieving tinnitus. Tricyclic antidepressants, such as amitriptyline and nortriptyline, have also been helpful for some people, but their use is limited by side effects.

If the problem is due to earwax or a side effect of medication, then it may be reversible. Tinnitus that is due to hearing loss or excessive noise exposure cannot be reversed, but there are a variety of lifestyle measures discussed below that can be helpful in coping.

Ask your doctor to measure your homocysteine level. Chronic tinnitus may be associated with an elevation in homocysteine levels. High homocysteine may also increase the risk of heart disease, high blood pressure, diabetes, and stroke.

SHERRY'S NATURAL PRESCRIPTION

Dietary Recommendations

Foods to include:

- Fruits, vegetables, whole grains, and legumes provide vital fibre, which helps reduce blood cholesterol levels. These foods are also lower in the glycemic index and can help improve blood sugar control and prevent type 2 diabetes. Refer to Appendix B for more information on the glycemic index.

- Drink plenty of water.

Foods to avoid:

- Alcohol increases the force of blood by dilating your blood vessels and causing greater blood flow to the inner ear area.

- Caffeine constricts blood vessels, increasing the speed of blood through your veins and arteries.

- Trans fats and saturated fat elevate cholesterol levels and contribute to atherosclerosis, which can cause or worsen tinnitus.

- High-glycemic foods (processed grains such as white bread and rice) increase insulin levels and can worsen tinnitus.

FOOD FLARES

Many people with tinnitus find that certain foods and/or drinks will worsen their symptoms. There is no simple test to determine which foods can worsen tinnitus. Keeping a food diary or trying an elimination diet can be helpful in pinpointing foods that trigger tinnitus. Refer to Appendix D for more information on food allergies and the elimination diet.

Lifestyle Suggestions

- Don't smoke: Smoking causes blood vessel damage and can worsen tinnitus.

- Protect your ears: Wear earplugs or earmuffs if you work in a noisy environment or are exposed to loud noise at home.

- Mask the noise: Using a fan or low-volume, soft music can help mask the noise from tinnitus. There are also special devices that emit white noise (low-tone sound that neutralizes other sounds).

- Consider a hearing aid: If you have hearing loss, amplifying outside sounds can make the tinnitus less noticeable.

- Reduce stress levels: Stress can worsen tinnitus. Try breathing techniques, yoga, and massage to promote relaxation.

- Exercise regularly to improve blood flow, reduce stress, and improve blood sugar control.

- Get adequate sleep, which will help with coping and reduce stress.

- Acupuncture and hypnosis may be helpful for reducing tinnitus and promoting relaxation. Biofeedback treatments can also help relieve tinnitus.

Top Recommended Supplements

Ginkgo biloba: Improves circulation to the brain and inner ear. Three small studies found reduction in symptoms while one larger study showed no benefit. It appears that ginkgo works for some people and not for others, likely depending upon the underlying cause. As well, it may take several weeks to months to detect a benefit. Dosage: 120 mg daily of a product standardized to contain 24 percent flavone glycosides and 6 percent terpene lactones.

Zinc: Highly concentrated in the inner ear; a deficiency of this mineral can cause tinnitus. Some studies have found improvement in symptoms with zinc supplements in those who are deficient in this mineral. Blood tests can detect zinc deficiency. High dosages were used in studies (90-150 mg daily); levels should be monitored by a doctor. It is important to take copper (2 mg) along with zinc because zinc interferes with copper absorption.

Complementary Supplements

Magnesium: Essential for nerve health and hearing. A deficiency of magnesium can cause blood vessels to constrict, which can reduce circulation to the brain and inner ear. Dosage: 100 mg three times daily with meals.

Melatonin: Shown in some studies to improve symptoms of tinnitus and also improve sleep quality. Dosage: 3 mg one hour before bed.

Vitamin B12: Essential in the manufacture of myelin, a fatty substance that covers and shields the nerves and allows them to function normally. Some research has found that those who are deficient are at greater risk of developing tinnitus. In studies, B12 injections reduced the severity of symptoms. Sublingual B12, which is better absorbed than oral B12, may offer similar benefits, although it has not been studied. Take B12 along with a B-complex that contains folic acid and vitamins B1, B3 and B6 as these other B-vitamins also play a role in proper nerve function and together they may help reduce tinnitus. Dosage: 5 mg B12 and 50-100 mg of the other B-vitamins daily.

FINAL THOUGHTS

To reduce the symptoms of tinnitus, consider the following:

1. Minimize caffeine, alcohol, trans fats, and processed and refined grains.
2. Don't smoke; get regular exercise and adequate sleep.
3. Avoid being around loud noise and protect your ears with earplugs or earmuffs.
4. Try masking the noise with music or a fan.
5. Consider supplements of ginkgo biloba and zinc.

ULCERS

Peptic ulcers are sores that develop on the inside lining of the stomach, upper small intestine, or esophagus, causing significant pain and discomfort. Their name is derived from pepsin, an enzyme secreted by glands in the stomach. Along with pepsin, acids are secreted in the stomach to aid digestion. Other glands in the stomach and intestine secrete mucus, which functions to protect the lining of the digestive tract from the corrosive effect of pepsin and acid. If there is damage to the lining of the stomach or intestine and the mucous layer breaks down, an ulcer can develop.

It is estimated that about one in 10 Canadians develops an ulcer at some time in his or her life. Ulcers generally affect people over the age of 30, but children can get them as well.

Years ago stress and poor diet were thought to be the cause of ulcers. In recent years, however, it was discovered that infection with a bacterium called *Helicobacter pylori* (*H. Pylori*) is responsible for causing most ulcers. This bacterium lives within the mucous layer that covers and protects the lining of the stomach and small intestine. *H. Pylori* is a normal inhabitant of this area, and does not always cause problems. However, in certain individuals and under certain conditions, it can disrupt the mucous layer, erode the lining of the digestive tract, and lead to an ulcer.

Stress and diet may still contribute to the problem, causing damage to the lining and making it easier for bacteria to invade and damage the sensitive tissues. Ulcers can also be caused by taking non-steroidal anti-inflammatory drugs (NSAIDs), which erode and inflame the lining of the stomach and intestines.

It is estimated that one in five people under 40 years and half of people over 60 are infected with *H. Pylori*. It is not known how it spreads, but it may occur with close contact, such as kissing, or through contaminated food and water.

TYPES OF ULCERS

Ulcers have different names, depending on their location:

Duodenal ulcers develop in the duodenum (first part of the small intestine), which is the most common location.

Esophageal ulcers are located in the lower section of the esophagus, and are often associated with chronic gastroesophageal reflux disease (GERD).

Gastric ulcers occur in the stomach.

SIGNS & SYMPTOMS

- Chest pain
- Dark blood in stools
- Loss of appetite
- Nausea or vomiting
- Pain, which is often worse when the stomach is empty and at night, and is temporarily relieved by eating or taking antacids

- Weight loss

Note: If left untreated, ulcers can lead to serious problems such as bleeding, obstruction of the digestive tract (due to scarring), or serious infection due to leaking of the intestinal contents into the belly.

In addition to *H. Pylori*, other factors that increase the risk of ulcers include:

- Alcohol: Irritates and erodes the mucous lining of the stomach and increases the amount of stomach acid that is produced

- Food allergies: May cause damage to stomach lining, increasing the risk of ulcers

- NSAIDs (non-steroidal anti-inflammatory drugs)

- Smoking: Nicotine increases the volume and concentration of stomach acid.

- Stress: May aggravate symptoms and delay healing

NON-STEROIDAL ANTI-INFLAMMATORY DRUGS AND ULCERS

Non-steroidal anti-inflammatory drugs inhibit production of an enzyme (cyclooxygenase) that produces prostaglandins, hormone-like substances that protect the stomach lining. Without this protection, stomach acid can damage the lining, causing bleeding and ulcers. Examples of these drugs include aspirin, Motrin and Advil (ibuprofen), Naprosyn (naproxen), and Indocid (indomethacin). Taking these drugs with meals may help reduce stomach upset, but will not prevent ulcers. Take only when absolutely necessary at the lowest dosage.

DOCTOR'S ORDERS

For ulcers caused by *H. Pylori* bacteria, a seven to 14-day course of antibiotics is prescribed to kill the bacteria. Antibiotics commonly used include Amoxil (amoxicillin), Biaxin (clarithromycin), or Flagyl (metronidazole). Two of these are typically prescribed along with an acid-blocking drug, such as Prevacid (lansoprazole), to allow the area to heal. Some companies put the three drugs together in one package, such as the HP-Pak.

Depending on the severity of the ulcer, acid-reducing drugs may be needed for several weeks to months to allow healing. Histamine (H-2) blockers reduce the amount of hydrochloric acid released into the stomach. They work by blocking the action of histamine, a substance that signals acid secretion into the stomach. Examples include Zantac (ranitidine), Pepcid (famotidine), and Tagamet (cimetidine).

Proton pump inhibitors shut down the pumps that secrete acid into the stomach. Examples include Prevacid, (lansoprazole), Nexium (esomeprazole), or Losec (omeprazole).

Antacids may be used along with the above drugs or alone. They provide rapid relief and work by neutralizing stomach acid. Examples include Tums, Rolaids, and Maalox.

Cytoprotective drugs protect the lining of the stomach and intestine. Examples include Sulcrate (sucralfate) and Cytotec (misoprostol). They may be given to protect the stomach when NSAIDS are being used.

SHERRY'S NATURAL PRESCRIPTION

Ulcers caused by *H. Pylori* infection will most likely require medical treatment. The following suggestions may help improve healing and reduce the risk of developing an ulcer.

Dietary Recommendations

Foods to include:

- Cultured and fermented foods such as kefir and yogurt provide friendly bacteria that help to combat *H. Pylori*.

- Cabbage and aloe vera juice may help improve healing.

- Foods rich in vitamin K (leafy green vegetables) and zinc (whole grains and seeds) can improve healing.

- Bananas are protective to the stomach.

- Drink herbal teas with marshmallow, slippery elm, and chamomile, which can soothe the irritated lining.

- Cranberry juice can prevent the adhesion of *H. Pylori* to the stomach wall.

Foods to avoid:

- Alcohol, caffeine, and spicy foods can irritate and increase stomach acid.

- Sugar and salt increase stomach acidity and may aggravate symptoms.

Lifestyle Suggestions

- Don't smoke, as nicotine is very irritating to the stomach lining and slows healing.

- Elevate your pillow to prevent stomach acid from flowing up your esophagus.

- Reduce stress by trying massage, yoga, breathing exercises, or meditation.

Top Recommended Supplements

Deglycyrrhizinated licorice (DGL): Soothes inflamed and damaged mucous lining, promotes healing, and may inhibit growth of *H. Pylori*. Some research suggests that it might help protect the stomach against NSAID usage. Dosage: 500 mg 15 minutes before meals and at bedtime. Look for a chewable product.

Probiotics: Several studies have found that probiotics (especially those in the Lactobacillus family) can inhibit the growth of *H. Pylori*. They also improve the ability of antibiotics to destroy bacteria and reduce antibiotic side effects such as diarrhea and yeast overgrowth. Dosage: One to three capsules daily of a product providing 1 billion live cells per capsule or tablet.

Complementary Supplements

Glutamine: An amino acid that provides energy for the cells that line the intestine and stomach. Levels may be depleted in those with ulcers, and supplementing has been shown to offer some benefits to promote healing. Dosage: 500–1,000 mg three times daily.

Zinc: Required for tissue repair. Some evidence suggests that it can promote healing of ulcers. Dosage: 25–50 mg daily. Take copper (1–3 mg) to prevent copper deficiency.

FINAL THOUGHTS

To reduce your risk of ulcers and improve healing:

1. Don't smoke, reduce stress, and avoid taking NSAIDs.
2. Eat fermented and cultured foods and drink cranberry juice to inhibit *H. Pylori*.
3. Cabbage, aloe vera juice, and green vegetables promote ulcer healing.
4. Probiotic supplements can inhibit *H. Pylori*, improve antibiotic treatment of *H. Pylori*, and reduce antibiotic side effects.
5. Promote healing of an ulcer with zinc, glutamine, and DGL.

VAGINITIS AND YEAST INFECTIONS

Vaginitis is an inflammation of the vagina that can cause discharge, itching, and pain. Vaginitis often results from irritation, infection, or hormonal changes, such as low estrogen levels in menopause. Most women will experience vaginitis at some point in their lives, and while it is unpleasant, it can be dealt with effectively with both conventional and natural approaches.

There are many different types of bacteria and yeast normally present in the vagina. However, when the numbers of these organisms become out of balance, infection can occur, causing vaginitis.

The most common cause of vaginitis is an overgrowth of the naturally occurring yeast *Candida albicans*. An estimated three out of four women will have a yeast infection in their lifetime. A yeast infection isn't considered a sexually transmitted disease because this yeast is naturally occurring in a woman's body, but it can spread from one partner to another.

Bacterial vaginosis is another common cause of vaginitis. There are several bacteria that can cause these infections, most commonly, *Gardnerella*. These infections can spread during sexual intercourse, but it also occurs in people who aren't sexually active.

Trichomoniasis is an infection caused by a parasite, which is commonly transmitted by sexual intercourse.

Vaginitis can also result from reduced estrogen levels after menopause, which causes the vagina to become thinner and drier, which may lead to itching, burning, or pain. Use of vaginal sprays, douches, perfumed soaps, and spermicidal products can also cause vaginal irritation, burning, and itching.

SIGNS & SYMPTOMS

- Change in your normal vaginal discharge and odour
- Light vaginal bleeding
- Pain during intercourse or urination
- Vaginal itching or irritation

Bacterial vaginosis typically causes a greyish-white, fishy-smelling discharge. Yeast infections cause a thick, white discharge that resembles cottage cheese. Trichomoniasis causes a greenish-yellow, sometimes frothy discharge in women while men often have no symptoms.

RISK FACTORS

Risk factors vary depending upon the type of vaginitis.

Yeast infections

- Hormonal changes (pregnancy)
- Medications such as antibiotics, steroids, and birth control pills
- Stress, lack of sleep

- Uncontrolled diabetes
- Use of vaginal contraceptives or feminine hygiene products
- Weakened immune system (HIV, chemotherapy, diabetes)
- Wearing damp or tight-fitting clothing

Bacterial vaginosis

- Douching
- Use of an intrauterine device (IUD)
- Women with new or multiple sex partners

Trichomoniasis

- Sexual contact with an infected partner

••

Women who have diabetes are at greater risk of developing vaginitis caused by *Candida albicans* due to impaired immune function.

••

DOCTOR'S ORDERS

There are various medications for vaginitis, depending on the underlying cause. Bacterial vaginosis is treated with metronidazole (Flagyl) or clindamycin (Dalacin). The latter drug is also used to treat Trichomoniasis.

Yeast infections are usually treated with miconazole (Monistat) or clotrimazole (Canesten) creams or vaginal suppositories, which are available over the counter. Your doctor may also prescribe a drug called fluconazole (Diflucan), which is a single-dose oral treatment. Many women prefer this as it is easy and provides rapid relief. However, it requires a prescription and is more expensive than the other products.

For women with vaginitis in menopause, doctors sometimes prescribe estrogen vaginal creams or rings, which help to thicken the vaginal area. Some estrogen still gets absorbed into the bloodstream, so these products should not be used by women with a history of breast cancer or who are at high risk.

SHERRY'S NATURAL PRESCRIPTION

Dietary Recommendations

Foods to include:

- Eat natural (organic) yogurt with live cultures daily. Studies have shown that daily consumption of yogurt can reduce the occurrence of BV and yeast infections.

- Garlic and onions have antifungal properties.

Foods to avoid:

- Alcohol, aged cheese, and fermented foods (vinegar and soy sauce) contain yeast and moulds, which can be a problem.

- Sugar allows yeast to thrive, and can increase the likelihood of yeast infections in susceptible women. Cut down on all sugar-containing foods.

Food allergies are believed to be a contributory factor in some cases of recurrent irritant vaginitis. See Appendix D for more information on food allergies and the elimination diet.

Lifestyle Suggestions

- Wear cotton underwear and minimize or avoid wearing pantyhose. Do not wear pants that are tight at the crotch.

- Do not use deodorized products, such as tampons, douches, and feminine deodorant sprays.

- Wash the vaginal area with a mild, unscented soap.

- Douche with 2 tsp of powdered acidophilus in a quart of warm water daily.

Top Recommended Supplements

Aged garlic extract: Supports immune function and has antibacterial and antifungal properties. Studies have shown that it can reduce *Candida albicans*. Dosage: Two capsules twice daily.

Boric acid: A substance with antiseptic and antifungal properties. One study found significant benefits with use of 600 mg boric acid capsules inserted into the vagina twice per day for two to four weeks. It is available at compounding pharmacies. Boric acid suppositories should not be used during pregnancy, and it is very toxic if taken orally.

Lactobacillus acidophilus: A type of friendly bacteria (probiotic) that is part of the normal vaginal flora and helps prevent overgrowth of Candida. Many supplements contain another probiotic called Bifidobacterium. Dosage: Two or three capsules daily of a product that provides at least one billion vaible cells per capsule, such as Kyo-Dophilus. Capsules can also be inserted vaginally at bedtime.

Complementary Supplements

Tea tree oil: Has antibacterial and antifungal properties. Studies have found topically applied tea tree oil helpful for Trichomoniasis, *Candida albicans*, and other vaginal infections. This should only be done under a doctor's supervision. Tea tree oil must be diluted to a 5 percent solution when used as a douche.

Vitamin C: Helps support immune function. One study found vitamin C vaginal tablets helpful for vaginitis. Dosage: 250 mg vaginally or 1,000 mg orally daily.

Vitamin E: When used orally or vaginally, it may help relieve itching and irritation and soothe the delicate vaginal tissue. Dosage: 400 IU orally, or apply the oil topically.

V

Vaginitis and Yeast Infections

FINAL THOUGHTS

To reduce the risk and promote healing of vaginitis, consider the following:

1. Eat yogurt with live cultures daily; reduce sugar, alcohol, and fermented foods.
2. Wear cotton underwear and loose-fitting pants.
3. Avoid using deodorized feminine hygiene products.
4. Take a probiotic supplement and aged garlic extract daily.
5. Consider supplements of vitamins C and E

VARICOSE VEINS

Varicose veins are dilated, bulging, discoloured veins that you can clearly see through the skin. It is estimated that at least 15 percent of the adult population in Canada suffers from varicose veins.

The heart pumps oxygenated blood from the lungs through the arteries to the cells throughout the body. Oxygen exchange takes place and blood returns up to the heart through the veins. Tiny one-way valves inside our veins function as trapdoors opening and closing with each muscle contraction to prevent the backflow of blood.

Varicose veins result from damage to the valves or vein walls, leading to pooling of blood, vein swelling, and increased venous pressure. Spider veins are a similar condition that affects the smaller veins. These veins spread out on the surface of the skin in a web-like fashion, hence their name.

SIGNS & SYMPTOMS

- Cramping
- Fatigue
- Heavy aching in the legs
- Itching and burning
- Swelling of leg or ankle
- Tenderness and pain

Note: If left untreated, varicose veins can worsen over time and cause skin changes such as rash, redness, and sores. Varicose veins are not life threatening; however, they can increase the risk of developing a blood clot, which is a serious concern.

RISK FACTORS

- Age: Most common in those over 50 years (but can occur earlier)
- Diet: A low-fibre diet and constipation can contribute to varicose veins.
- Family history
- Gender: Women are affected approximately four times more often than men.
- Lifestyle/occupation: Prolonged sitting or standing with little activity causes pooling of blood and damage to the valves.
- Obesity: Weight gain can increase venous pressure and cause the veins to enlarge.
- Pregnancy: Hormonal changes can weaken vein walls; weight gain increases venous pressure; veins enlarge from increased blood volume; and the growing uterus can compress the veins and increase pressure.

Other factors that may contribute to or worsen varicose veins include: exposure to excessive heat, use of birth control pills or estrogen, and wearing high-heeled shoes.

DOCTOR'S ORDERS

Depending on the severity, one of the following medical treatments may be recommended:

Ablation/sclerotherapy/laser: These procedures destroy the affected vein. Blood is rerouted through other veins and the damaged vein is absorbed by the body.

Bypass: An artificial or transplanted vein is connected to the damaged vein to help improve blood flow.

Compression stockings: These specially designed stockings provide firm support to improve blood flow back to the heart and prevent swelling in the legs. They are available for both men and women, and are custom ordered.

Stripping: This is a surgical procedure to remove the damaged vein.

··

DID YOU KNOW?

The incidence of varicose veins is higher in developed (Western) countries due to lifestyle factors: poor diet (low fibre), lack of activity, and obesity.

··

SHERRY'S NATURAL PRESCRIPTION

Dietary Recommendations

Foods to include:

- A high-fibre diet is essential to prevent constipation and straining. Aim for 25–35 g of fibre daily. The best food sources are fruits, vegetables, whole grains (oats and bran), legumes, nuts, and seeds (flaxseed and sunflower seeds).

- Berries and grapes provide flavonoids, which strengthen the walls of the veins and help circulation.

- Buckwheat contains rutin, a flavonoid that is beneficial for vein health.

- Fish, nuts, and seeds contain essential fatty acids, which help reduce inflammation, prevent clotting, and improve circulation.

Foods to avoid:

- Saturated fats (animal fats) and trans fats (fast food and processed food) can impede circulation in both the veins and arteries, cause free radical damage, and trigger inflammation.

- Reduce sodium intake from foods such as soda pop, chips, crackers, and deli meats, as sodium can increase fluid retention and swelling.

- Minimize caffeine and alcohol, as they are dehydrating and may worsen symptoms.

Lifestyle Suggestions

- Exercise regularly. Activities that involve movement of the calf muscle will help pump blood back to the heart. Try walking, cycling, and swimming.

- Avoid standing or sitting in the same spot for a long time. Move around, flex your ankles, circle your foot, do calf raises, and shift your body weight.

- Lose excess weight, which will reduce pressure on your legs.

- Avoid excessive heat on your legs (sunbathing and hot baths), which can cause the veins to dilate, thus worsening the problem.

- Elevate your legs when sitting and resting. Don't cross your legs, which hampers circulation and can worsen leg aching.

- Minimize or avoid wearing high heels and tight shoes, as they impair circulation.

- Don't wear tight clothing, especially around the waist.

- Avoid constipation and straining on the toilet as this can increase vein pressure.

- Don't smoke, as smoking damages the veins and blood vessels, increases blood pressure, and impairs circulation.

Top Recommended Supplements

Diosmin: A flavonoid that improves the tone and strength of the blood vessels, reduces swelling, fights free-radical damage, and stimulates lymphatic flow. Over 30 clinical studies have found it effective for improving vein disorders. Diosmin has a quick onset of action (one to two weeks) and is not associated with any side effects or drug interactions. Dosage: 600 mg once daily. Look for a product standardized to 95 percent diosmin and 5 percent hesperidin.

Horse chestnut seed extract: Promotes circulation, improves vein wall tone, and relieves swelling. It offers modest benefits and may take six to eight weeks to notice results. It may cause nausea and upset stomach and can enhance the effect of blood-thinning medications. Avoid it if you have kidney or liver disease. Dosage: 300 mg twice daily, standardized to 50 mg of aescin.

Pine bark extract: A flavonoid that offers antioxidant activity, strengthens capillaries, improves circulation, and supports the integrity of collagen and elastin (proteins in connective tissue that support organs, joints, blood vessels, and muscles). A few small studies have shown benefits. Dosage: 100–300 mg daily; no known side effects or drug interactions.

Complementary Supplements

Antioxidants: Help improve circulation and vein health. In addition to diosmin and pine bark, other antioxidants to consider are vitamins C and E, bilberry, and grape seed extract.

Butcher's Broom: Improves the strength and tone of the veins, acts as a mild diuretic, and has mild anti-inflammatory effects. Dosage: 100 mg three times daily.

FINAL THOUGHTS

To improve vein health, consider the following:

1. Boost intake of fibre and antioxidant-rich foods, and reduce your intake of saturated fats, processed foods, and sodium.
2. Exercise regularly, elevate your feet when resting, and avoid standing or sitting in the same spot.
3. Don't smoke.
4. Wear compression stockings.
5. Consider a supplement of diosmin, horse chestnut, or pine bark.

SECTION IV

APPENDICES

APPENDIX A

DETERMINATIONS FOR BODY FAT AND WEIGHT

Carrying extra body weight or being obese greatly increases the risks of developing health problems such as heart disease, diabetes, and certain cancers. While the words "obese" and "overweight" are used synonymously, there is a great difference between these terms in both definition and associated health risk.

"Overweight" is defined as a body weight above an acceptable weight in relation to height. This term can be misleading because it does not distinguish between body fat and lean muscle mass. For example, it is possible to be overweight without being obese, such as a bodybuilder. Having a greater proportion of muscle mass would make this individual appear overweight according to standard weight/height charts, yet this person could have low body fat and be in good physical shape.

So how do you know if you are overweight or obese? There are several methods that are used to determine overweight, obesity, and the level of associated health risks. They include the body mass index (BMI), percentage of body fat, and waist circumference.

BODY MASS INDEX

The most commonly used tool to determine weight is the body mass index (BMI), which compares your height and weight to a standard. To calculate your BMI, take your weight in kilograms and divide that by your height in meters squared (Kg/m2).

- BMI less than 18.5 is *underweight*
- BMI of 18.5–24.9 is *normal weight*
- BMI of 25.0–29.9 is *overweight*
- BMI of 30.0–39.9 is *obese*
- BMI of 40.0 or higher is *severely (or morbidly) obese*

Since the BMI does not take into consideration body composition or gender differences (women have a higher amount of body fat), there are limitations with this method. However, studies have shown that the greater the BMI, the greater the risk of developing health problems, such as heart disease and diabetes.

BODY COMPOSITION

While we often look at our weight on the scale, knowing your body composition is actually more important as this reflects the level of body fat versus lean body mass (tissue, bone, and muscle), and it is excess body fat that is dangerous to health.

Body composition can be measured by:

Bioelectric impedance: A machine is used to measure an electric signal as it passes through lean body mass and fat. The higher the fat content, the greater the resistance to the current. This method is more effective than skin-fold caliper testing, but is not 100 percent accurate.

DEXA (dual energy X-ray absorptiometry): Uses two X-ray energies to measure body fat, muscle, and bone mineral. This method is highly accurate, but also the most expensive and time consuming.

Near infrared technology: Infrared light is shone on the skin (usually bicep area). Fat absorbs the light, while lean body mass reflects the lights back. The reflected light is measured by a special sensor, transmitted into the computer, and translated into percentage of body fat. This method is highly accurate, comparable to underwater weighing, but slightly more expensive than the above two methods.

Skin-fold calipers: Measures the thickness of subcutaneous fat at various locations on the body. The measurements obtained are used in special equations to obtain an estimated percent fat value. This method is not very accurate and is dependent upon the skills and judgment of the person performing the test.

Below are recommended body fat ranges for women and men along with the ranges considered to be overweight or obese:

	Women	*Men*
Normal	15–25 percent	10–20 percent
Overweight	25.1–29.9 percent	20.1–24.4 percent
Obese	Over 30 percent	Over 25 percent

WAIST CIRCUMFERENCE

Just as the degree of obesity is correlated with health risk, so is the location of the fat. Studies have shown that an apple-shaped body, which is defined by abdominal obesity or having a potbelly, greatly increases the risk of type 2 diabetes, high cholesterol and blood pressure, heart disease, stroke, and early death. In fact, waist circumference measurements have been shown to be a better predictor of health risk than the body mass index (BMI). Following are the waist measurements and their corresponding level of risk:

For men:
- Increased risk: Waist more than 38 inches (97 cm)
- Substantially increased risk: Waist more than 40 inches (102 cm)

For women:
- Increased risk: Waist more than 32 inches (81 cm)
- Substantially increased risk: Waist more than 35 inches (89 cm)

Men often deposit weight in the waist region, whereas women tend to gain weight around the hips and buttocks, giving them the pear shape. Fat deposited primarily around the hips and buttocks does not carry the same risk as that gained around the midsection. In recent years, researchers have found that abdominal fat, which surrounds our internal organs, secretes compounds that trigger inflammation and insulin resistance, thus increasing the risk of heart disease, diabetes, and other problems.

The tendency to deposit fat around the midsection is influenced by a number of factors, including genetics and lifestyle choices. Physical activity, not smoking, and using unsaturated fat over saturated fat have been shown to decrease the risk of developing abdominal obesity.

For recommendations on weight loss, refer to the obesity section in this book.

GLYCEMIC INDEX TABLE

The glycemic index or GI is a ranking of carbohydrates based on how quickly they are broken down and affect blood sugar. Also called blood glucose, blood sugar is the fuel used by the cells in the body for energy. Carbohydrates that are rapidly digested and broken down quickly into blood glucose are ranked as "high GI." These include refined starches such as white bread and highly processed foods. Carbohydrates that are more slowly digested and broken down into blood glucose have a "low GI." Examples include most vegetables, non-tropical fruits, and unprocessed grains. Low-GI foods have a less dramatic impact on blood sugar and help keep levels more balanced.

Eating high-GI foods can lead to blood sugar imbalances, which may result in fatigue, increased appetite, and food cravings, particularly for sweets. Furthermore, numerous studies have linked diets that include large amounts of high-GI foods to obesity, increased belly fat, insulin resistance, type 2 diabetes, high cholesterol, and increased risk of cardiovascular disease. On the other hand, research indicates that a low-glycemic diet can promote better blood sugar control. A low-GI diet can help facilitate weight loss by reducing hunger and cravings and increasing metabolic rate. This healthy way of eating can also improve mood and energy levels and, over the long term, may cut the risk of several chronic diseases such as type 2 diabetes, heart disease, and certain cancers. For all of these reasons, it is best to minimize your intake of high-GI foods and maximize your intake of low-GI foods. Following is a table that includes low-, moderate-, and high-GI foods.

Low Glycemic (55 or Less)	Moderate Glycemic (56–69)	High Glycemic (70 and over)
Apples (fresh and dried)	Arrowroot biscuit	Bagel (white)
Apple juice	Beer	Bread stuffing
Apricots (dried)	Beets (canned)	Broad beans
Banana (ripe)	Breton® crackers	Cereal (Cheerios™, Crisp-ix™, Corn Flakes®, Corn Pops®, Grapenuts™, Rice Krispies®, Total™)
Barley	Buckwheat	
Beans (haricot, lima, kidney, mung, navy, and pinto)	Cantaloupe	
Bean sprouts	Cereal (Shredded Wheat, Just Right, Nutrigrain, and Raisin Bran)	Corn cakes (puffed)
Broccoli		Corn chips, Dates
Carrots (raw)	Corn (sweet)	Doughnut (cake type)
Cereals (All-Bran™)	Cornmeal	English muffin
Chapati (bread)	Couscous	French baguette
Cherries	Cranberry juice cocktail	French fries
Chickpeas	Croissant (white)	Fruit Roll-ups®
Chocolate (dark)	Digestive biscuits	Glucose
Grapefruit	Figs	Graham wafers
Grapes	Flan cake	Instant mashed potatoes
Kiwi fruit	Hamburger bun (white)	Jellybeans
Lentils	Honey	Kaiser roll
Milk	Jam (strawberry)	Life Savers®
Oat bran bread	Mango (ripe)	Melba toast
Oatmeal (slow-cook oats)	Muesli	Pancake syrup
Oranges	Pancakes	Parsnips
Pasta (al dente/firm)	Papaya	Pasta (corn, rice)
Peaches (fresh and dried)	Pasta (white, soft)	Popcorn
Pears (fresh and dried)	Pineapple	Pop-Tarts™
Peppers	Pita bread	Potato (baked)
Plums	Porridge (rolled oats)	Pretzels
Pumpernickel bread	Potatoes (mashed or boiled)	Rice (instant, jasmine, sticky)
Rice (long grain, converted, wild)	Raisins	
Sourdough bread	Rice (basmati, brown)	Rice bread
Soybeans	Rye bread	Rice cakes (white)
Soy beverages	Split pea/green pea soup	Rice crackers
Split peas	Sugar (sucrose)	Rutabagas
Sushi	Taco shells (corn)	Scone
Sweet potatoes	Water crackers	Soda crackers
Syrup (pure maple)	Wheat Thins™	Sports drinks
Taro	Whole wheat bread	Tapioca (boiled)
Yam		Watermelon
Yogurt (plain)		White bread

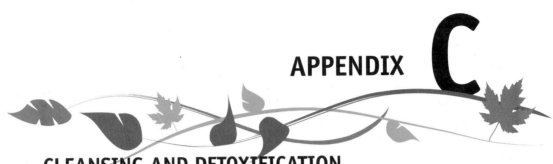

APPENDIX C

CLEANSING AND DETOXIFICATION

The purpose of doing a cleanse or detoxification (detox) program is to enhance the body's elimination of wastes and aid the reparative processes. This practice has been used for thousands of years for the treatment of a variety of health conditions. While cleansing is not widely embraced by mainstream medicine, it is highly popular and routinely recommended by natural health care practitioners.

Our bodies work hard every day eliminating toxins. Toxins are produced in the body during normal functions such as the digestion, but we also get toxins from eating foods containing chemicals (preservatives, dyes, pesticides, and hormones), taking drugs, being exposed to pollution and smoke, and from contact with household cleaners, heavy metals, and other chemicals. There is an intricate system in our bodies that transforms toxins into less harmful compounds. The liver, kidneys, colon, skin, lungs, and lymphatic system are all involved in this process. Toxins are eliminated through our sweat, stools, and urine.

WHY DO WE NEED TO CLEANSE AND DETOXIFY?

Under ideal circumstances, our bodies are capable of detoxifying chemicals that we ingest and are exposed to, but a poor diet, poor digestion or elimination, and exposure to excessive amounts of toxins can create a burden on our natural detoxification system. As well, fat-soluble chemicals that we ingest, such as pesticides and hormones from the food we eat, can deposit and be stored in our fat cells and build up over time. This can result in health problems and increased risk of disease, so by doing a cleanse, we support and enhance the body's ability to eliminate toxins.

HOW DO YOU KNOW IF YOU ARE TOXIC?

Early on, the signs of toxin overload may be subtle, such as fatigue, poor digestion, and skin problems. However, there are possible serious consequences associated with some of these chemicals. Pesticides and compounds found in certain plastics contain chemicals (xenoestrogens), which are hormone disrupters. These chemicals have been linked to various cancers and other hormone-related problems such as PMS, fibroids, and thyroid disturbances. Excessive toxins are also associated with impaired immune function, nutritional deficiencies, and impaired cognitive function.

There are various lab tests that can be done to check for toxins and also to assess your body's detoxification system. These tests may involve checking urine, blood, stool, hair, and liver function. It is best to consult with a naturopathic doctor or medical doctor who practises natural and environmental medicine, as many mainstream doctors are not familiar with these tests.

HEALTH BENEFITS OF CLEANSING AND DETOXIFICATION

Most people who do a cleanse or detox program notice that they have more energy, improved concentration and memory, improved digestion and bowel function, reduced pain and inflammation, and clearer skin. It is also possible to lose some weight when doing a cleanse. Each person reacts differently.

TYPES OF CLEANSING AND DETOXIFICATION PROGRAMS

A cleanse or detox diet program may include a special diet, fasting or drinking juice only, taking herbs and supplements, colonics, exercise, chelation, and sauna therapy. There are various programs or kits available that target the organ systems involved in detoxification: the skin, liver, kidneys, colon, lungs, and lymphatic system.

A natural health care practitioner can design a program that suits your needs by targeting specific organ systems. For people trying a cleanse for the first time, a detox diet is recommended. This involves making dietary changes to avoid ingesting high-toxin foods. Fasting is another method of cleansing that is highly effective, yet more challenging to do. Below are some general guidelines for a detox diet and fasting.

Detox Diet

Eat three to four meals with the recommended foods below, which are rich in nutrients that help support detoxification. Choose organic foods as much as possible to avoid ingesting toxins. Chew your food thoroughly and eat small portions. Drink lots of purified water—at least eight to 10 glasses daily between meals. Water helps to eliminate wastes from the body. The length of time that you follow this diet will depend on your existing health. You may want to do a detox diet once or twice a year to improve overall health and prevent disease. Consult with your health care provider for further recommendations.

Foods to include:
- Beans
- Condiments: celery salt, sea salt, cider vinegar, naturally fermented soy sauce
- Extra-virgin olive oil
- Fresh fruits and vegetables, especially artichokes, beets, broccoli, cauliflower, onions, garlic, peppers, and leafy green vegetables
- Herbal teas, including green tea
- Nuts and seeds: almonds, cashews, walnuts, flaxseed, pumpkin seeds, sesame seeds, and sunflower seeds
- Whole grains: brown rice, quinoa, millet, and amaranth

Foods to avoid:
- Alcohol
- Coffee, soft drinks, and other caffeinated beverages
- Dairy products
- Fast foods, processed foods, and refined foods (white flour products)
- Food additives and preservatives
- Gluten (found in wheat, rye, barley, spelt, and kamut)
- Sugar (white or brown) and any foods with added sugar or containing artificial sweeteners
- Yeast

Fasting

Fasting is one of the oldest and most effective ways to detoxify. It gives the body a period of rest from digestion and dealing with the continual intake of toxins. It allows the body to focus on elimination of wastes and to enhance the reparative processes. Fasting has been practised for thousands of years and is commonly done in cultures around the world to improve various health conditions and to simply aid detoxification.

If this is your first fast, it is important to talk with your health care provider first. The length of a fast will depend on your health status. Many practitioners recommend one- to three-day fasts. The ideal time to do a fast is when you can get lots of rest. Do not exercise or do vigorous activities while fasting. A leisurely walk and stretching is fine.

Some people drink only water during a fast, while others drink juices, such as elderberry or vegetable juices (carrot, beet, celery, wheat grass, and barley grass). It is very important to ensure that your body gets adequate fluids because that is necessary to help flush toxins out of the body and to prevent dehydration. Drink fluids throughout the day as dictated by thirst, but be sure to have at least eight to 10 glasses of water a day. Eat lightly for a few days before starting a fast; have small meals of fruits and vegetables only. The day before the fast, eat foods that are easy to digest such as soups, fruits, salads, and herbal teas. After finishing a fast, eat small, light meals, and gradually resume a healthy diet.

PRECAUTIONS

Consult with your health care provider before starting a cleanse or detox program to ensure it is appropriate for you. These programs are not recommended for pregnant or nursing women or children. Those with serious health conditions such as cancer, diabetes, epilepsy, heart disease, kidney disease, liver disease, hypothyroidism, low blood pressure, ulcers, ulcerative colitis, should not try a fast or detox program unless recommended and supervised by a doctor. Fasting or restrictive detox diets are not recommended for the long term as they can result in nutrient and protein deficiencies.

Medication should never be stopped or reduced without first consulting with your health care provider.

Possible Adverse Effects

As the body is eliminating toxins, it is common to experience headache, fatigue, bad breath, dizziness, nausea, skin rash or eruptions, and mild flu-like symptoms. These symptoms often occur within the first few days and then go away. If you are currently drinking coffee or other caffeine-containing drinks, you will likely have withdrawal symptoms, such as headache and irritability when you stop consuming caffeine. This also goes away within a few days. If you are drinking a high amount of caffeinated beverages (more than 3 cups per day), it would help to gradually wean down before starting a detox diet or fast.

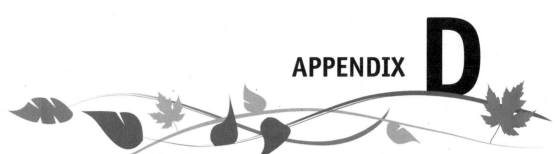

APPENDIX D

FOOD ALLERGIES AND THE ELIMINATION DIET

Allergic reactions to food, also called food hypersensitivities, are an increasingly common problem today. Hippocrates wrote about adverse food reactions and their link to various health problems back in 400 BC. However, it wasn't until the twentieth century that food allergies became understood and well documented. Today it is estimated that over 5 percent of the population suffer with some type of food allergy. Food reactions are also suspected to play a role in many health problems such as attention-deficit hyperactivity disorder, arthritis, asthma, eczema, fatigue, irritable bowel syndrome, migraine headache, and recurrent otitis media. As a result, a growing number of health care practitioners are using elimination diets to identify food allergies and food intolerances in their patients.

The elimination diet and food challenge test are tools that can help identify food allergies and intolerances. The elimination diet involves removing specific foods or ingredients from your diet that you and your doctor suspect may be causing your allergy symptoms. These foods are then gradually reintroduced. Some of the most common allergy-causing foods include milk, eggs, nuts, wheat, soy, and shellfish.

WHY ARE FOOD ALLERGIES ON THE RISE?

There are several reasons or theories as to why food allergies are on the rise, including:

Antibiotic usage: Antibiotics destroy the normal bacteria (flora) in the intestine, which leads to an overgrowth of fungi. Fungi secrete chemicals that alter normal immune function and cause allergic reactions. Antibiotic use also leads to increased intestinal permeability.

Genetics: There are genetic tendencies toward food allergies and intolerances. Studies indicate that if both parents have allergies, their children have a 67 percent chance of developing food allergies. When only one parent is allergic, the child has a 33 percent chance of developing food allergies.

Poor digestive function: The digestive tract plays a vital role in preventing illness and disease by providing a protective barrier. When the integrity of the intestinal barrier is broken down or compromised, a condition coined *leaky gut syndrome* develops. In a person with leaky gut syndrome, partially digested dietary protein can cross the intestinal barrier and be absorbed into the bloodstream. These large molecules can cause allergic reactions in the intestines or throughout the body. There are many factors that can break down the intestinal barrier such as stress, antibiotic use (which destroys beneficial bacteria), and parasitic infections.

Poor immune function: Stress, environmental toxins, pesticides, and other chemicals can alter immune function and cause our immune system to react inappropriately to certain foods.

Repeated consumption of certain foods: Eating the same foods over and over can be taxing to the immune system. For example, wheat, which is a common food allergen, is found in many commonly consumed food products such as breakfast cereals, bread, pasta, sauces, coatings, and fillers. Milk and eggs are other common allergens that are frequently eaten and found as ingredients in many foods, especially baked goods.

FOOD ALLERGIES VS. INTOLERANCES

Food allergies occur when your immune system mistakenly identifies a specific food or a component of food as a harmful substance. In response your immune system triggers certain cells to produce immunoglobulin E (IgE) antibodies to fight the food (allergen). The next time you eat even the smallest amount of that food, the IgE antibodies sense it and signal your immune system to release histamine and other chemicals into your bloodstream.

Food allergies are classified as either immediate or delayed. Immediate hypersensitivity reactions occur within minutes to hours after a food is eaten and cause symptoms such as a rash, hives, a running nose, or a headache. In some cases these immediate hypersensitivity reactions can be life-threatening, causing anaphylactic shock, a condition in which the throat swells and blocks the airways. These reactions are most commonly associated with milk, eggs, peanuts, tree nuts (walnuts), soy, strawberries, wheat, fish, and shellfish. People who get this type of reaction must be diligent in avoiding contact with the allergen and also carry an Epi-pen with them at all times in case they have a reaction. An elimination diet is not recommended for those with immediate hypersensitivity reactions.

Delayed hypersensitivities do not appear right after consuming an allergen, making them difficult to pinpoint. These reactions may not appear for days and can cause a wide range of symptoms such as dark circles or puffiness under the eyes, fluid retention, skin rash, sinus congestion, fatigue, abdominal pain or bloating, joint inflammation, mood swings, indigestion, headaches, chronic ear infections, asthma, poor memory, anxiety, and depression. It is thought that over half of the population suffers with delayed food hypersensitivities. An elimination diet can be very helpful for determining the offending food(s).

Food intolerances are food reactions that are not caused by an immune system reaction. "Food intolerance" is an umbrella term that refers to any abnormal physiological response to a food that is not caused by an immune system reaction.

These reactions may be caused by enzyme deficiencies, poor function of the digestive tract, or by sensitivity to a natural or synthetic chemical. For example, sulphites are a common food preservative added to dried fruits, wine, and processed foods that can cause severe reactions, particularly in those with asthma. Some people react to food dyes, such as tartrazine or the flavour enhancer, monosodium glutamate (MSG), which is often added to Asian food.

The most common food intolerance is lactose intolerance, which occurs when the body does not produce enough of the digestive enzyme called lactase, which breaks down the milk sugar (lactose) found in dairy products. When too much undigested lactose makes its way into the large intestine, people suffer from gas and/or diarrhea. It is estimated that about 30 percent of adults are lactose intolerant. This is particularly common among Africans and Asians.

Another common source of food intolerance is gluten, a protein found in wheat, barley, and rye. Celiac disease is one condition associated with gluten intolerance. In people with celiac disease, gluten damages the absorptive surface of the intestine. Symptoms include diarrhea or constipation, gas, bloating, fatigue, weight loss, anemia, hair loss, and depression. It is estimated that about one in 100 Canadians have gluten intolerance.

There are also naturally occurring substances in foods that can cause reactions in some people, such as salicylates, which are found in many vegetables, herbs, spices, fruits, and chocolate. Salicylates have been associated with various mental health problems such as attention deficit hyperactivity disorder, depression, and headaches.

ELIMINATION DIET
Food allergies and food intolerances are a major source of undesirable symptoms that negatively impact the quality of life of many people. Many health care practitioners believe that the only definitive way to identify and manage adverse food reactions is through the use of an elimination diet followed by carefully organized food challenges. This can be a difficult process to follow as it requires strict dietary changes. However, it can be incredibly rewarding to identify foods that are causing unpleasant reactions.

Below are some guidelines for a standard elimination diet. It is best to work with your health care provider during this process.

Foods to include:
- All vegetables and fruits except those listed below
- Beans
- Brown rice, quinoa, amaranth, buckwheat, tapioca, and flours made of these grains
- Chicken, turkey, lamb, and cold-water fish; choose organic/free-range as much as possible
- Clarified butter (ghee)
- Nuts except soy and peanuts
- Olive, sunflower, safflower, and flaxseed oil
- Salt, pepper, garlic, and fresh herbs
- Water, herbal teas, rice milk, vegetable juice, and fruit juice (drink sparingly and avoid orange juice)

Foods to avoid:
- Alcohol, soft drinks, juice cocktails, coffee, and chocolate
- Beef, pork, veal, and deli meats
- Citrus fruit (oranges, orange juice, and grapefruit), apples, and strawberries
- Dairy products (milk, cheese, yogurt, butter, ice cream) and eggs
- Eggplant, corn, potatoes, tomatoes, and bell peppers
- Foods containing yeast (breads and baked goods unless yeast and gluten-free)
- MSG, food dyes, preservatives, and artificial sweeteners
- Soy products (soy nuts, soy milk, tofu) and peanuts
- Sugar (white and brown) and foods containing sugar
- Trans fatty acids (hydrogenated oils, which are found in margarines and many baked goods and processed foods)
- Wheat (found in bread, pasta, cereals, sauces, thickeners, and as a filler in processed meats)

If salicylates and/or amines are a suspected allergen, then you will also need to avoid tomatoes, broccoli, olives, spinach, mushrooms, avocado, all dried fruit, smoked meats, canned fish, soy sauce, miso, and vinegars.

Follow these dietary guidelines for at least one month to cleanse the body of the offending food. Take time to plan your meals, and eat a variety of the allowed foods. Stock your cupboard and refrigerator with the allowed foods. Read food labels and find out about food ingredients and preparation methods when dining out. Keep a food diary, noting what you are eating and any symptoms that you experience.

It is not uncommon to experience withdrawal symptoms within the first week, such as headaches, food cravings, and changes in bowel function. This occurs as the body detoxifies and adjusts to your new diet. Coffee drinkers typically experience more severe symptoms such as headache and a foggy-headed feeling when caffeine is stopped.

After following the diet for 30 days, reintroduce one food item at a time into your diet. This re-addition of foods is called the "challenge" phase of the diet. On the first day of food challenges, a food is eaten one to three times during the day. Over the next few days, return to the elimination diet, and watch for the return of any symptoms. If any symptoms develop, it is possible that you are allergic or intolerant to that reintroduced food.

It can take several months to complete an elimination and challenge diet. It is best to do this only if you can commit to following the strict guidelines. Cheating will defeat the purpose and hinder your ability to detect potential allergens or intolerances. Keep in mind that if you've had a severe (anaphylactic) reaction to certain foods, this method can't be used. It is advisable to work with a health care professional when considering an elimination diet so that you can get proper nutritional advice, recommendations on supplements, and monitoring throughout this process.

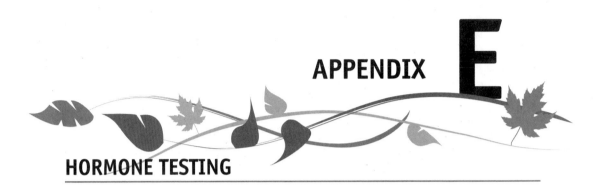

APPENDIX E

HORMONE TESTING

Throughout this book there are discussions about the importance of proper hormone balance and the impact of imbalanced hormones on health. Imbalanced hormones can affect many areas of health and cause problems such as depression, sleep disturbances, weight gain or loss, bone loss, breast swelling and tenderness, fibroids, low libido, sexual dysfunction, and many other aspects of health.

While blood tests are most commonly done to check hormone levels, testing saliva for hormones is becoming increasingly popular. In fact, if you're experiencing hormone-related symptoms, a saliva hormone test is possibly the best way to uncover hormone causes of symptoms. Generally, the best test for hormone balance involves testing the 'big five'" sex steroid hormones: cortisol, DHEA, estradiol, progesterone, and testosterone. The balance between these hormones is critical to good health. For example, Rocky Mountain Analytical, a Canadian saliva hormone testing lab, has data that shows that 7 out of 10 women with self-reported symptoms of depression and 4 out of 5 women with hot flashes and/or low sex drive had laboratory-confirmed hormone imbalance. This tells us that saliva hormone test results correlate very well with how patients feel. Unfortunately, blood tests do not look at symptoms, nor do they test all the same hormones.

There are basically three ways to test for hormones: in blood, in saliva, or in urine. Blood testing is the standard method most doctors use to test for hormones. There are some drawbacks with blood tests for hormones. For example, blood or serum is less accurate for the measurement of testosterone in women because the test is calibrated for the high testosterone levels seen in men. As well, hormones in blood are often bound to proteins and may or may not be available to the tissues that require them. Consequently, blood and serum levels of hormones may not give the best picture of how hormones are behaving at the tissue level. This means that blood test results often don't match up with the symptoms you are experiencing.

Saliva, on the other hand, measures the amount of hormone that actually gets into tissue because salivary hormones have already passed through tissue (the saliva gland) to get into saliva. Saliva hormone levels tend to correlate well with symptoms. Saliva samples are also easier to collect—it can be done at home and samples can be mailed in. There are suggested ranges for women who are supplementing with hormones. In addition, there are some hormones that are not routinely measured in blood.

Saliva hormone testing has been in the scientific literature for over 50 years and is rapidly becoming the test method of choice for hormone monitoring for many practitioners. Nevertheless, saliva testing is not without controversy. Some saliva hormone-testing facilities claim that the tests can be used to determine the "right" dose of hormones for a patient, and that supplementing to achieve specific ratios of one hormone level to another is ideal. Unfortunately, there is no test—blood, saliva, or urine—that tells a doctor exactly how much hormone to give or what dose is right for you. The tests can help guide the doctor in choosing the dose (and in choosing which hormones to supplement with), but you still need to work with a doctor who understands hormone balance and hormone testing. Saliva testing is still the best choice to help uncover the cause of hormone symptoms. You are best to choose an accredited laboratory that includes symptom information in its analysis of your saliva specimen.

Hormone imbalance contributes to many common health conditions. For example, PMS is often due to estrogen dominance (or a lack of progesterone) in the last half of the menstrual cycle. Endometriosis, fibrocystic breast disease, and uterine fibroids have also been associated with estrogen dominance. And even bone loss can arise from hormone imbalance, specifically a lack of testosterone or lack of estrogens or both. In other words, keeping your hormones in balance is an important part of good health, and saliva hormone testing is a great way to find out if you're in balance.

Urine testing is less common because a 24-hour specimen is needed, which makes collection more challenging. Urine testing may be particularly helpful for determining thyroid status. Low thyroid (hypothyroidism) is very common and also commonly undiagnosed. This is because it is possible to have blood results within the normal range, yet have inadequate thyroid function. Symptoms of low thyroid include weight gain, depression, dry skin, feeling cold all the time, low libido, and hair loss.

Typical blood tests for thyroid include measuring levels of the thyroid hormones T3, T4, and TSH (thyroid-stimulating hormone). Urinary thyroid assessments may be helpful for people who have normal serum TSH levels, but who still have symptoms of low thyroid function. Research from Europe has shown that the urinary thyroid test results match patient symptoms better than the serum TSH. What this means is that many people who have normal TSH results register low on a urinary thyroid assessment and this matches their symptoms.

The urinary thyroid assessment involves collecting all your urine for a full 24 hours. The sample is sent away to the laboratory and is analyzed for T3, T4, and selenium, which is a very important mineral for proper thyroid function. The results are reported to your doctor along with an interpretation based on your results and the symptoms you reported.

In Canada, Rocky Mountain Analytical is an accredited laboratory that collects symptom information and provides a complete interpretation of results. Located in Calgary, Alberta, they specialize in saliva hormone testing and other prevention-focused tests, including: urinary thyroid assessment, food allergy testing, omega-3 fatty acid testing, testing for insulin resistance, and many others. Rocky Mountain Analytical is unique in that they collect symptom information prior to testing, and they use the symptoms along with the test results to provide an interpretation to your doctor. They do this because it is important to look at test results as being part of, not separate from, the person. And symptoms provide information about how a person is doing, so even if the results look fairly normal, if the symptoms are severe, the interpretation gives some suggestions as to why those symptoms might be prominent.

For more information on saliva hormone testing, visit www.rmalab.com or call (403) 241-4513.

INDEX